Microincision Vitrectomy Surgery

Developments in Ophthalmology

Vol. 54

Series Editor

F. Bandello Milan

Microincision Vitrectomy Surgery

Emerging Techniques and Technology

Volume Editors

Hideyasu Oh Hyogo
Yusuke Oshima Osaka

145 figures, 124 in color, and 10 tables, 2014

KARGER

Basel · Freiburg · Paris · London · New York · Chennai · New Delhi · Bangkok · Beijing · Shanghai · Tokyo · Kuala Lumpur · Singapore · Sydney

Hideyasu Oh
Hyogo Prefectural Amagasaki Hospital
Higashidaimotsu-cho 1-1-1
Amagasaki 660-0828 (Japan)

Yusuke Oshima
Vitreoretina & Cataract Surgery Center
Oshima Eye Clinic
1-12-8 Nishikanmuri, Takatsuki-city
Osaka 569-0055 (Japan)

Library of Congress Cataloging-in-Publication Data

Microincision vitrectomy surgery : emerging techniques and technology / volume editors, Hideyasu Oh, Yusuke Oshima.
p. ; cm. -- (Developments in ophthalmology ISSN 0250-3751 ; vol. 54)
Includes bibliographical references and index.
ISBN 978-3-318-02660-3 (hard cover : alk. paper) -- ISBN 978-3-318-02661-0 (electronic version)
I. Oh, Hideyasu, editor. II. Oshima, Yusuke, editor. III. Series: Developments in ophthalmology ; v. 54. 0250-3751.
[DNLM: 1. Vitrectomy--instrumentation. 2. Vitrectomy--methods. 3. Eye Diseases--surgery. 4. Microsurgery--instrumentation. 5. Microsurgery--methods. 6. Vitreous Body--surgery. W1 DE998NG v.54 2014 / WW 250]
RE86
617.7'460598--dc23

2014022827

Bibliographic Indices. This publication is listed in bibliographic services, including Current Contents® and Index Medicus.

www.karger.com
Printed in Germany on acid-free and non-aging paper (ISO 9706) by Kraft Druck, Ettlingen
ISSN 0250–3751
e-ISSN 1662–2790
ISBN 978–3–318–02660–3
e-ISBN 978–3–318–02661–0

Contents

List of Contributors

Luis A. Acabá
University of Puerto Rico
140 de Diego Ave
00909 San Juan (Puerto Rico)
E-mail lacaba@me.com

J. Fernando Arévalo
The King Khaled Eye Specialist Hospital
Al-Oruba Street
PO Box 7191
Riyadh 11462 (Saudi-Arabia)
E-mail arevalojf@jhmi.edu

Francesco Barca
U.O. Chirurgia Oftalmica
Azienda Ospedaliero Universitaria Pisana
via Paradisa 2
IT–56124 Pisa (Italy)
E-mail barcaf@hotmail.com

Maria H. Berrocal
Department of Ophthalmology
University of Puerto Rico
140 de Diego Ave
00909 San Juan (Puerto Rico)
E-mai mariahberrocal@hotmail.com

Anniken Burés-Jelstrup
Instituto de Microcirugía Ocular (IMO)
C Josep María Lladó, no 3
ES–08035 Barcelona (Spain)
E-mail nekinna13@hotmail.com

R.V. Paul Chan
Weill Cornell Medical College
New York Presbyterian Hospital
1305 York Avenue, 11th Floor
New York, NY 10021 (USA)
E-mail roc9013@med.cornell.edu

Steve Charles
Hamilton Eye Institute
University of Tennessee
6401 Poplar Avenue
Memphis, TN 38119 (USA)
E-mail scharles@att.net

David R. Chow
University of Toronto
St. Michaels Hospital
Toronto Retina Institute
Toronto, ON M5B 1W8 (Canada)
E-mail davidrchow@me.com

Carl Claes
Speelhofdreef 8
BE–2979 Schilde (Belgium)
E-mail claes.md@skynet.be

Yousef J. Cruz-Iñigo
Department of Ophthalmology
University of Puerto Rico
Rio Piedras Medical Center
00909 San Juan (Puerto Rico)
E-mail yousef.cruz@upr.edu

Manuel Díaz-Llopis
Faculty of Medicine
University of Valencia
Av Blasco Ibañez 17
ES–46010 Valencia (Spain)
E-mail manuel.diaz@uv.es

Rosa Dolz-Marco
Department of Ophthalmology
University and Polytechnic Hospital La Fe
Av Fernando Abril Martorell, 106
ES–46026 Valencia (Spain)
E-mail rosadolzmarco@gmail.com

Pravin U. Dugel
Retinal Consultants of Arizona
1101 E. Missouri Ave.
Phoenix, AZ 85014 (USA)
E-mail pdugel@gmail.com

Renaud Duval
Maisonneuve-Rosemont Hospital
5415 Boulevard de l'Assomption
Montréal, QC H1T 2M4 (Canada)
E-mail renaud.duval@gmail.com

Fiona J. Ehlies
Murray Ocular Oncology and Retina
6705 Red Road, Suite 412
Miami, FL 33143 (USA)
E-mail fehlies@murraymd.com

Ehab N. El Rayes
Retina Department
Institute of Ophthalmology
35 Salah Salem Street
Cairo 11371 (Egypt)
E-mail erayes1@hotmail.com

Hiroshi Enaida
Department of Ophthalmology
Saga University Faculty of Medicine
5-1-1 Nabeshima
Saga 849-8501 (Japan)
E-mail enaida2002@yahoo.co.jp

Roberto Gallego-Pinazo
Department of Ophthalmology
University and Polytechnic Hospital La Fe
Av Fernando Abril Martorell, 106
ES–46026 Valencia (Spain)
E-mail robertogallegopinazo@gmail.com

Enrico Giacomotti
Vitreoretinal Service Igea Clinic
IT–20122 Milan (Italy)
E-mail giacomotti@tin.it

Aaron S. Gold
Murray Ocular Oncology and Retina
6705 Red Road, Suite 412
Miami, FL 33143 (USA)
E-mail agold@murraymd.com

María Gómez-Resa
Instituto de Microcirugía Ocular (IMO)
C Josep María Lladó, no 3
ES–08035 Barcelona (Spain)
E-mail mariagomezresa@hotmail.com

Jeffrey S. Heier
Ophthalmic Consultants of Boston
50 Staniford St., Ste. 600
Boston, MA 02114 (USA)
E-mail jsheier@eyeboston.com

Toshio Hisatomi
Department of Ophthalmology
Graduate School of Medical Sciences
Kyushu University
3-1-1 Maidashi, Higashi-ku
Fukuoka 812-8582 (Japan)
E-mail hisatomi@med.kyushu-u.ac.jp

Yasuhiro Ikeda
Department of Ophthalmology
Graduate School of Medical Sciences
Kyushu University
3-1-1 Maidashi, Higashi-ku
Fukuoka 812-8582 (Japan)
E-mail ymocl@patnol1.med.kyushu-u.ac.jp

Maiko Inoue
Department of Ophthalmology
Yokohama City University Medical Center
4-57 Urafune-cho, Minami-ku
Yokohama, Kanagawa 232-0024 (Japan)
E-mail maicoo@urahp.yokohama-cu.ac.jp

Makoto Inoue
Kyorin Eye Center
Kyorin University School of Medicine
6-20-2 Shinkawa, Mitaka
Tokyo 181-8611 (Japan)
E-mail inoue@eye-center.org

Tatsuro Ishibashi
Department of Ophthalmology
Graduate School of Medical Sciences
Kyushu University
3-1-1 Maidashi, Higashi-ku
Fukuoka 812-8582 (Japan)
E-mail ishi@eye.med.kyushu-u.ac.jp

Pravin Jain
Retina Foundation
Shahibag
380004 Ahmedabad (India)
E-mail jainpravin74@hotmail.com

Kazuaki Kadonosono
Department of Ophthalmology
Yokohama City University Medical Center
4-57 Urafune-cho, Minami-ku
232-0024 Yokohama, Kanagawa (Japan)
E-mail kado@med.yokohama-cu.ac.jp

Peter K. Kaiser
Cole Eye Institute
Cleveland Clinic
9500 Euclid Avenue
Cleveland, OH 44195 (USA)
E-mail pkkaiser@gmail.com

P. Ayumi Kawakami-Campos
Hospital Dr. Luis Sanchez Bulnes
Asociacion para Evitar la Ceguera en Mexico
Vicente Garcia Torres 46
Mexico City 04030 (Mexico)
E-mail ayumika@gmail.com

Michael A. Klufas
Weill Cornell Medical College
New York Presbyterian Hospital
1305 York Avenue, 11th Floor
New York, NY 10021 (USA)
E-mail mak2049@med.cornell.edu

Hiroshi Kunikata
Department of Ophthalmology
Tohoku University Graduate School of Medicine
1-1 Seiryo-machi, Aoba-ku
Sendai 980-8574 (Japan)
E-mail kunikata@oph.med.tohoku.ac.jp

Anna Paula Lafetá
Speelhofdreef 8
BE-2979 Schilde (Belgium)
E-mail ap.lafeta@gmail.com

Timothy Y.Y. Lai
Department of Ophthalmology and Visual Sciences
The Chinese University of Hong Kong
Hong Kong Eye Hospital
147K Argyle Street
Kowloon, Hong Kong
E-mail tyylai@cuhk.edu.hk

Azeema Latiff
Murray Ocular Oncology and Retina
6705 Red Road, Suite 412
Miami, FL 33143 (USA)
E-mail alatiff@murraymd.com

Thomas C. Lee
Children's Hospital Los Angeles
4650 W. Sunset Blvd
Los Angeles, CA 90027 (USA)
E-mail ThLee@chla.usc.edu

Tamer H. Mahmoud
Department of Ophthalmology
Duke University Medical Center
2351 Erwin Road
Durham, NC 27710 (USA)
E-mail tamer.mahmoud@duke.edu

Carlos Mateo
Instituto de Microcirugía Ocular (IMO)
C Josep María Lladó 3
ES-08035 Barcelona (Spain)
E-mail carlosmateo@me.com

Virgilio Morales-Canton
Hospital Dr. Luis Sanchez Bulnes
Asociacion para Evitar la Ceguera en Mexico
Vicente Garcia Torres 46
Mexico City 04030 (Mexico)
E-mail vmoralesc@mac.com

Marco Mura
Academic Medical Center
University of Amsterdam
Meibergdreef 9
NL-1105AZ Amsterdam (the Netherlands)
E-mail m.mura@amc.uva.nl

Timothy G. Murray
Murray Ocular Oncology and Retina
6705 Red Road, Suite 412
Miami, FL 33143 (USA)
E-mail tmurray@murraymd.com

Manish Nagpal
Retina Foundation
Shahibag
38004 Ahmedabad (India)
E-mail drmanishnagpal@yahoo.com

Shintaro Nakao
Department of Ophthalmology
Graduate School of Medical Sciences
Kyushu University
3-1-1 Maidashi, Higashi-ku
Fukuoka 812-8582 (Japan)
E-mail shintaro.nakao@yahoo.com

Hideyasu Oh
Hyogo Prefectural Amagasaki Hospital
Higashidaimotsu-cho 1-1-1
Amagasaki 660-0828 (Japan)
E-mail hideyasu@kuhp.kyoto-u.ac.jp

Shunsuke Osawa
Okanami General Hospital
1734 Uenokuwamachi, Iga
Mie 518-0842 (Japan)
E-mail s.osawa1108@gmail.com

Yusuke Oshima
Vitreoretina & Cataract Surgery Center
Oshima Eye Clinic
1-12-8 Nishikanmuri, Takatsuki-city
Osaka 569-0055 (Japan)
E-mail yusukeoshima@gmail.com

Samir N. Patel
Weill Cornell Medical College
New York Presbyterian Hospital
1305 York Avenue, 11th Floor
New York, NY 10021 (USA)
E-mail snp2002@med.cornell.edu

Fabio Patelli
Head Vitreoretina Service Igea Clinic
Director Milano Retina Center
Carones Ophthalmology Center
Via Pietro Mascagni 20
IT–20122 Milan (Italy)
E-mail Fabio@patelli.it

Paolo Radice
Vitreoretina Service Fatebenefratelli Ophthalmic Hospital
IT–20122 Milan (Italy)
E-mail p.radice@hotmail.it

Kourous A. Rezaei
Illinois Retina Associates
Ingalls Hospital Professional Building
71 West 156th Street
Harvey, IL 60426 (USA)
E-mail karezaei@yahoo.com

Stanislao Rizzo
U.O. Chirurgia Oftalmica
Azienda Ospedaliero Universitaria Pisana
via Paradisa 2
IT–56124 Pisa (Italy)
E-mail stanislao.rizzo@gmail.com

Hiroyuki Shimada
Department of Ophthalmology
Surugadai Hospital of Nihon University
Surugadai, Kanda, Chiyodaku
Tokyo 101-8309 (Japan)
E-mail sshimada@olive.ocn.ne.jp

Peter Stalmans
Department of Ophthalmology
University Hospitals Leuven
Kapucijnenvoer 33
BE–3000 Leuven (Belgium)
E-mail peter.stalmans@uzleuven.be

George Trichonas
Cole Eye Institute
Cleveland Clinic
9500 Euclid Avenue
Cleveland, OH 44195 (USA)
E-mail gtrichonas@gmail.com

Victor M. Villegas
Murray Ocular Oncology and Retina
6705 Red Road, Suite 412
Miami, FL 33143 (USA
E-mail vvillegas@murraymd.com

Andrea C. Wildner
Murray Ocular Oncology and Retina
6705 Red Road, Suite 412
Miami, FL 33143 (USA)
E-mail awildner@murraymd.com

Matthew T. Witmer
Retinal Consultants of Arizona
1101 E. Missouri Ave.
Phoenix, AZ 85014 (USA)
E-mail mwitmer@retinalconsultantsaz.com

S. Chien Wong
Moorfields Eye Hospital
162 City Road
London EC1V 2PD London (UK)
E-mail chien22@yahoo.com

Glenn Yiu
Department of Ophthalmology
Duke University Medical Center
2351 Erwin Road
Durham, NC 27710 (USA)
E-mail gyiu@post.harvard.edu

Shigeo Yoshida
Department of Ophthalmology
Graduate School of Medical Sciences
Kyushu University
3-1-1 Maidashi, Higashi-ku
Fukuoka 812-8582 (Japan)
E-mail usyosi@gmail.com

Preface

Since Robert Machemer, MD, first pioneered closed-eye vitrectomy, the evolution of vitrectomy surgery has rapidly progressed. Numerous advances in the technologies and techniques have been made for the establishment and refinement of this surgical modality. Of these, enormous advances in minimizing the size of the surgical equipment for carrying out sutureless vitrectomy may be the most remarkable advancement in modern vitrectomy surgery. Visualization techniques have also made huge progress, i.e. the introduction of wide-viewing systems in conjunction with chandelier illumination and the utilization of vital dyes to better visualize transparent intraocular tissue such as the vitreous and membranes. Thanks to the recent advancements, we can now routinely achieve less invasive surgery and consequently have earlier recovery with improved safety.

This volume starts with the fundamentals of microincision vitrectomy surgery by introducing both the mechanics and the physics of the newer-generation vitrectomy machines. The following chapters describe the discrete gauge systems, namely the 23-, 25-, and – the latest – 27-gauge systems. In the second section, both individualized and requisite settings, techniques, and technology are discussed in detail. These include illumination, wide-viewing systems, and surgical adjuvants. The third section focuses on the practical management of specific diseases, and includes more than 10 chapters dedicated to giving surgeons thorough plans with concrete strategies.

Since the development of microincision vitrectomy surgery continues at a dizzying pace, our principal endeavor is to encompass all of the recent advancements obtained in this field so that both comprehensive ophthalmologists and vitreoretinal specialists can quickly review and catch up with the most up-to-date knowledge and have some surgical pearls as well. We wish all readers enjoyment with this book, which can be used as a quick reference for specific diseases and as a sophisticated guide to understand the latest advances in vitreous surgery technology.

Hideyasu Oh, Amagasaki
Yusuke Oshima, Osaka

Acknowledgments

The publication of this book is made possible by a number of key opinion-leading authors as well as the dedicated support of the publisher. I am extremely grateful for my colleague (and also co-editor) Dr. Yusuke Oshima for allowing me to share and invite his unrivaled network of leading surgeons from all over the world as well as for his critical review of the manuscript.

I was fortunate enough to start my career as a vitreoretinal fellow at Tenri Yorozu Hospital (Nara), where I could learn from and be trained by so many outstanding surgeons, not only specialized in vitreoretinal diseases, but also in cataract and glaucoma. I would also like to thank Prof. Nagahisa Yoshimura (Kyoto), Prof. Satoki Ueno (Kanagawa), Prof. Ryoji Yamakawa (Fukuoka), Prof. Hitoshi Takagi (Kanagawa), Dr. Morio Okada (Okayama), and Dr. Mihori Kita (Kyoto) for giving me the opportunity to work with and share their knowledge with me. Although the progress in this field is rapid and the advancements are huge, one thing they all taught me was the importance of safe and less invasive surgery. With this principle we will not be easily lost even in hard cases, and it is also the principle which we still rely on to find our way through the myriad of information. Finally, my special thanks go to my colleagues, Dr. Shunsuke Osawa, Dr. Makoto Inoue, and Dr. Hiroshi Kunikata, for their insightful discussions.

Hideyasu Oh, Amagasaki

Oh H, Oshima Y (eds): Microincision Vitrectomy Surgery. Emerging Techniques and Technology.
Dev Ophthalmol. Basel, Karger, 2014, vol 54, pp 1–7 (DOI: 10.1159/000360442)

Machines and Cutters: Constellation®

Matthew T. Witmer · Pravin U. Dugel

Retinal Consultants of Arizona, Phoenix, Ariz., USA

Abstract

The Alcon Constellation® provides state-of-the-art technology for vitrectomy surgery. Its innovative features include utilization of high-speed and small-gauge vitrectomy systems, surgeon-controlled duty cycle, fine intraocular pressure control, and integrated laser and intraocular gas mixing capabilities. The goal of vitrectomy surgery is the safe and efficient removal of vitreous while avoiding iatrogenic retinal tears or iatrogenic incarceration of retinal tissue. This requires the removal of vitreous in a controlled manner while maintaining safe levels of intraocular pressure. The Alcon Constellation contains improvements in technology that allow a surgeon to consistently accomplish these goals.

High-Speed Cutting

For the past two decades, many vitreoretinal surgeons have intuitively assumed that a faster cut rate allows for safer surgery. The vitreous is highly viscous, and without a cutting action the aspiration from the vitrectomy probe would unintentionally pull on collagen within the vitreous cavity. This vitreous pull could cause retinal traction and subsequent tears or retinal incarceration. We can assume that the greater the length of collagen pull, the greater the vitreous traction and the greater the likelihood of iatrogenic retinal tears and retinal incarceration. In other words, the greater the length of collagen pull, the less safe the surgery. Conversely, the shorter the length of collagen pull, the less vitreous traction and the safer the surgery. This relationship is described in a surprisingly simple mathematical formula: the length of traction (collagen pull, in cm) equals flow rate (in ml/min) divided by the internal lumen area of the probe (in cm^2), divided by the cut rate (in cuts/min), as shown in equation 1.

$$\text{Length of traction} = \frac{\text{aspiration flow rate} \div \text{internal lumen area of probe}}{\text{cut rate}}. \quad (1)$$

The internal lumen area is related to the inner radius of the vitrectomy probe, r, by the equation: area = πr^2. When the internal lumen area is held constant, only the aspiration flow and the cut rate affect the length of the traction pull (which is related to the viscosity of the aspirated liquid).

Equation 1 tells us that increasing the flow rate will increase the length of collagen pull. That relationship makes it evident that a very high flow rate is not necessarily beneficial and may, in fact, be dangerous. High flow rates increase the vitreous traction and the subsequent potential for retinal tears and incarceration. Especially when working near the retina, the slowest flow rate possible in order to get the job done would be desired. On the other hand, the higher the cut rate, the less the length of collagen pull, the less the viscosity of the vitreous, and the less the vitreous traction. Therefore, the highest cut rate possible would be desirable.

Increasing the cut rate not only reduces the length of pull, but also reduces the 'bite size', or the size of a piece of aspirated vitreous. Bite size, or discrete aspirated volume, is another way to consider viscosity. A fluid composed of large pieces would be highly viscous, while a fluid composed of tiny pieces would have low viscosity. The discrete aspirated volume is defined as the volume aspirated in a single cycle of the vitreous cutter opening and closing, and is calculated by dividing the flow rate by the cut rate. Figure 1 shows the results of our modeling to reveal how bite size decreases as cut rate increases. The reduction in bite size is dramatic at high cut rates. At 5,000 cuts/min, the discrete aspirated volume is only 1.6 μl. As the cut rate doubles, the discrete aspirated volume is reduced twofold.

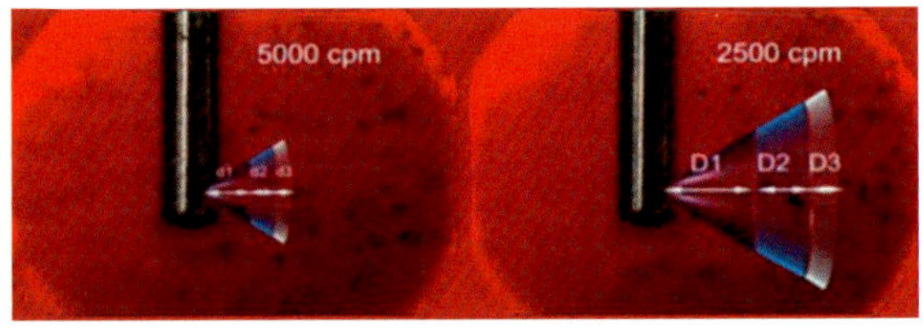

Fig. 1. The length of pull of each bite (D) decreases with cut rate and with distance from the cutter. cpm = Cuts/min.

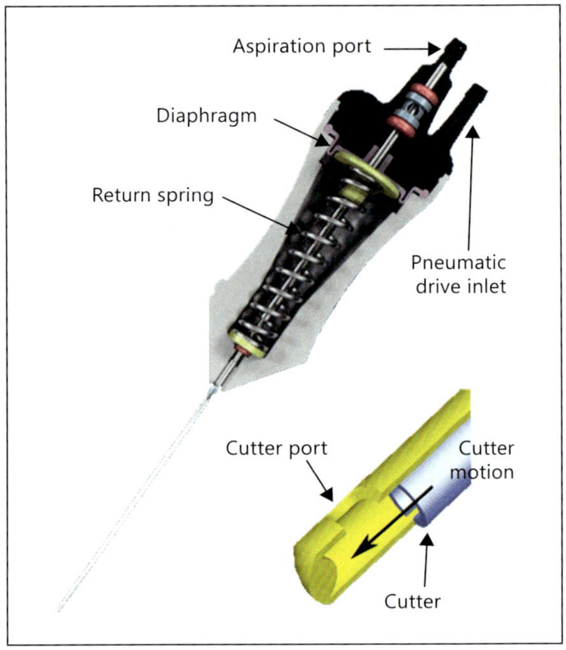

Fig. 2. A typical first-generation vitrectomy probe.

The Alcon Constellation® is compatible with high-speed vitrector probes, which can deliver up to 7,500 cuts/min. This is possible through the use of dual pneumatic drive probes.

First-generation pneumatic vitrectomy probes typically relied on a spring mechanism to recoil the cutter following a pneumatic pulse. A typical first-generation pneumatic vitrectomy probe is shown in figure 2. A pressure pulse entered the rear cavity of the probe and acted upon a diaphragm, which in turn compressed a spring. Attached to the diaphragm is an inner lumen that is forced across the probe port opening, thus producing the guillotine-like cutting action. When the pneumatic pulse is vented, the return spring pushes the diaphragm back, opening the cutter port. The repetition of this drive sequence defines the cut rate. The cut rate of first-generation pneumatic cutters was limited by the drive pulse rising edge, venting of the pressure pulse, and mechanical characteristics of the spring.

The Alcon Constellation employs recent advancements in dual pneumatic drive cutter technologies, which have replaced the return spring used in single-drive pneumatic vitrectomy probes with a second pneumatic drive. Figure 3 shows a cutaway view of a dual pneumatic drive probe. A pneumatic pulse enters the chamber behind the diaphragm, driving the cutter port closed. A second pulse, the return pulse, then acts on the front side of the diaphragm to return the cutter to the open position.

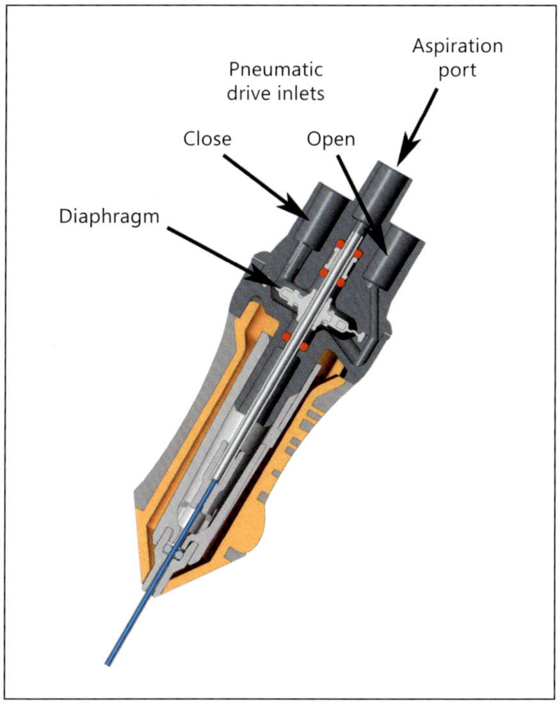

Fig. 3. A dual pneumatic drive vitrectomy probe.

Small-Gauge Vitrector Probes

The Constellation also allows the use of small-gauge vitrectomy systems, including 23, 25, and 27 gauge. This increases the safety of the procedure because of the port-based limit to flow during the surgery.

The relationship defined by the Hagen-Poiseuille law applies to flow through the vitreous cutter. The Hagen-Poiseuille law defines the flow through a tube (or, in terms of intraocular surgery, the vitrectomy probe) in terms of flow rate, pressure drop (ΔP), and resistance to flow, as shown in equation 2:

$$\text{Flow rate} = \Delta\text{P}/\text{resistance factor}. \quad (2)$$

This equation is analogous to Ohm's law for electrical circuits. The resistance inside the tube is affected by the length of the tube (L) and the internal radius of the tube (r), as shown in figure 4.

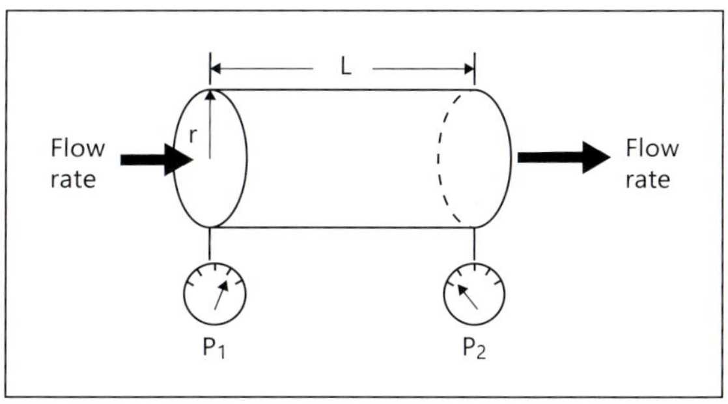

Fig. 4. Flow rate is dependent upon the pressure difference across the tube, the length, and the radius of the tube.

The resistance is also affected by the viscosity of the aspirated liquid (η), so equation 2 can be rewritten in more detail, as follows:

$$\text{Flow rate} = \frac{\text{pressure difference}}{\dfrac{\eta\, L\, 8}{\pi\, r^4}}. \quad (3)$$

Here π is a mathematical constant (3.14). By rearranging terms, equation 3 can be rewritten as follows:

$$\text{Flow rate} = (\pi r^4 \Delta\text{P})/(8\,\eta\,\text{L}). \quad (4)$$

Equation 4 shows some important dependencies of flow rate on several factors. First, the flow rate is proportional to the fourth power of the inner radius of the tube. In terms of vitrectomy instruments, larger-gauge vitrectomy cutters have

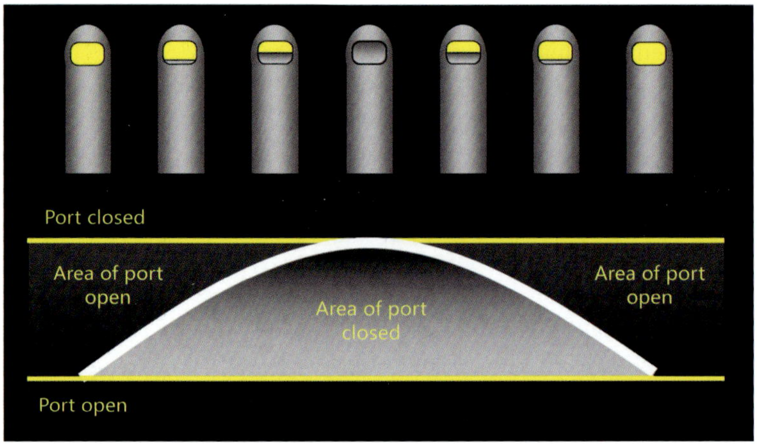

Fig. 5. Duty cycle.

higher flow rates than smaller-gauge instruments under similar conditions and vacuum levels. Secondly, the viscosity directly impacts the flow rate: lower viscosities allow higher flow rates at any given pressure differential. Consequently, during vitrectomy, the flow rates increase when the probe port leaves the vitreous face and enters clear fluid, and flow decreases when the probe port leaves clear fluid and enters the vitreous.

The flow through the port is limited due to design characteristics of the probe [1, 2]. The inner lumen radius of the probe has a fourth-order effect on the flow (see equation 4). Consequently, smaller-gauge probes (e.g. 25-gauge probes), have a far slower flow than 20-gauge probes at any aspiration vacuum setting. The probe port dimensions only restrict the flow if the port area is smaller than the inner lumen area. Most modern probes have port openings that exceed the inner lumen area and do not geometrically restrict the flow.

Surgeon-Controlled Duty Cycle

The Constellation allows more precise control of the vitrectomy by the surgeon. This is accomplished partly through a concept known as duty cycle. Since the cutter must physically close off the port to create the guillotine-like cutting action, the port cannot remain open 100% of the time. To fully understand this flow restriction, surgeons must understand the concept of the port duty cycle.

The cutting action of most vitrectomy probes is generated as the inner lumen of a vitrectomy probe moves across a port opening. When the cutter is in action, the inner lumen is repeatedly forced past the port opening, which generates a shearing action. Tissues are drawn into the port by the pressure differential when the port is in the open configuration. When the inner lumen is forced across the port opening, the tissues are sheared and aspirated through the inner lumen. During the time the port is closed by the inner lumen, no flow can pass through the probe port. Aspiration flow rates match the duty cycle: the higher the duty cycle, the higher the aspiration flow at any given vacuum level.

The amount of time the port remains open is referred to as the 'port duty cycle', which is represented graphically in figure 5. Duty cycle is frequently misunderstood as the amount of time the port remains open divided by the amount of time closed. The correct definition of duty cycle is the amount of time the port is open divided by the

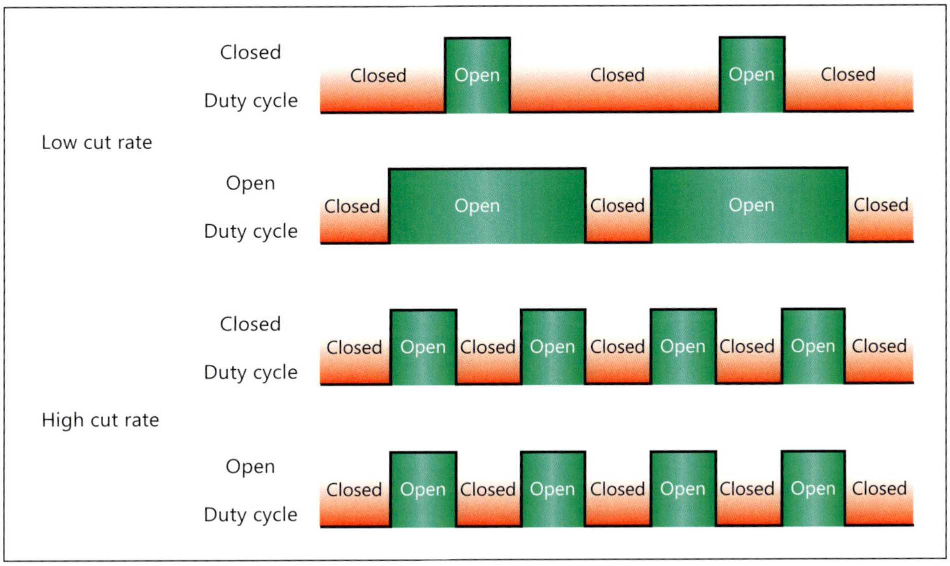

Fig. 6. Duty cycles at slower (low) and faster (high) cut rates. With a biased-closed duty cycle, the amount of time closed is reduced at a faster cut rate. With a biased-open duty cycle, the amount of time the port is open is reduced at a faster cut rate.

time of one complete cut cycle, as shown in equation 5:

$$\text{Duty cycle} = \frac{\text{duration port open}}{\text{duration of total cutting cycle}}. \quad (5)$$

The duty cycle of an electrically driven cutter is constant at just below 50%. The linear motion of the guillotine-like cutter is tied mechanically to the rotary motion of an electric motor. The duty cycle is slightly less than 50% because the cutter must over-travel across the port. While the duty cycle remains constant across cut rates, the cutter velocity decreases with slower cut rates due to the reduced speed of the rotary motor driving the cutter.

Certain physical phenomena related to the cut rate of pneumatically driven vitreous cutters affect the duty cycle, such as how quickly the pneumatic pulse is vented, the frictional forces within the probe, and inertial forces as the cut rate increases. Typically, the duty cycle of pneumatic cutters decreases as the cut rate increases. At slower cut rates, duty cycles of 80% or more are common. At faster cut rates, duty cycles can drop to 40% or lower. By increasing the width of the pneumatic pulse that opens the port, the amount of time the port is open is increased, resulting in a biased-open duty cycle. When the pneumatic pulse closing the port is increased, the duty cycle of the port is biased-closed.

Since the time required to open and close the port is somewhat fixed by the physical phenomena described above, the duty cycle is affected by the cut rate. When the duty cycle is biased-open, the cutter closes as fast as physically possible and then immediately returns open as fast as physically possible. In order to increase the cut rate, the only time segment that can be reduced to accommodate an increased number of cut cycles is the dwell open time. Consequently, the duty cycle is reduced. Likewise, to increase the cut rate of a biased-closed duty cycle, the amount of time the port dwells closed is reduced and the duty cycle increases. Figure 6 shows the effects of cut rate on duty cycle. As the cut rate is increased, both biased-open and biased-closed duty cycles approach a 50% duty cycle.

Intraocular Pressure Control

During vitreoretinal surgery, intraocular pressure (IOP) depends on the fluid flow rate into the eye from the infusion line and out of the eye through the vitrectomy probe. If the fluid flow into the eye is faster than the fluid removal by the probe, hypertony can occur. When using high infusion pressures (30–40 mm Hg) while operating on eyes with poor blood flow, such as the eyes of diabetics or glaucoma patients, hypertony may cause the blood vessels of the optic nerve to pulsate or lack perfusion [3]. Conversely, if fluid flow into the eye is slower than the fluid removal by the probe, hypotony can occur. Intraoperative hypotony during vitreoretinal surgery has been associated with choroidal detachment [4] and suprachoroidal hemorrhage [5, 6]. Corneal folds due to intraoperative hypotony can make visualization difficult for the surgeon and can damage the patient's corneal endothelium [3].

Traditional vitreoretinal instrumentation makes regulation of intraoperative IOP difficult for surgeons. The measurable applied infusion pressure at the console does not necessarily equal the resultant IOP, and the multiple factors described earlier that affect flow rate out of the eye through the vitrectomy probe are not apparent from the instrumental settings. Recent advancements in IOP compensation have removed these unknown parameters and uncertainties. An IOP compensation feature on the Constellation maintains the IOP at the desired IOP regardless of flow conditions. This feature is intended to reduce IOP fluctuations while the surgeon is exchanging instruments and to reduce the chance of globe collapse during deep scleral depression or when using high flow rates. Instead of applying 30 mm Hg at the bottle, hoping for 15 mm Hg at the eye after adjusting for pressure drop, a surgeon can apply 20 mm Hg and expect to get 20 mm Hg with the IOP compensation feature.

Integrated Laser and Gas Mixing Capabilities

Earlier vitrectomy platforms typically required the use of an external laser system to provide endolaser during vitrectomy surgery. The Constellation provides an integrated laser for use during surgery. The laser port also allows for the use of illuminated lasers for visualization during portions of the surgery that require endolaser.

In addition, the Constellation offers the option of mixing the typical intraocular gases used during vitrectomy surgery. The gas tanks are simply attached to the back of the machine and the gas can be drawn into a syringe in the front of the machine. The exact percentage of gas is inputted into the console and the Constellation mixes the pure gas with room air to provide the desired concentration.

Conclusion

The Constellation represents several advancements in vitreoretinal surgical technology and technique. These improvements offer safer and more efficient surgical procedures with the potential for improved outcomes and fewer complications.

Disclosure Statement

Dr. Witmer has no financial interests to disclose. Dr. Dugel is a paid consultant for Alcon.

References

1 Charles S: Debating the pros and cons of 23-g vs 25-g vitrectomy: the pros of 25-g vitrectomy. Retin Physician 2006;3:24–25.
2 Deboer C, Fang S, Lima L, McCormick M, Bhadri P, Kerns R, et al: Port geometry and its influence on vitrectomy. Retina 2008;28:1061–1067.
3 Packo K, Ho A, Dugel P, Pollack J, Rizzo S, Murray T: Rethinking intraocular pressure requirements. Retin Physician 2009;Suppl:12–13.
4 Verma L, Venkatesh P, Chawla R, Tewari HK: Choroidal detachment following retinal detachment surgery: an analysis and a new hypothesis to minimize its occurrence in high-risk cases. Eur J Ophthalmol 2004;14:325–329.
5 Lakhanpal V, Schocket SS, Elman MJ, Dogra MR: Intraoperative massive suprachoroidal hemorrhage during pars plana vitrectomy. Ophthalmology 1990; 97:1114–1119.
6 Chu TG, Green RL: Suprachoroidal hemorrhage. Surv Ophthalmol 1999;43: 471–486.

Pravin U. Dugel, MD
Retinal Consultants of Arizona
1101 E. Missouri Ave.
Phoenix, AZ 85014 (USA)
E-Mail mwitmer@retinalconsultantsaz.com

Oh H, Oshima Y (eds): Microincision Vitrectomy Surgery. Emerging Techniques and Technology.
Dev Ophthalmol. Basel, Karger, 2014, vol 54, pp 8–16 (DOI: 10.1159/000360443)

Machines and Cutters: Stellaris PC

Timothy Y.Y. Lai[a, b]

[a]Department of Ophthalmology and Visual Sciences, The Chinese University of Hong Kong, Hong Kong Eye Hospital, and [b]2010 Retina and Macula Centre, Hong Kong, SAR, China

Abstract

The Stellaris PC (Bausch & Lomb) is a versatile platform that allows surgeons to perform both anterior segment and posterior segment surgeries. It was developed based on the Stellaris microincision cataract surgery system and can therefore perform <2-mm coaxial or bimanual microincision cataract surgery in combination with posterior segment surgery. Similar to Millenium, its predecessor, the Stellaris PC has an open architecture with modular design that allows products and instruments manufactured by other companies to be used with the system. Vitrectomy can be performed using the traditional 20-gauge system or with microincision 23- or 25-gauge transconjunctival sutureless vitrectomy systems. The special design of the vitreous cutter with increased port area, improved fluidics, and optimized port open time makes the Stellaris PC an efficient system for performing microincision vitrectomy surgery. This article will describe the design, features, and details of various components of the Stellaris PC, including machine controls, entry site alignment trocar/cannula system, fluidics, and high-speed vitreous cutter, as well as its unique illumination system.

The Stellaris PC (Procedure Choice) is a vitrectomy system developed by Bausch & Lomb (Aliso Vieji, Calif., USA) that was launched commercially in 2010 (fig. 1). The system was developed from the Stellaris Vision Enhancement System, which has been available since 2007 as a microincision cataract surgery system that allows coaxial or biaxial phacoemulsification via a wound size down to 1.8 mm. The Stellaris PC surgical platform allows surgeons to have the versatility to perform phacoemulsification surgery alone, posterior segment surgery alone, or combined phacoemulsification and posterior segment surgery. Vitrectomy can be performed using conventional 20-gauge instruments, or with microincision 23- or 25-gauge transconjunctival sutureless vitrectomy instruments.

Design of the Stellaris PC

The Stellaris PC machine adopts an open architecture modular design similar to Millennium, the previous generation of vitrectomy systems manufactured by Bausch & Lomb [1]. Since the

Stellaris PC is based on the Stellaris phacoemulsification system, it allows an easy transition between microincision cataract surgery and vitrectomy during combined cataract and posterior segment surgeries. The open architecture also allows surgeons to use various instruments made by other manufacturers with the system and enables easier maintenance and future upgrades of the system. For instance, when it first went on the market in 2010, the Stellaris PC did not have a built-in laser as it was still under development. A fully integrated laser system was subsequently introduced in late 2013 and this can be installed easily into the drawer slot below the surgical tray in the middle of the Stellaris PC machine.

As with the previous Millennium system, the Stellaris PC is a Venturi-based system. Nonetheless, the redesigned Venturi pump in the Stellaris PC has led to significant improvement in the fluidics of the system. It has a pinch valve within the system which completely stops venting in the aspiration line and therefore passive aspiration which might be associated with the Millennium system does not occur [2]. Pressurized air to drive the system can be provided by wall air, bottled compressed air, or an air compressor, and the airline is plugged to the back of the machine.

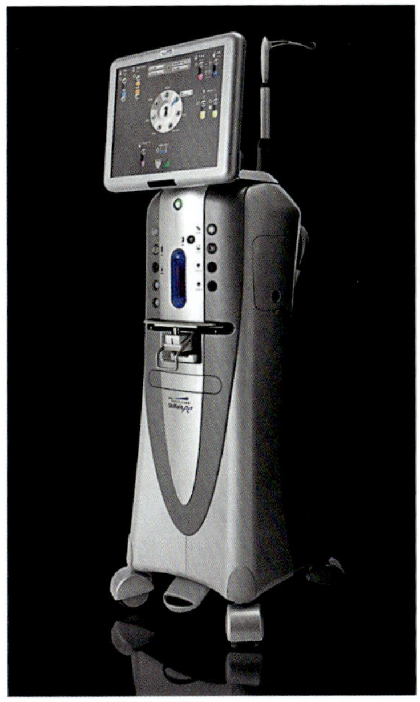

Fig. 1. The Stellaris PC machine. A touch-screen LCD provides the control interface for the machine in the top section. In the middle section, cassette and various devices can be connected to the machine. The lower portion has a movable surgical tray and a drawer in which a laser system can be installed.

Machine Controls and Foot Pedal

The main control interface of the Stellaris PC machine is via a touch-screen liquid crystal display (LCD) monitor occupying the upper portion of the system (fig. 2). The touch-screen interface has been specially designed for user-friendliness, and different functions and settings of the system can be navigated and operated easily. The brightness of the LCD screen can be controlled via the touch screen and adjusted to match the ambiance light environment during different steps of the surgery.

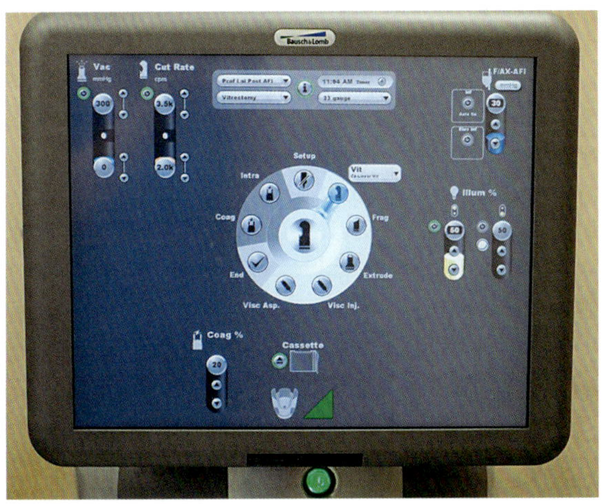

Fig. 2. LCD touch-screen interface of the Stellaris PC. All parameters required for the surgery can be accessed easily on a single screen.

For the operating surgeon, similar to the Millennium vitrectomy system, the Stellaris PC also features a dual-linear foot pedal (fig. 3). This allows the surgeon to control different surgical pa-

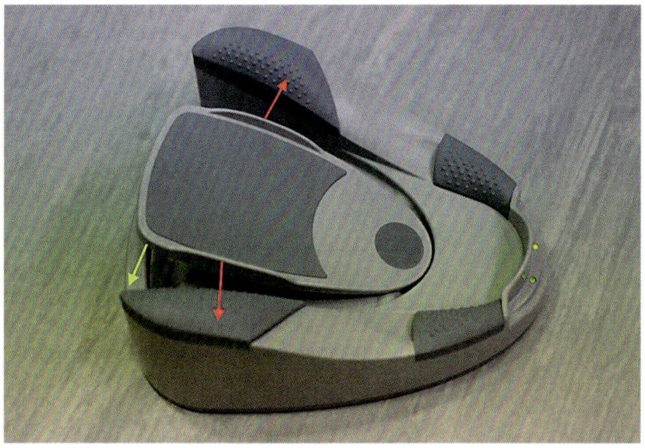

Fig. 3. Stellaris PC foot pedal. The wireless foot pedal has a special dual-linear design in which the pitch (green arrow – up and down) and yaw (red arrow – left and right) axes can be moved independently. This allows the surgeon to change the vacuum, cut rate, or phacoemulsification parameters simultaneously.

rameters by adjusting the pitch (up and down movement) and yaw (left and right movement) axes of the pedal simultaneously. The surgeon can control the pitch axis for changing the amount of vacuum and alter the yaw axis for changing the cutting rate or phacoemulsification power, or vice versa. The foot pedal connects wirelessly to the main machine and therefore eliminates the potential of cord clutter or accidental tripping of operating room personnel by the cable. The wireless foot pedal battery needs around 6 h to fully charge, and the foot pedal can operate for up to 12 working hours after charging. In case the foot pedal runs out of power, a cable can be used to connect the foot pedal to the machine for controlling the machine and for battery charging. Four auxiliary buttons are also available in the four corners of the foot pedal and they can be programmed to perform all the functions of the vitrectomy machine based on the surgeon's preference.

Entry Site Alignment Trocar/Cannula System

Vitreoretinal procedures with the Stellaris PC system can be performed using the conventional 20-gauge system, or with microincision transconjunctival sutureless vitrectomy 23- or 25-gauge systems. Each vitrectomy procedural pack contains a vitrectomy cutter, handheld light pipe, scleral plugs, and MVR blade (for 20-gauge) or entry site alignment (ESA) trocar/cannula system (for 23-gauge and 25-gauge). The disposable cutters and other instruments are color-coded for easy recognition, with 20-, 23-, and 25-gauge systems being coded gray, green, and blue, respectively (fig. 4). Scleral markers are available at the blunt end of the trocar for measuring the sclerotomy site.

When the Stellaris PC was launched initially, some surgeons found that extra force might be needed to insert the trocar/cannulas through the sclera [3]. Bausch & Lomb has subsequently redesigned and modified the ESA trocar/cannula system and the current design provides excellent wound construction and sealing. Instead of a hollow needle-type blade, the ESA now utilizes a solid round-tip blade design which provides a longer taper for more cutting surface and easier penetration into the eye (fig. 5) [3]. This also allows a more shallow wound entry and therefore better retention of the cannula. The 23-gauge ESA cannula is 4 mm in length and is made of polyamide material, which might allow better retention compared with stainless steel cannula. The cannula has a beveled chamfer on the leading edge located very close to the edge of the blade, which allows the cannula to slide tissue away from the entry site during insertion (fig. 5). A study in simulated eyes has demonstrated that the force required to insert the 23-gauge ESA trocar/cannula is comparable with products from other manufacturers (fig. 6) [3].

Since late 2013, 23- and 25-gauge titanium ESA cannulas with self-sealing valves have also become available (fig. 5). These valved cannulas eliminate the need for scleral plugs when instruments are removed from the eye and therefore allow maintenance of constant pressure within the globe (fig. 7). This is particularly useful for complex vitreoretinal surgery such as proliferative di-

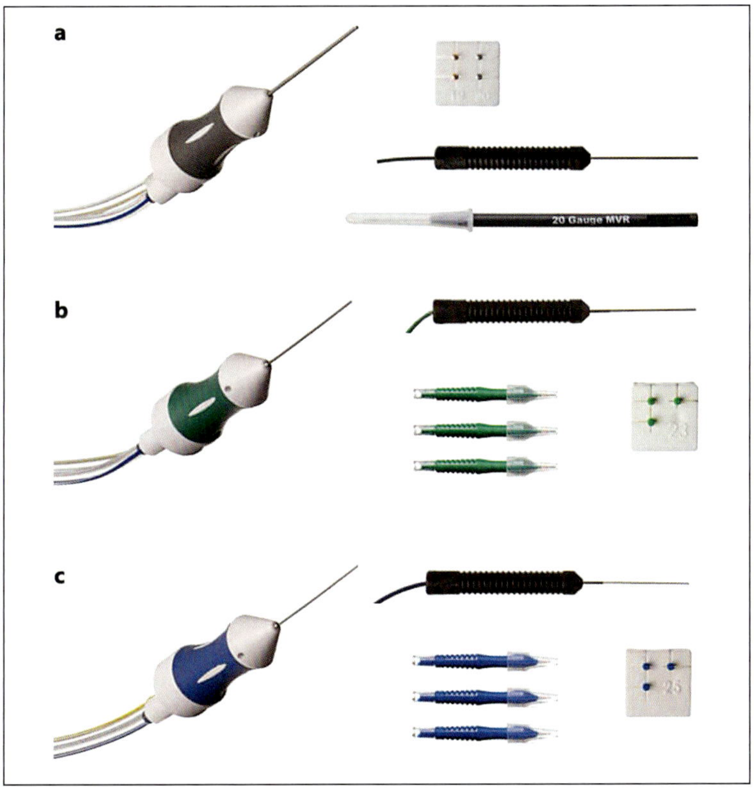

Fig. 4. Color-coded Stellaris PC posterior segment procedural pack. **a** Black color for 20-gauge cutter, MVR blade, handheld light pipe, and scleral plugs. **b** Green color for 23-gauge cutter, ESA trocar/cannulas, handheld light pipe, and scleral plugs. **c** Blue color for 25-gauge cutter, ESA trocar/cannulas, handheld light pipe, and scleral plugs.

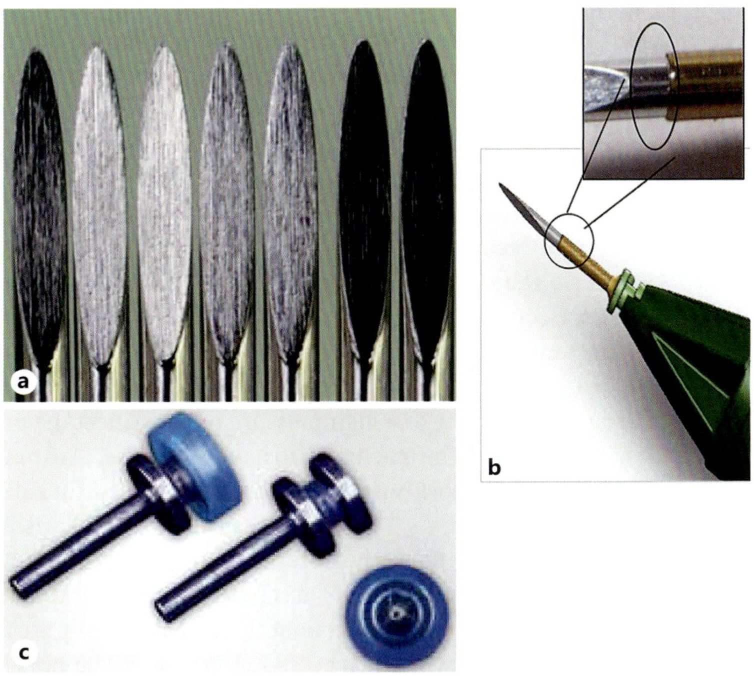

Fig. 5. ESA trocar/cannula system. **a** The trocar uses a tapered round-tip solid blade design. **b** The polyamide cannula has a bevel edge which allows tissue displacement during site insertion. **c** The 25-gauge titanium ESA trocar and cannula with removable valve.

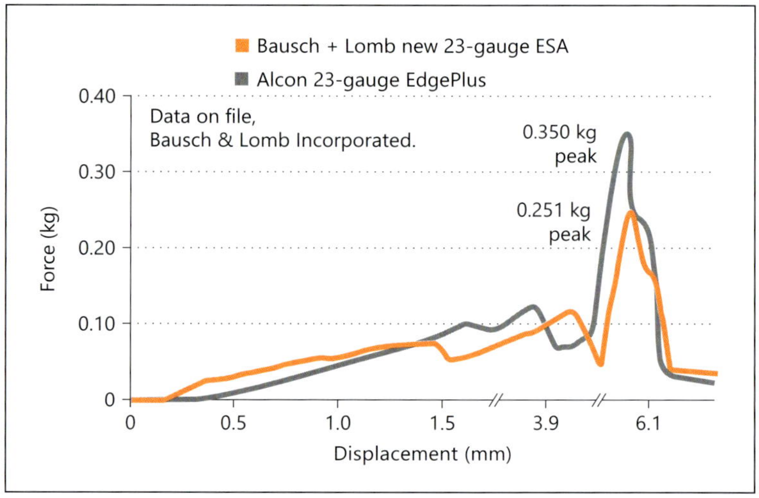

Fig. 6. Comparison of force required for inserting the 23-gauge ESA trocar/cannula and other entry system.

abetic retinopathy or tractional retinal detachment as bleeding from blood vessels can be reduced due to less fluctuation of intraocular pressure associated with change of instruments. The valve is also removable for easier use with soft-tip instruments.

Fluidics: Infusion and Vacuum

The infusion of fluid into the vitreous cavity in the Stellaris PC can be performed either by gravity passively or by pressure actively via vented air-forced infusion (AFI), in which air is injected into the infusion bottle to pressurize the bottle via a vault tube (fig. 8). A standard infusion pressure of 30–35 mm Hg is used during vitrectomy for most settings. The vented AFI infusion allows a much faster change in infusion pressure compared with gravity-assisted infusion with an automated intravenous pole, and the surgeon can quickly elevate the infusion pressure from around 40 mm Hg to a high pressure of 60 mm Hg within 0.5 s [4]. The machine also has an independent pump which does not rely on external pressurized air. In addition, the system also has a power failure mode that temporarily preserves the globe's intraocular pressure in case of electricity power loss, which allows more time to seal the globe and restore electric power [5].

The vacuum created by the Stellaris PC can be controlled precisely by the surgeon and can go down to as low as 2 mm Hg. The system has a high responsiveness and with the foot pedal, the surgeon can change the vacuum from 0 to 600 mm Hg within 1.5 s [4]. The system also has a reflux function that allows continuous flow of infusion fluid via the cutter to blow blood or other debris away from the retinal surface at a preset pressure. This reflux function is particularly useful when operating cases of proliferative retinopathy, as blood can be cleared away from the bleeding site for further treatment with intraocular diathermy or endolaser.

High-Speed Vitreous Cutter

The pneumatic vitrectomy cutter in the Stellaris PC system has a maximum cut rate of up to 5,000 cuts/min. A pneumatic line and an aspiration line connect the proximal end of the cutter to the machine. An optional extension handle can be installed for vibration dampening and better grip. The Stellaris PC cutter has a preset port opening time (duty cycle) which has been optimized for safety and performance for all the cutting speeds, and the port is open at least 50% of time (fig. 9) [4]. The port has been moved closer to the tip of

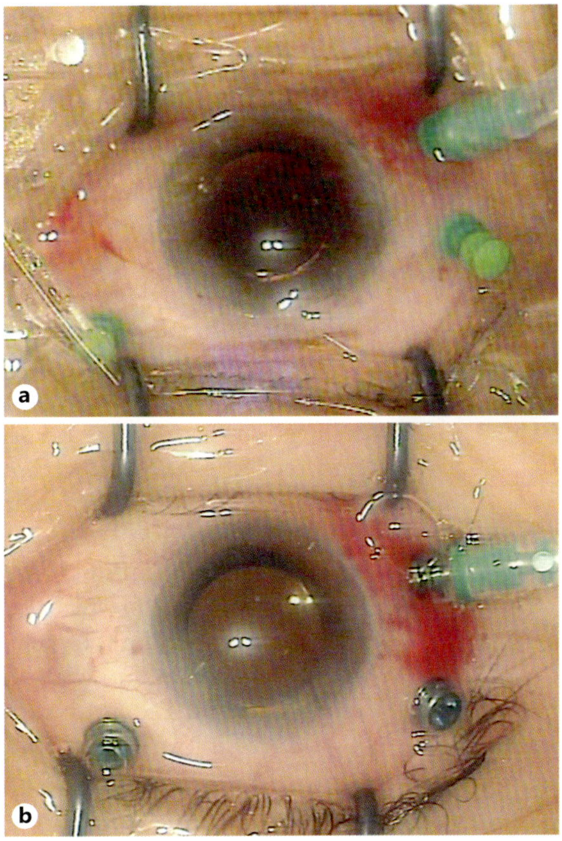

7

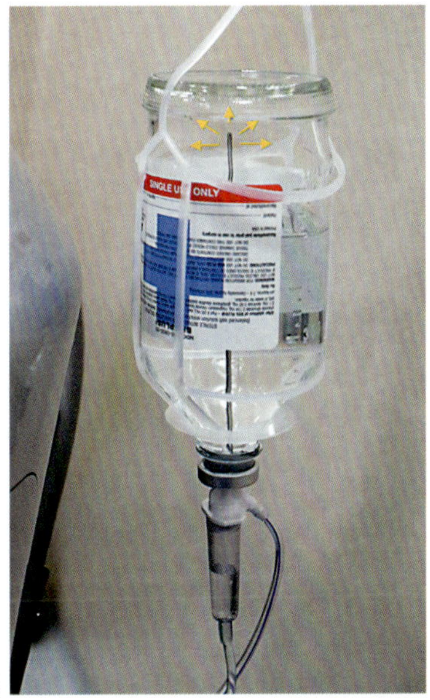

8

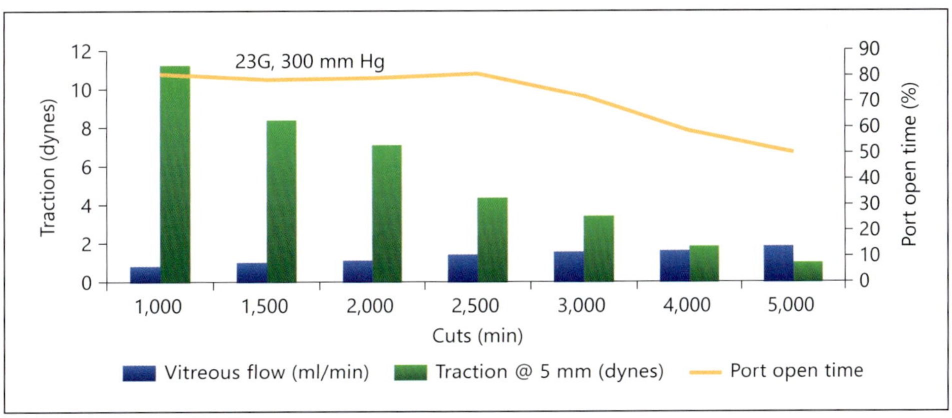

9

Fig. 7. Intraoperative photo with 23-gauge ESA nonvalved (**a**) and 23-gauge ESA valved (**b**) trocar/cannula inserted with infusion line connected. The self-sealing valves eliminate the need for scleral plugs and allow for better maintenance of intraocular pressure during introduction and removal of instruments.

Fig. 8. AFI in which air is actively pumped into the upper part of the infusion fluid bottle (arrows); this can provide more stable and rapid changes in infusion pressure required.

Fig. 9. Graph of vitreous flow, traction, and port open time vs. cutting rate for 23-gauge cutter at a 300-mm Hg fixed vacuum.

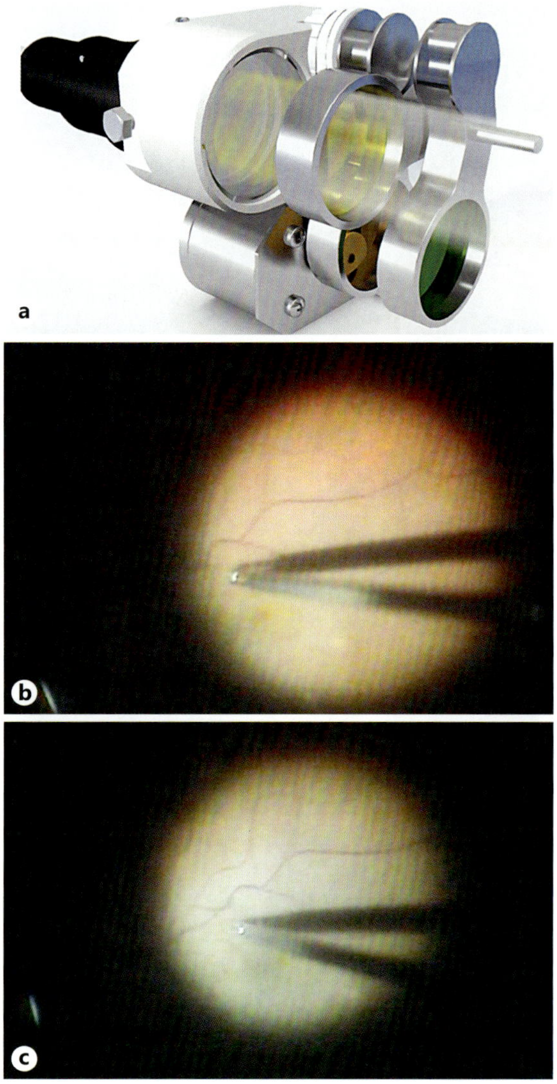

Fig. 10. a Diagram of xenon light source with colored filters for changing different illumination environment. Intraoperative view of epiretinal membrane peeling under normal xenon white light (**b**) and with green light from the xenon source (**c**).

the cutter probe compared with previous systems, allowing the surgeon to work closer to the retina [5]. This also enables safer removal of epiretinal fibrosis by the cutter without using a forceps or scissors. In addition, the port opening area of the cutter in the Stellaris PC is relatively larger than some other systems, and the combination of a high cut rate and large port area allows an efficient vitrectomy.

Priming of the Stellaris PC cutter is performed with a hands-free automatic function. To start priming, the scrub nurse or assistant can place the cutter and the infusion line in the disposable priming tray provided in the procedural pack, and the entire cutter and tubing system can be primed in about 45 s following the press of the button. Following priming, various vitrectomy settings can be used according to the surgeon's preferences. These settings can include the dual-linear mode in which the vacuum and cut rate can be altered by the foot pedal independently, a fixed maximum cutting rate and variable vacuum, or a colinear '3D' mode in which the surgeon can alter the vacuum with the foot pedal and the cutting rate is at a maximum when the vacuum is at a minimum, and the cutting rate is reduced in higher vacuum.

Illumination

The Stellaris PC has an illumination function which allows the installation of two light sources. The light sources can be two xenon lamps or a xenon lamp and a mercury vapor lamp. These two light sources can be used independently or simultaneously and various illuminated instruments such as a chandelier and illuminated picks can be connected to these light sources. The xenon light source has a cutoff filter at 435 nm to give a standard white light illumination. In addition, it also has a colored filter system that alters the color of the light being emitted and the illumination color can change from white to yellow, green, or amber (fig. 10). Changing the color of illumination can provide safer illumination and also enable better visualization of different structures within the eye [4, 6]. For example, the green light has been suggested to improve the visualization during membrane peeling in macular surgery and the amber light can greatly enhance safety by prolonging the

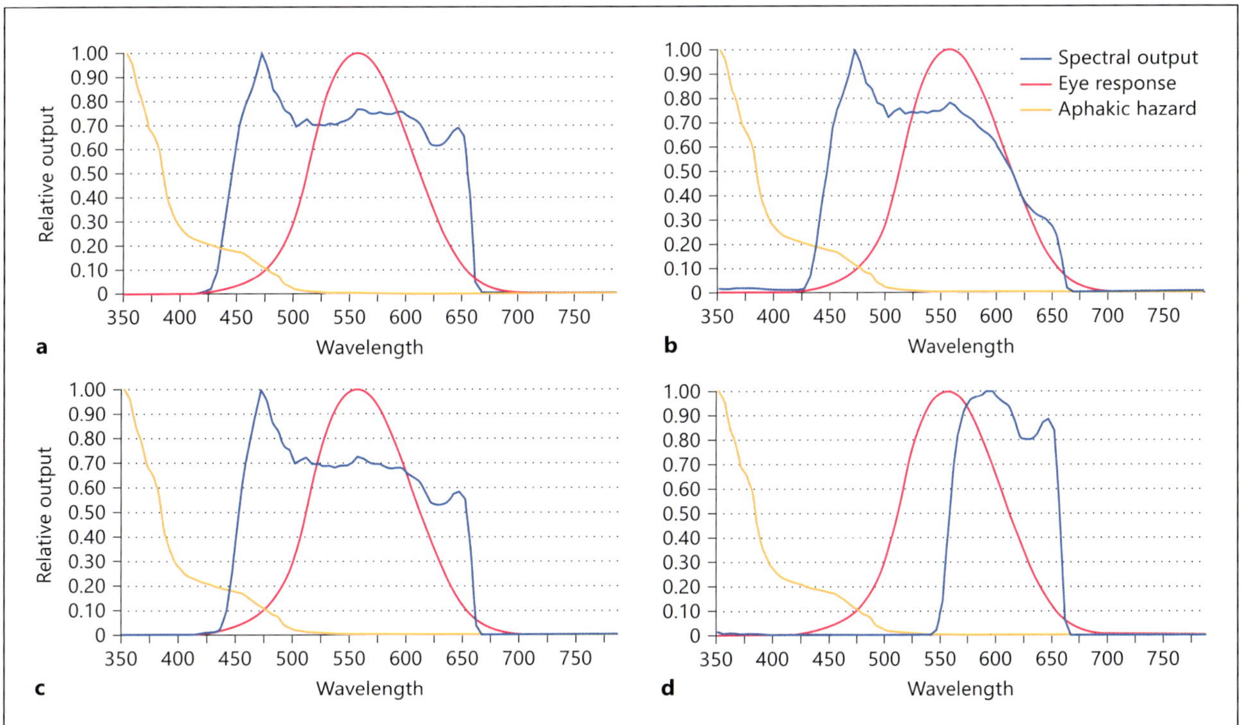

Fig. 11. Spectral output curves at various wavelengths of the Stellaris PC built-in xenon illumination: without filter (**a**), with green filter (**b**), with yellow filter (**c**), and with amber filter (**d**). The amber filter has the highest safety margin due to the least overlap with the aphakic hazard curve.

threshold duration of retinal light phototoxicity (fig. 11). The mercury vapor light source also incorporates a blue filter which gives a slight yellow and green tint to the illumination color. This light source is particularly suitable for connecting the chandelier due to its high brightness, and for longer surgical procedures due to enhanced safety by reducing phototoxicity [2]. For standard handheld illumination, a focal illuminator is available to provide a focused field of illumination of around 50° and is suitable for macular and most vitreoretinal surgery. When a more uniform diffuse illumination is required, a handheld wide-field illuminator is also available to provide a wide-angle illumination of 115°. It also has a shield around the tip of the light pipe to prevent glare from affecting the surgeon during surgery.

Other Additional Features

As with most other vitrectomy systems, infusion of air or silicon oil can be performed with the Stellaris PC. The system has a secondary infusion line for fluid-air exchange and the process can be triggered by the scrub nurse on the LCD screen or by the surgeon with the foot pedal. Silicon oil infusion and removal can also be performed using the viscous fluid injection and viscous fluid extraction kits, respectively. Thermal coagulation can be performed using monopolar or bipolar diathermy connected to the machine. Finally, since late 2013, an integrated double-frequency Nd:YAG 532-nm laser module is also available and can be operated with the wireless foot pedal when switched to the laser mode.

Conclusion

The Stellaris PC is a fully integrated combined phacoemulsification and vitrectomy machine which incorporates the ability to perform <2-mm microincision cataract surgery and advance microincision posterior segment surgery with good efficacy. Surgeons can operate and switch efficiently and quickly from cataract surgery to vitreoretinal surgery using a single machine. In addition, new features such as high-speed cutting, pressurized AFI infusion, ESA trocar/cannula system, color-filtered illuminations and a user-friendly interface are beneficial features of the Stellaris PC system.

Disclosure Statement

Dr. Lai has received honorarium for lecture fees from Bausch & Lomb Inc.

References

1 Chow DR: PC = Procedural Choice. Retinal Physician 2011;Suppl:4.
2 Awh CC: System enables today's most advanced technique. Retin Physician 2011;Suppl:5–7.
3 Ferrone P: Advanced wound management with a new trocar/cannula entry system. Retin Physician 2011;Suppl: 10–11.
4 Awh CC: Stellaris PC: next generation vitrectomy technology. Innov Ophthalmol 2011, pp 44–45.
5 Hassan T: State-of-the-art vitreous cutting and fluidics. Retin Physician 2011; Suppl:8–9.
6 Huang SS: Novel illumination with an eye on the future. Retin Physician 2011; Suppl:12–14.

Timothy Y.Y. Lai, MD, FRCS, FRCOphth
Department of Ophthalmology and Visual Sciences
The Chinese University of Hong Kong, Hong Kong Eye Hospital
147K Argyle Street
Kowloon, Hong Kong, SAR (China)
E-Mail tyylai@cuhk.edu.hk

Oh H, Oshima Y (eds): Microincision Vitrectomy Surgery. Emerging Techniques and Technology.
Dev Ophthalmol. Basel, Karger, 2014, vol 54, pp 17–22 (DOI: 10.1159/000360444)

Machines and Cutters: VersaVIT – Potential and Perspectives of Office-Based Vitrectomy

Virgilio Morales-Canton · P. Ayumi Kawakami-Campos

Retina Department, Hospital Luis Sanchez Bulnes, Asociacion para Evitar la Ceguera en México, Universidad Nacional Autonoma de Mexico, Mexico City, Mexico

Abstract

The concept of office-based vitrectomy has been a topic for several years; however, the large size of the vitrectomy machines has limited the options for many years. Today, though, smaller machines can offer adequate performance regarding vitrectomy. As a result, we can now make more arguments for this type of surgery to be performed in the office environment, despite the limitations these machines may still have.

Since Fujii et al. [1] first introduced the new concept of transconjunctival sutureless vitrectomy using a trocar technique and 25-gauge instrumentation, the term microincision vitrectomy has evolved and dramatically changed the way vitrectomies are performed globally over the last decade. The main advantages of these developments are reduced corneal astigmatism, less scarring in the conjunctiva, better patient comfort, and (more importantly) better instrumentation [2–4].

Today, we know that retinal surgery is never constant – different procedures call for different technologies. Some procedures will be time-consuming and require more equipment, while others will be quick and easy to solve. It is left to the surgeon to discern which variant the procedure is likely to be. The equipment used for each procedure should be chosen as part of the protocol prior to bringing the patient into the operating room.

As vitrectomy systems have become more efficient, technologically superior, and individualized to the performing surgeon, they have consequently become more expensive. Venturi-based or peristaltic systems, as well as other systems that combine these two in order to meet the surgeon's expectations and simplify the procedure, are now commercially available [5]. One of the most widely used Venturi-based systems is Alcon's Accurus, one of the first machines available for anterior and posterior segment surgery with disposable ready-to-use consumables previously selected and preordered in an Alcon pack. The same packs were used for both easy and difficult cases (i.e. the same expense), and since the unused material could not be resterilized, no savings in terms of equipment expense could be seen for easy and uncomplicated cases.

Other companies recognized this weakness of Accurus and the potential in developing a more

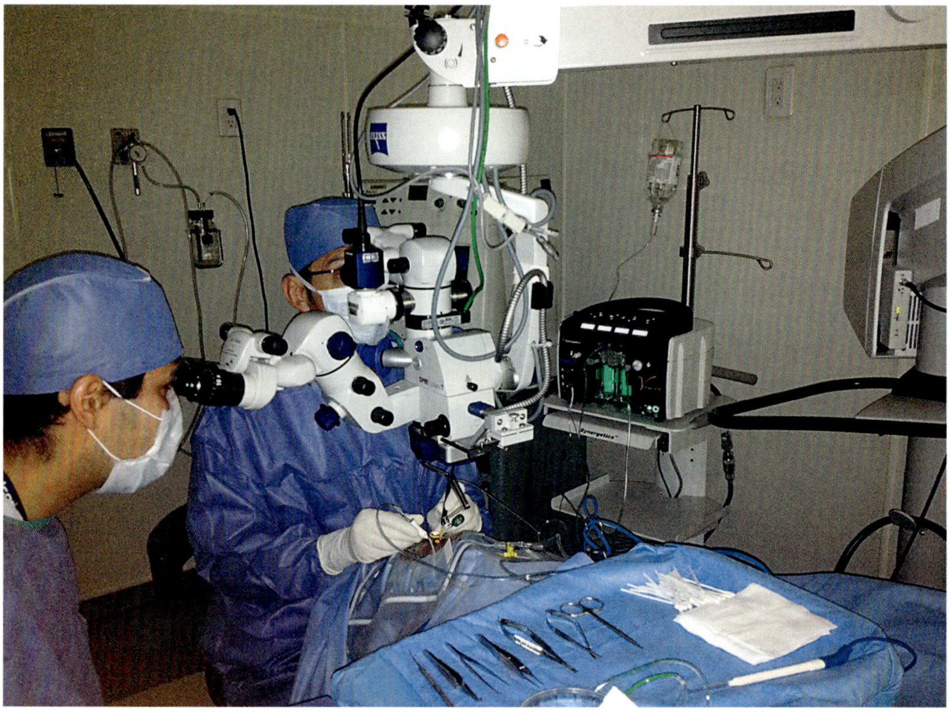

Fig. 1. The small size of the VersaVIT machine.

customizable approach to this type of surgery. Synergetics USA Inc. developed a Venturi pump-based vitrectomy system with fluidics similar to Alcon's Accurus, but utilized costumizable packs available in 20, 23, 25, and 27 gauge, and compatible with the Accurus system as well. As a result, it is still possible to use Accurus as your primary vitrectomy machine with selected features in personalized packs according to personal necessities, such as chandelier, widefield, midfield, or focal illumination; steel versus polyimide cannulas; curved versus straight laser probe, and valved versus open trocar entry.

Office-Based Vitrectomy Limitations

Excluding teaching-hospital settings, most operating rooms tend to constrict the space intended for ophthalmic surgery as it is considered part of ambulatory procedures. On the other hand, some surgeons have two or more facilities at their disposal at distant locations, making it more cost-effective to transport a vitrectomy machine between them instead of fulfilling the needs of each center individually.

Vitrectomy systems such as the Stellaris PC, Constellation, and Accurus, although having great performance, require wide spaces, infrastructure, and specially trained personnel. Having observed these drawbacks, some competitors realized the need for smaller, portable, and use-friendly interfaces in vitrectomy systems; developers such as Oertli and Synergetics came up with the OS3/FAROS and VersaVIT machines, respectively, as alternatives.

Synergetics' VersaVIT provides a small yet effective vitrectomy system (fig. 1, 2), which can easily be stored in a travel case to be safely trans-

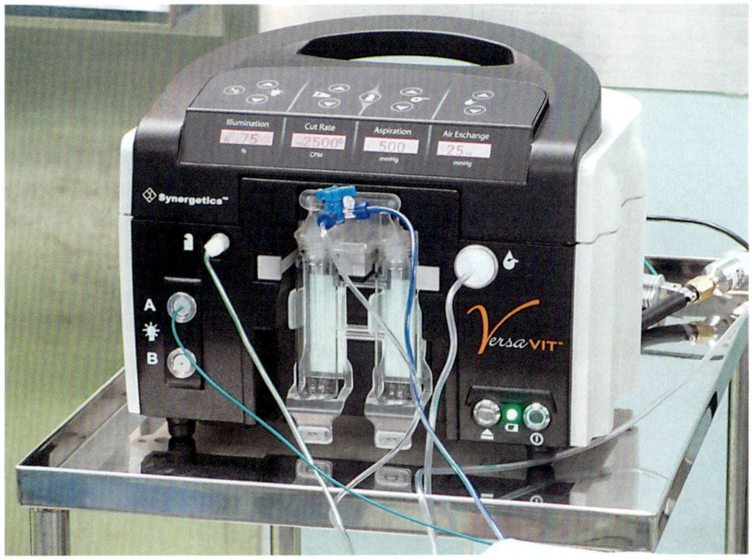

Fig. 2. The system has controls for illumination (2 ports), cut rate, vacuum, and air pressure for air-fluid exchange.

ported between settings with a weight slightly over 25 lbs (11 kg). Its quick startup helps reduce wasted time inside the operating room, and in case of technical difficulties it can run on an electrical power source or inner rechargeable battery. As not all operating rooms are the same, you may use VersaVIT powered on CO_2, compressed air, or nitrogen, expanding the availability of multiple facilities for one single surgeon.

Procedure and Machine Pairing

Most vitreoretinal surgeons claim to select the machine according to the procedure intended; however, not every surgery goes as planned and diversity in functionality is a mandatory specification when it comes to vitrectomy systems. Older systems such as Accurus offer a 2,500-cuts/min (cpm) rate with a nonoptimal pneumatic vitreous cutter, which leads to underachievement in challenging situations. Newer systems, like the Stellaris PC and Constellation can achieve up to 5,000–7,500 cpm while delivering stable fluidics and expected performance during surgery. The

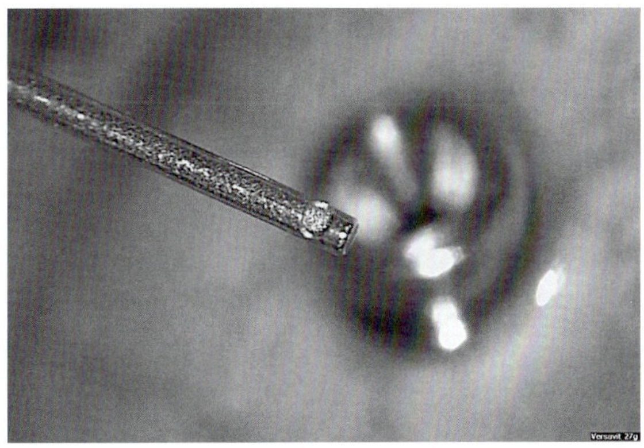

Fig. 3. 27-gauge vitrectomy probe. The port is located 0.04 mm to the tip of the instrument.

VersaVIT vitrectomy probe with the Ultimate Vit Enhancer is an exclusive system, available in 23- and 25-guage versions, with a pneumatic cutter that can perform up to 8,000 cpm at a 500-mm Hg vaccum level; this advance comes with a reasonable change in cutter opening location and extension. It is placed 0.04 mm closer to the tip of probe and it has a 0.02 mm wider opening compared to Constellation's 25-guage probe (fig. 3). The tro-

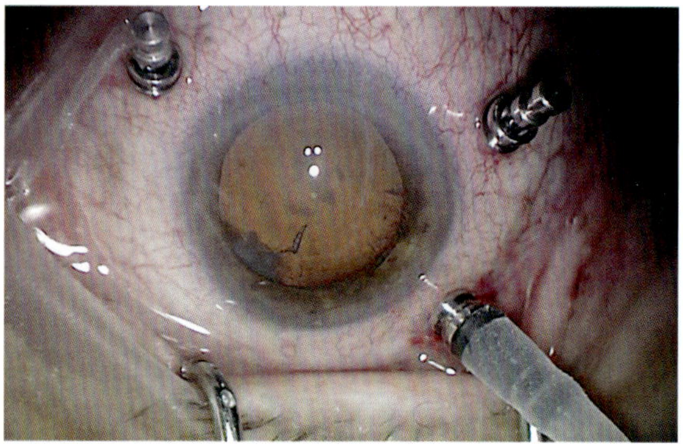

Fig. 4. 27-gauge trocars inserted with metal plugs.

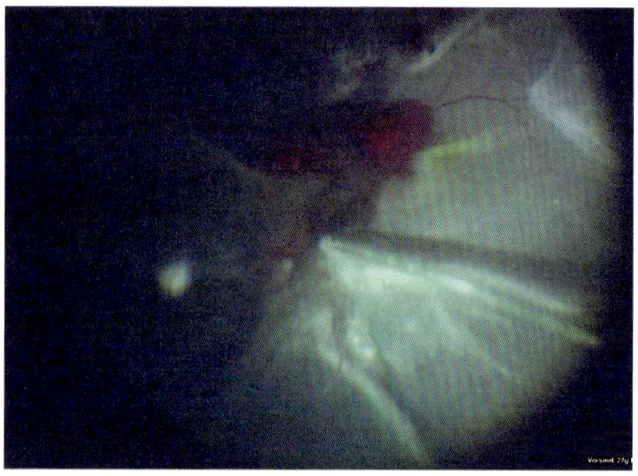

Fig. 5. The 27-gauge probe can be introduced between the retina and the membranes facilitating their removal.

car insertion of this equipment is very smooth and controlled thanks to very sharp stilettos that are on the trocars (fig. 4).

In our opinion, the VersaVIT 27-gauge probe is an excellent instrument in complicated cases of tractional detachments secondary to proliferative diabetic retinopathy. The adequate fluidics and the proximity of the port to the tip of the instrument facilitates the cutting of the fibrous tissues. The tip can be introduced between the retina and the membranes, and the cutting action removes the tissue in an adequate manner. This surgical approach has been performed previously by Oshima et al. [6] (fig. 5).

Although VersaVIT comes with an air-fluid exchange feature, it does not include a preset silicon oil injection or extraction function as many other systems do. The lack of such a feature causes some surgeons to doubt the multitasking capabilities of VersaVIT. In some centers, such as ours, silicon oil extraction and injection can be performed manually using a surgeon-selected syringe (best results with 4 or 5 syringes of 1 ml) and either a silicon tip or a peripheral venous catheter whose length is modified by the surgeon to fit around the trocar in use. For obvious reasons this last technique is only useful when using nonvalved trocars. Either way, the lack of an oil injection feature does not diminish the multiple procedure versatility of this vitrectomy system.

Basic Surgical Aspects

Retina surgery has one aspect that is different from some other ophthalmic procedures: we need more time to do a complete job and the clear media to do so. However, since the latter tends to restrain the former, time is actually invaluable. To reduce some of the preparation time, Synergetics has now released the Express 3-in-1 port entry system, which allows the surgeon to introduce all three ports without trading dangerous multiple blades with his/her assistant, as they all are preloaded in a single handle. After placing the first cannula, the surgeon only has to press a button to advance the next one to be inserted.

All experienced surgeons agree that vitreoretinal surgery requires an assistant – this does not mean it cannot be done without one, but is just a lot easier. In many countries (both developed and underdeveloped), retina specialists are not evenly distributed – there may be some cities crowded with them, while other places do not have any.

Some surgeons will occasionally travel to perform surgery in different facilities. They generally prefer to have a surgical assistant come along, but may not always be able to find one for these trips. With this in mind, many technologies have been developed to increase surgeon independency when it comes to vitrectomy. Synergetics has developed illuminated laser probes, with a 20-gauge light pipe intensity that makes it perfect for self-scleral depression and peripheral retinal laser ablation. Another product is the Microfiber Illuminated Vitrector Sleeve, which can increase the diameter of the latter but allows the surgeon to use the other hand freely without the need of a chandelier. Another handy item in Synergetics' catalogue is the Illuminated Infusion Chandelier, which achieves not only 20- to 25-guage panoramic lighting, but also keeps the solution flow going.

Since illumination during surgery is a vital, if not the most essential, issue for a retina specialist, a special mention of endoilluminators' characteristics is in order. For starters, every surgeon becomes used to seeing things in a certain way during surgery, whether it is xenon versus filtered light, wide- versus middlefield, or focal versus chandelier. As with many companies, Synergetics has different options for different types of surgeries and surgeons.

The traditional Accurus add-on endoilluminator has close to a 79° angle with a xenon source, allowing surgery under a safe and adequate intensity of light. This is the starting point for illuminators available on VersaVIT, which can achieve up to 135–140° (widefield), or 100–110° (midfield). When bimanual surgery is attempted, a chandelier is the best way to achieve maximum endoillumination on a widefield concept without sacrificing the use of the second surgeon's hand. Synergetics' 25- and 29-gauge chandelier accomplishes widefield, safe, and unanimous light on a preloaded cannula in a self-retaining fashion, reducing the risk of unnoticed extrusion and sclerotomy leak after removal.

Endolaser has been one of the biggest advances in retina surgery in the last decades – it is hard to believe that we once did not have it. Once a surgeon has tried a curve laser probe, one of two things will happen: he/she will never look at the same straight probe with excitement, or he/she decides it is not bad as a spare probe. Whatever the case, the Directional II Laser probe can keep both of them satisfied, starting as a straight endolaser probe, it has a slide button that retrieves the straight coating, allowing it to curve in an adaptable fashion up to 90°. The probe can stop its angling at any time by releasing the button on the handle, which can come in handy when the peripheral retina is reached and eye wall curvature is adverted.

Disadvantages

The small size of the machine limits the amount of vitreous and fluid collected on the cassette. This can be a problem in long cases where the surgeon needs to perform several maneuvers. When using this machine, the surgeon must have an external bipolar machine for cauterization. We think that the VersaVIT would be more complete if it would come with a bipolar module.

Conclusions

VersaVIT is a very solid vitrectomy machine (despite its small size) that can offer portability, adequate fluidics, and good cutting features. There is no doubt that it lacks some of the advantages the bigger machines have; however, for uncomplicated cases and due to limitations in the operating room, is a very nice machine to work with.

References

1 Fujii GY, et al: A new 25-gauge instrument system for transconjunctival sutureless vitrectomy surgery. Ophthalmology 2002;109:1807–1812, discussion 1813.

2 Recchia FM, et al: Small-gauge pars plana vitrectomy: a report by the American Academy of Ophthalmology. Ophthalmology 2010;117:1851–1857.

3 Okamoto F, et al: Changes in corneal topography after 25-gauge transconjunctival sutureless vitrectomy versus after 20-gauge standard vitrectomy. Ophthalmology 2007;114:2138–2141.

4 Rizzo S, et al: 25-gauge, sutureless vitrectomy and standard 20-gauge pars plana vitrectomy in idiopathic epiretinal membrane surgery: a comparative pilot study. Graefes Arch Clin Exp Ophthalmol 2006;244:472–479.

5 Magalhaes O Jr, et al: Perspective on fluid and solid dynamics in different pars plana vitrectomy systems. Am J Ophthalmol 2011;151:401–405.e1.

6 Oshima Y, et al: A 27-gauge instrument system for transconjunctival sutureless microincision vitrectomy surgery. Ophthalmology 2010;117:93–102.e2.

Virgilio Morales-Canton, MD
Hospital 'Dr. Luis Sanchez Bulnes', Asociacion para Evitar la Ceguera en Mexico
Vicente Garcia Torres 46
San Lucas Coyoacan, Coyoacan, Mexico City 04030 (Mexico)
E-Mail vmoralesc@mac.com

Oh H, Oshima Y (eds): Microincision Vitrectomy Surgery. Emerging Techniques and Technology.
Dev Ophthalmol. Basel, Karger, 2014, vol 54, pp 23–30 (DOI: 10.1159/000360445)

Enhancing Visual Acuity

Peter Stalmans
Department of Ophthalmology, University Hospitals Leuven, Leuven, Belgium

Abstract
The Enhancing Visual Acuity (EVA) System (Dutch Ophthalmic Research Centre International B.V.) features a unique fluid control system – VacuFlow Valve Timing Intelligence (VTi®) – and represents the next-generation evolution of pump machines. VacuFlow VTi® overcomes the limitations of existing Venturi and peristaltic pumps and provides the potential to enable safer, faster, and more precise techniques. Alongside many other innovative and functional features, such as a light-emitting diode light source, integrated laser, high cutting speed with twin duty cycle cutting, automated infusion compensation, wireless foot pedal, phaco module with thresholding, and viscous fluid module, EVA could make a major contribution to advancing ophthalmology.

Vitrectomy is fundamental in treating patients affected by retinal detachment, retinopathies, macular diseases, vitreous hemorrhage, and several other vitreoretinal diseases. More than 500,000 vitrectomy procedures are performed globally by physicians every year, and this number is rising. Despite its widespread use and great potential, it is still considered a delicate surgery with intraoperative and postoperative risks for patients. Specialists generally welcome advances in surgical tools that offer opportunities for added precision, safety, and security.

The Enhancing Visual Acuity System

The Enhancing Visual Acuity (EVA) system was developed by the Dutch Ophthalmic Research Centre International B.V. (fig. 1). It features a unique fluid control system – VacuFlow Valve Timing Intelligence (VTi®) – and represents the next-generation evolution of pump machines. EVA induces an aspiration flow effect by implementation of a displacement pump, providing precise flow and fast vacuum, eliminating the risk of unwanted pulsation or alterations in flow, and increasing the control that the surgeon has over the procedure. The system received CE approval on March 3, 2013 and became commercially available in June 2013.

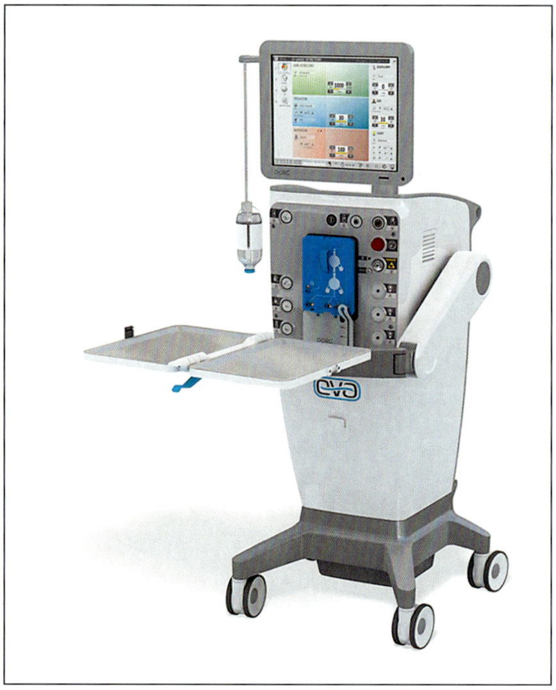

Fig. 1. DORC EVA device. The blue front cap on the middle of the machine is the disposable cassette of the VTi fluidics system. The infusion bottle can be toggled from left to right. The instrument tray can be mounted on the left or right. Instrument connectors are color coded. Menu changes can be selected using the foot pedal or using the touch screen.

Development

EVA's unique flow control system, the VacuFlow VTi®, was developed to overcome two main limitations of existing Venturi and peristaltic pumps. The first is the time lag created by dispelling large volumes of air from the (typically ≥250 ml) cartridge of many Venturi systems before the desired vacuum level is attained. VacuFlow VTi offers a significant improvement by combining a series of very precise computer-controlled operating pistons and valves working in very small flow chambers (volume: 6 ml). Secondly, the weaknesses of both the Venturi and peristaltic pumps have been compensated with EVA's combined flow and vacuum system. Venturi pumps have never enabled precise, viscosity-independent flow control, whereas the peristaltic system characteristically produces mild flow fluctuations inherent to the rotary compression of flexible tubing. In addition, with advances in vitrectomy procedures, including peripheral vitrectomy and using smaller-gauge instrumentation, new options in vitrectomy systems were essential.

VacuFlow VTi® technology was introduced in 2012 by DORC with the prototype EVA platform and has since been used to perform vitrectomy, phaco procedures, and combined phaco-vitrectomy procedures. DORC made EVA available to a selected number of retina surgeons worldwide during its development and worked in close collaboration with them, incorporating their feedback to modify the final product design.

The EVA system allows the user to decide between two different modes: vacuum or flow control mode. In vacuum mode, the pistons work at high speed to build and maintain the desired vacuum value. In flow control mode, the valves operate at a precalculated speed to achieve the desired flow. The result is a perfectly synchronized system that enables exact control of aspiration and flow with a precision never achieved before. Moreover, a desired switch from vacuum to flow mode or vice versa is instantaneous since no mechanical changes are involved in this transition.

Features

Fluidics (fig. 2)

Better flow control allows for faster, more efficient cutting and a higher safety profile. In addition, with techniques, such as peripheral vitrectomy and smaller-gauge procedures on the rise, precise flow management is becoming even more critical to reduce the risks of this type of procedure.

The main limitation of the Venturi pump is the control of the depression generated by the pump that affects aspiration control. The Venturi pump can only create a depression of vacuum, increasing the gradient of pressure required to

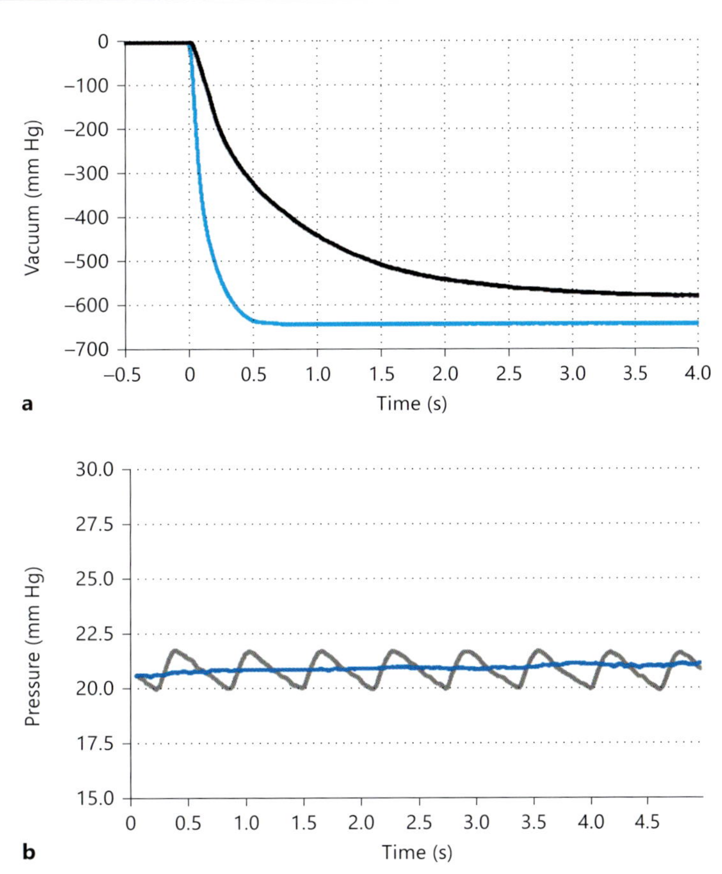

Fig. 2. DORC EVA VTi fluidics system. **a** Compared to a Venturi system, the rise time of the EVA VTi in vacuum mode is much faster, hence the desired vacuum is obtained with a shorter response time. Black line: vacuum response of a Venturi vitrectomy system. Blue line: vacuum response of the VTi system. **b** Compared to a rotary peristaltic system, the pressure output generated by the EVA VTi in flow mode does not show any oscillations, resulting in a more stable fluidics system. Gray line: pressure variation of a peristaltic vitrectomy system. Blue line: pressure variation of the VTi system.

maintain flow. A typical vacuum pump has a minimum outflow, based on the pressure gradient and the instrumentation size, which rules out the possibility to control the aspiration flow below. Since Venturi pumps cannot work with positive pressure at the pump level, many surgeons compensate by setting the cut rate as high as possible to provide partial compensation for this issue. Peristaltic systems generate a gradient of pressure so that flow remains stable independent of the fluid's viscosity. The European Vitreoretinal Society (EVRS) Retinal Detachment Study, published in 2013, showed that retinal detachment surgery performed with vacuum-based venturi systems had a 2.9 times higher failure rate compared to the same surgery performed with flow-based peristaltic systems [1, 2]. A failure rate of 0.7% with 23-gauge surgery and 1.1% with 20-gauge surgery was achieved with peristaltic pumps, which rose to 1.4% with 23-gauge surgery and 2.5% with 20-gauge surgery when a Venturi system was used.

EVA's unique flow control system eliminates the need for a conventional large-size cartridge. It is replaced with a microchamber system, in which computer-controlled pistons and valves work in harmony with high-precision pressure sensors. The two synchronized operating pistons compensate for changes in pressure, as recognized by the high-sensitivity pressure sensors. Two valves allow filling and emptying of the microchambers without disruption of flow or pressure. Optimal pressure balance blocks any fluctuations in aspiration pressure, with the ability to create a vacuum from 0 to 650 mm Hg in less than 0.3 s. EVA is a synchronized system that enables the exact control of aspiration and flow with a precision that has never been achieved before. In flow mode, EVA can control flow to within 0.1 ml accuracy – equivalent to 1,000% more precision than former machines. The vacuum response time is four times faster than previous pump technologies.

High-Speed Cutting with Twin Duty Cycle Control

Choosing an optimal cut rate and duty cycle are critical elements for safe and effective surgery. They also influence the control of flow in Venturi pumps, with higher cutting speed increasing safety. However, using these systems at too-high cutting speeds can hamper aspiration of the vitreous. EVA enables a high cutting speed with optimal aspiration. The maximum cutting speed attainable with EVA is 8,000 cuts/min (cpm). Using high cut speeds with controlled aspiration can offer advantages for many procedures, such as core vitrectomy for retinal detachments in which the retina is mobile because there is less traction. Switching to flow mode to shave the vitreous base, using 8,000 cpm, paired with a lower duty cycle (port open 40% of the time), is ideal for vitreous removal close to the retina. In combination with 8,000-cpm high-speed and high-flow technology, the vitreous can be removed up to the vitreous base virtually without any traction, avoiding the creation of (additional) retinal breaks. In core vitrectomy, working with EVA in vacuum mode at relatively low cutting speeds (1,500–3,000 cpm) with a higher duty cycle (port open 60% of the time) enables the core vitreous to be removed quickly, usually in the setting region of 0–4 ml/min and precisely controlled by the foot pedal.

A new cutter type is available that is equipped with an opening in the vitrectome blade [twin duty cycle (TDC) cutter]. This feature offers two advantages: (1) each time the blade moves forwards and backwards, two cuts are made, which effectively produces cut rates up to 16,000 cpm, and (2) even when the blade is in the forwards position, the port is not occluded, which enhances the flow through the system. As a result, even at maximal cut rates and using flows around 4 ml/min, there is almost no buildup of a vacuum in the aspiration line, which provides precision control of the flow in the tubing.

Small-Gauge Instrumentation

Smaller-gauge instruments enable greater precision in procedures, and offer less tissue manipulation, reduced inflammation, sutureless surgery, and decreased postoperative pain with more rapid visual recovery. However, working with smaller gauges requires a higher level of understanding of flow characteristics because all material must travel through an instrument with a smaller diameter. Higher infusion and aspiration pressures are needed to remove the vitreous when working with 23- and 25-gauge probes. In addition, smaller-gauge instrumentation has increased flexion, rendering it more appropriate for certain procedures and not others.

The enhanced flow control offered by EVA makes smaller-gauge surgery more feasible. The TDC vitrectome – for use with 23-, 25-, and 27-gauge instrumentation in EVA – features a larger rectangular aperture in the inner tube and a blade with two sharp cutting edges. The vitreous is brought into the inner aperture and cut in a forward and backward movement, increasing the amount of vitreous that is cut in a single motion. The aperture in the inner tube results in almost constant aspiration flow into the port. The inner port on the new cutter is larger than previous designs, which should enable a larger amount of material to be taken per cut and increase the speed of surgical procedures. The TDC vitrectome removes 2–3 times more vitreous than a standard cutter. Even at the highest cutting rates possible, the vibration of the TDC vitrectome is minimal.

Automatic Infusion Control

High intraocular pressure during vitrectomy compromises vascularization in the eye. Ideally, the intraocular pressure should be constant at 20 mm Hg. However, when aspirating with the vitrector in vacuum mode at a relatively high vacuum of 350 mm Hg, the volume of fluid removed from the eye will be larger than the volume of liquid flowing into the eye, which can cause the eye to collapse. Automatic infusion control, as featured on EVA, compensates this and elevates the pressure settings by generating higher air pressure in the infusion bottle as the aspiration of the vitrector increases and prevents collapse. When the aspiration from the cutter stops, the air pressure in the bottle is vented back to baseline (e.g. 20 mm Hg) to prevent a rise in intraocular pressure.

Illumination

EVA includes LEDStar technology incorporating a light-emitting diode (LED) light source, which produces a white light within the safest range of the phototoxicity curve. It has a similar curve to the spectral sensitivity of the eye. The EVA has three independent LED light ports, all of which are equipped with two light sources: a white and a yellow LED. By changing the balance between the white and the yellow LED, any variation between bright white and full yellow light temperature can be selected. Used together with a yellow setting of 20%, the light source presents virtually no photochemical toxicity and emits a light that is distinctly yellow, comparable to the light temperature of a halogen light. If the yellow color is dialed down to 10, there is still relatively no photochemical toxicity and the light is a brighter white with a small amount of yellow color. LED bulbs in the light offer robustness and durability, with a 10,000- to 20,000-hour lifetime and break resistance. Compared to the 400 h of service from metal-halide bulbs, the longevity of LED lights is a significant advantage in terms of maintenance. In addition, LEDStar lighting offers a safe, brighter option, which is particularly important when working with 27-gauge fibers. It is even bright enough when used at 30–40% of its maximum output for 23-gauge vitrectomy with a standard illuminating fiber. Used in conjunction with widefield fibers, a typical output of 70–80% is used.

Integrated Laser

EVA has an integrated 532-nm laser with outstanding ergonomics. It is controlled via a wireless foot pedal. The integrated laser reduces the need for an additional instrument on the floor of the operating room or additional responsibilities for operating room staff. Control of the laser power from the foot pedal, as well as the possibility to switch the laser on or off using the foot pedal, are definite advantages.

Combined Procedures

EVA offers optimum versatility, allowing use of the vacuum mode for core vitrectomy with the opportunity to switch to flow mode for work in the periphery. An increasing proportion of clinical cases require combined phaco-vitrectomy. The system has a built in phaco module featuring thresholding. EVA's fast vacuum rise time provides a quick and powerful attraction of lens particles during segment removal, which reduces the amount of phaco power required by around 30%. The integral vacuum thresholding rapidly reduces the amount of aspiration when occlusion of the phaco tip breaks, eliminating a surge in aspiration that can induce collapse of the anterior chamber. In phaco mode, the machine typically allows a set vacuum of 400 mm Hg when the phaco tip is occluded. Before occlusion and after the lens particle is emulsified (resulting in a break in occlusion), the vacuum can be set to automatically return to 200 mm Hg. Using a higher vacuum also allows reduced use of phaco power for lens removal, providing extra safety for the endothelium. During core vitrectomy, working in vacuum mode in combination with relatively low cutting speeds (1,500–3,000 cpm), the core vitreous can be removed very quickly. For vitreous base shaving,

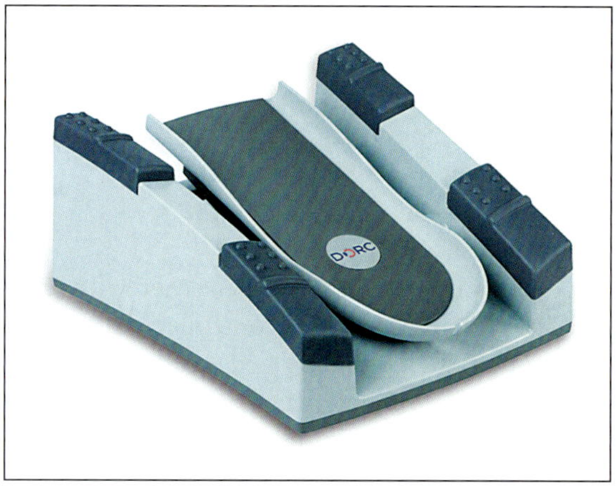

Fig. 3. DORC EVA wireless foot pedal. The foot pedal can be used in linear mode (vertical movement control) or dual-linear mode (horizontal and vertical movement controls different functions). The 4 rocker switches can be programmed according to the surgeon's preferences.

EVA can be set to flow mode with a very low fluid displacement (in the region of 0–4 ml/min), and can be precisely controlled using the foot pedal.

Foot Pedal Control

EVA's wireless foot pedal can be adapted to the needs of individual surgeons (fig. 3). The foot pedal has four different rocker settings that can each be programmed individually. Whether the surgeon moves his/her foot on the left or the right, a personalized set of functions can be requested and programmed in. The foot pedal can be operated with single-linear, dual-linear, or 3D control. This can be switched between procedures, for example using the single-linear mode for phaco procedures, such as making a groove in the lens, and using the dual-linear mode for extracting lens fragments and core vitrectomy procedures.

Ergonomics

EVA has a number of innovative ergonomic advantages. The flexible arm can be adjusted to any preferred position required by the surgeon or scrub nurse. Its large touch screen can be encased in packed sterile foil, which is easily replaced by operating room staff, ensuring optimal sterility without the need of technical intervention (fig. 4). The balanced salt solution bottle can be mounted on the left or right side of the patient. No tools are required to switch between the two positions. In addition, the height of the surgical instrument tray is fully adjustable and provides the flexible option for use as a half or full tray. EVA's integral sound system informs the surgeon of important instrumentation developments during procedures, which aids in understanding what is happening during surgery, saves time, and enables greater precision. For example, audio indications communicate when there is no more vitreous in the tube or when the pressure pump is positive. Overall, EVA offers the surgeon optimal ergonomics that ensure comfort and enable the surgeon to be in full control of all instrumentation parameters themselves, with limited reliance on technical support.

Accessories/Packs

DORC offers a wide range of phaco and vitrectomy accessories and color-coded packs for EVA, covering all gauge requirements and surgical preferences.

Future Developments

DORC is currently exploring options to provide network connection with hospital picture archiving and communications systems via EVA's USB connector device.

Getting Acquainted with the Enhancing Visual Acuity System

Due to EVA's user-friendly features and extensive programming flexibility, training to use the system is minimal. The system is unique in that it can be configured to any surgeon's preferred settings. For those working previously with the Stellaris PC (Bausch & Lomb), the work format with the vacuum mode and dual foot pedal can be eas-

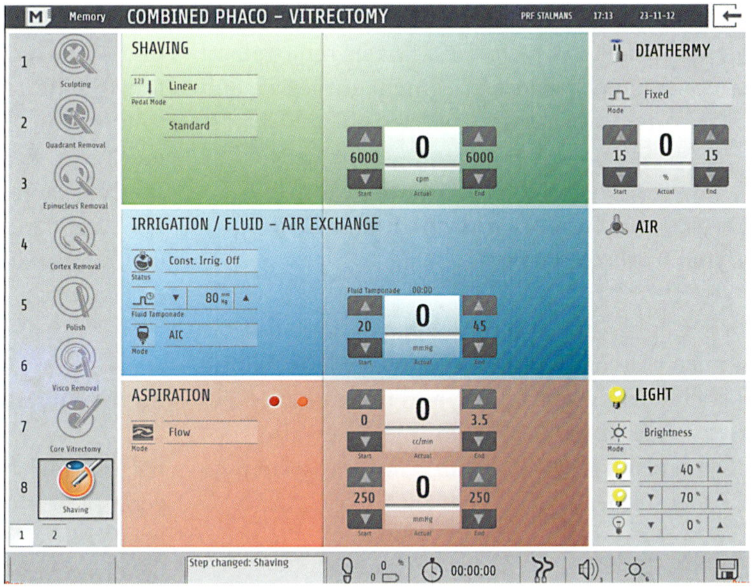

Fig. 4. DORC EVA user interface. The left column displays the current surgery mode. The green area shows the preset and actual cut rate (in vitrectomy) or phaco power (in phaco mode). The blue area displays the preset and actual irrigation pressure, while the lower orange area shows the VTi pump settings. Other essential functions such as diathermy power and light intensity can also be changed on the touch screen.

ily emulated in EVA by specific programming. For those more familiar with the foot pedal of the Constellation Vision System (Alcon), linear and 3D programming can be adjusted to emulate this work format. To get acquainted with EVA, surgeons can begin working with the system on their familiar settings and later explore and switch to other settings as their proficiency increases. They can also configure the system to start with 'non-aggressive' settings and build to more 'aggressive' settings to increase their surgery speed as familiarity with the system grows. Initial settings can be programmed by DORC's support experts following discussion with individual surgeons and examination of the hospital set up, or the required programming details can be shared by them so that configuration can be carried out by hospital staff. From my own experience, I found learning to use EVA to be similar to adapting to driving an upgraded model of a familiar vehicle. DORC regularly consults specialists using EVA for their feedback on the system and includes advanced training experiences for EVA customers at their facility in the Netherlands where they can expand on a basic working knowledge of using the system and ask specific questions. In addition, further information can be gained from transmission of live surgery using EVA to different symposia and congresses worldwide, as well as during on-invitation workshops. And for detailed discussion and debate on the use of EVA, specialists can join a new interactive platform at http://www.evabydorc.com/.

Results Achieved with the Enhancing Visual Acuity System

EVA was tested extensively as a surgical platform during the year prior to its launch. After wet lab surgical simulations by different experienced surgeons at the DORC facility, a variety of cases including vitrectomy, phaco procedures, and combined phaco-vitrectomy surgery were performed beginning in October 2012. EVA has been used successfully for surgical procedures in a wide variety of cases from simple to very difficult, such as trauma-induced injuries. Presently, more than 500 surgical cases were performed using the EVA platform at the University of Leuven covering macular pucker, macular holes, retinal detachments, diabetic vitrectomies, floater removal, oil removal, other posterior segment surgeries, and cataract removal cases.

Service and Support with the Enhancing Visual Acuity System

DORC provides a comprehensive and flexible service and support package for EVA including installation, programming, and maintenance elements, which reduces downtime. They also supply regular software updates for the system to EVA customers.

Comparison with Existing Technologies

Compared to the Stellaris PC (Bausch & Lomb), Constellation Vision System (Alcon), Accurus (Alcon), and OS3 (Oertli), EVA (DORC) offers many advantages. The reactivity and precision of flow control in combination with the TDC cutter on EVA is a considerable improvement. The automatic infusion control is simpler and more intuitive than the complex systems seen on other machines. Results achieved in accuracy, savings in time, and added safety are clearly evident. EVA's enhanced ergonomics and wireless, versatile foot pedal offers many operational advantages, too.

Implications for Industry

EVA's aspiration flow control system offers surgeons a new advanced option in a wide range of procedures. It has the potential to enable safer, faster, and more reliable techniques for all the different pathologies and conditions involving the vitreous by overcoming the limitations of previous-generation systems. By supporting current clinical developments in phaco-vitrectomy, EVA could make a major contribution to advancing ophthalmology.

References

1 European Vitreoretinal Society Retinal Detachment Study. http://www.evrs.eu/evrs-rd-study/.

2 Michalewska Z, Ducournau D, Adelman RA; the EVRS RD Study Group: How do vitrectomy parameters influence the results of rhegmatogenous retinal detachments repair? EVRS RD Study No. 3. Acta Ophthalmol 2013, Epub ahead of print.

Peter Stalmans, MD, PhD
University Hospitals Leuven, Campus Sint-Rafaël, Ophthalmology
Kapucijnenvoer 33
BE–3000 Leuven (Belgium)
E-Mail peter.stalmans@uzleuven.be

Oh H, Oshima Y (eds): Microincision Vitrectomy Surgery. Emerging Techniques and Technology.
Dev Ophthalmol. Basel, Karger, 2014, vol 54, pp 31–37 (DOI: 10.1159/000360446)

Fluidics and Cutter Dynamics

Steve Charles

Hamilton Eye Institute, University of Tennessee, Memphis, Tenn., USA

Abstract

An understanding of the physics and engineering principles underlying vitrectomy fluidics and cutter function is essential as we seek to improve outcomes by reducing iatrogenic retinal breaks and facilitate removal of all traction. One of the many challenges facing the vitreoretinal community working in collaboration with engineers developing new systems is the difficulty in moving forward from obsolete, less effective, and potentially higher-risk techniques and parameters. The notion that 20-gauge vitrectomy is the 'gold standard' and should be used for difficult cases is simply wrong. Similarly, the idea that huge flow rates are 'efficient' and beneficial when in fact they cause excessive vitreoretinal traction is a significant issue. The obsolete notion of combining vitrectomy with scleral buckling must be eradicated; patients do not want pain, long procedures, refractive error, or strabismus; vitbuckle outcomes are not better than vitrectomy alone.

An understanding of infusion and aspiration fluidics as well as cutter dynamics is essential to a rational approach to machine selection, gauge selection, and machine parameters [1–4]. Use of outdated machine parameters, 20-gauge technology, and even surgical techniques remains a significant barrier to improved outcomes. This chapter explains the engineering principles underlying these issues and the clinical implications.

Infusion System

Infusion systems available prior to the development of the Accurus (Alcon Inc., Ft. Worth, Tex., USA) were gravity based, i.e. IV poles. Gravity-based systems have significant disadvantages: there is no digital readout of infusion pressure and surgeons cannot mentally convert inches (or cm) of water to millimeters of mercury, and motorized IV poles are slower than the vented gas-forced infusion and the more advanced Alcon Constellation Vision System pressurized infusion system. The prior gas-forced infusion is only better than gravity-based systems because air-pressurized infusion produces a sensor-based direct digital readout of infusion pressure, not intraocular pressure, in the familiar mm Hg. Due to console-controlled venting, the vented gas-forced infusion implemented on the Accurus was better than gas-forced infusion because it allowed a rapid decrease as well as increase of infusion pressure via a surgeon foot pedal command [5].

The Constellation Vision System has an intraocular pressure compensation system which compensates for pressure drop in the infusion tubing and cannula. This system determines the fluidic resistance of the actual infusion tubing and cannula during push-priming by using a known pressure, sensed by dual pressure sensors and measuring fluid flow using an ultrasonic flow sensor. The system calculates fluid Ohm's law and adjusts infusion pressure according to the sensed flow rate to produce the selected intraocular pressure during surgical aspiration [6]. The Constellation Vision System posterior cassette utilizes dual, small infusion chambers in the cassette; one chamber infuses while the other chamber is refilling with infusion fluid. The very small chambers pressurized by a proportional air pressure valve plus dual pressure sensors enable a rapid response to commanded infusion pressure, both increases to stop bleeding and decreases because of perfusion deficits or corneal edema [5].

Aspiration Fluidics and Vitreous Cutting

Pars plana vitrectomy requires both infusion and aspiration, and infusion and aspiration fluidics are influenced by the same physical principles. Resistance to flow is determined by the internal diameter of a lumen or port, length of tubing, cannula, or tool, as well as the cutter port opening and closing, cyclically obstructing the port. Fluidic resistance is proportional to the 4th power of the diameter (Hagen-Poiseuille equation) and linearly related to the length. The impact of diameter is very significant because of the 4th power relationship and clinically relevant because of the transition from 20 gauge (0.89 mm) to 23 (0.75 mm), 25 (0.5 mm), or 27 gauge (0.41 mm). The flow is limited far more by the resistance of the cutter inner needle and the infusion port than the 84 inches of connected tubing. Ohm's law [voltage = current × resistance (E = IR)] is mathematically equivalent to Ohm's law for fluid flow (pressure gradient = flow × resistance) [5, 6].

'Port-based flow limiting' is a term coined by the author to describe the flow limiting resulting from smaller-diameter cutters as well as that caused by higher cutting rates and biased closed duty cycles. Higher cutting rates cyclically interrupt flow through the port, thereby increasing fluidic resistance when using single actuation pneumatic cutters [7, 8]. High cutting rates at the port are beneficial for all cases and all tasks because of increased fluidic stability, which in turn decreases pulsatile vitreoretinal traction on both detached and attached retinas and thereby reduces the incidence of iatrogenic retinal breaks. The author refers to the amount of fluid that passes through the port during an open-close cycle as 'pulse flow'. High cutting rates produce smaller pulses with much less pulsatile vitreoretinal traction than occurs using lower cutting rates [9, 10]. Small pulse flow means that the vitreous does not have time to accelerate and produce remote effects because of the force = mass × acceleration (F = MA) relationship [6].

Higher cutting rates have not been proven to cut collagen fibers significantly better, although theoretically there is an inertial cutting mechanism in addition to shearing. While the velocity of the UltraVit cutter increases with higher cutting rates, this is probably not the case with singe actuation cutters [11]. In addition, port-based flow limiting decreases surge and therefore iatrogenic retinal breaks after sudden elastic deformation of dense epiretinal membrane (ERM), lens material, or scar tissue through the port.

Furthermore, in addition to producing port-based flow limiting, high cutting rates reduce the travel of uncut vitreous collagen fibers through the port. 25 gauge provides more resistance than 23 gauge because fluidic resistance is proportional to the 4th power of the diameter. It has long been incorrectly taught that cutting rates should be reduced when removing dense ERM, scar tissue, and lens material, or performing core vitrectomy; in fact, the highest possible cutting rate should be used for all tasks and all cases unless all the vitreous has been removed and very dense tissue must be addressed [12]. Some surgeons incorrectly believe that 25-gauge vitrectomy is 'inefficient' or produces insufficient flow rates, when in fact it is safer because of less pulsatile vitreoretinal traction [6, 13]. Many surgeons incorrectly believe that 20-gauge systems should be used for straightforward and complex retinal detachments such as diabetic traction retinal detachments, proliferative vitreoretinopathy, giant breaks, and complex trauma. In fact, 25-gauge systems are safer and more effective than 20- or even 23-gauge systems for all cases [6, 14–16].

Port-based flow limiting relies on the same physical principles as the high-vacuum, low-flow phaco first implemented on the Alcon MicroFlare ABS and MicroTaper ABS phaco probes. High-vacuum, low-flow phaco has become the standard of care because it produces better anterior chamber stability and decreased fluid surge after an occlusion break, which is directly analogous to the advantages of port-based flow limiting for posterior vitrectomy [6].

Venturi versus Peristaltic Pumps

Peristaltic pumps directly control flow. Combining a flow-based system with vacuum sensors can only stop the pump when a preset vacuum level has occurred; it cannot proportionally control the vacuum if there are any bubbles or gas segments in the tubing. Peristaltic pumps are not optimal for vitrectomy for many reasons: transorifice pressure rises rapidly when dense ERM, dense vitreous hemorrhage, scar tissue, or lens material occludes the port, and when an aspiration surge occurring when dense material suddenly goes through the port causes retinal breaks. In addition, peristaltic pumps inherently produce a low-frequency pulsatile vacuum as the rollers compress; they do not produce constant flow rates as some surgeons incorrectly state. Peristaltic pump console-based flow control must interact through two-way transmission of the fluidic signal through 84 inches of compliant tubing with a very slow response time driven automatically by sensors in the console or surgeon foot pedal command while port-based flow limiting via small-diameter cutters and duty cycle control is instantaneous. Peristaltic pumps suffer from another major disadvantage: they do not function well in an air-fluid mixture. A common and useful technique is to remove residual vitreoretinal traction as fluid-air exchange is performed, one subtype of interface vitrectomy. Air dampens and restricts retinal motion and the visible air-vitreous interface helps identify the residual traction.

The Constellation Vision System aspiration subsystem utilizes a very small chamber emptied by a peristaltic pump. Optoelectronic level sensing provides a signal which drives the peristaltic pump fluid removal rate. The purpose of the small chamber is to produce a rapid response to a commanded vacuum decrease or increase in response to proportional (linear) foot pedal command. The vacuum-over-fluid aspiration chamber incorporates dual proportional vacuum valves and dual sensors enabling precise control at very low vacuum levels as well as maximum vacuum of 650 mm Hg. The aspiration system also has a proportional pressure valve which provides more precise and rapid response than simply venting unwanted high vacuum when the foot pedal is lifted.

Vitrectomy versus the Phaco Technique

The phaco technique is largely based on techniques to mobilize lens material away from the lens capsule to prevent capsular defects and vitreous loss. In marked contrast, the vitreous cutter port should be moved to the vitreous rather than the vitreous pulled to the port using excessive flow rates. Phaco surgeons doing vitrectomy must consciously focus on moving the port to the vitreous because their phaco experience teaches them the opposite approach. Engaging vitreous and applying vacuum while moving the cutter away from the retina inherently produces marked vitreoretinal traction [6].

Efficiency

Higher flow rates from larger-diameter cutters are not more or less efficient; efficiency is defined as the volume of vitreous removed per volume of infusion fluid. An overemphasis on higher flow rates incorrectly referred to as efficiency has produced the unintended consequence of increasing iatrogenic retinal breaks. Similarly, efficiency is not a function of cutting rate; efficiency is entirely driven by technique – keeping the port constantly immersed in vitreous produces efficiency. The author refers to the optimal technique as 'continuous engage and advance vitrectomy'. Emphasis on operating room efficiency and faster operating times can result in the unintended consequence of pulling the cutter away from retina while aspirating, and rapid cutter repositioning which produces vitreoretinal traction [6].

Vitrectomy Dynamics

Vitreous is a highly complex tissue with marked inhomogeneity; the physical properties vary widely from patient to patient, disease to disease, and change dramatically as the vitrectomy progresses. Vitreous hyaluronan acts as a non-Newtonian, pseudoplastic fluid similar to viscoelastic agents (OVDs) used in cataract surgery. This semisolid property resists deformation into the cutter port. Early in the vitrectomy, surgeons often believe that there is little or no flow when in fact hyaluronan is being removed and they may react by unsafely increasing flow rates, usually by unsafely decreasing the cutting rate. Hyaluronan acts as a dampening agent, reducing vitreoretinal traction from pulsatile flow through the port. Hyaluronan is diluted as the vitrectomy progresses, decreasing the dampening effect, which is an issue because vitrectomy near the vitreous base is performed after core vitrectomy. Furthermore, infusion fluid changes the electrochemical properties of the vitreous, dramatically decreasing viscosity; vitreous viscosity is reduced by a factor of five in minutes after removing it from the eye or enucleating an animal eye [6].

Cutter Technology

Pneumatic cutters are much lighter and more compact than electric cutters, which is a significant advantage because it improves dexterity and decreases hand fatigue. Disposable cutters reduce per case costs because they eliminate cleaning, rinsing, drying, wrapping, sterilization, storage, replacement, and spare parts. Cleanup of any tool with a lumen which includes cutters, scissors, forceps, and cannulas has the potential of creating a TASS-like (toxic anterior segment syndrome) inflammation from biological materials from previous patients, enzymes used in ultrasonic cleaning, autoclave water impurities, etc. In addition, vitreous cutters, scissors, and forceps, especially in smaller-form factors (23, 25, and 27 gauge) have fragile cutting and gripping surfaces which are easily damaged by the cleaning and sterilization process [6].

The author invented the InnoVit dual actuation scheme to eliminate the spring used to open the port after the pressure pulse on the single actuation diaphragm actuator closed the port. Elimination of the spring increased cutting rates as well as cutter velocity at the time of closure. The InnoVit utilized a limited angle rotary cutting scheme rather than an axial (guillotine) cutting action [17]. The UltraVit developed for the Alcon Constellation system uses a diaphragm-based, dual actuation, axial cutting design. Duty cycle is defined as the percentage of port open time versus total time. A lower duty cycle results in greater port-based flow limiting and therefore fluidic stability and less pulsatile vitreoretinal traction. A higher duty cycle produces greater flow suitable for core vitrectomy. The Alcon Constellation UltraVit currently cuts at 7,500 cuts/min and has variable duty cycle control enabling control of port-based flow limiting even at relatively high cutting rates. Higher cutting rates produce higher flow rates only with the UltraVit dual actuation scheme because the pulse flow remains constant [6]; single actuation cutters used by all of the manufacturers except Alcon produce a significant decrease in duty cycle and therefore flow rates when used at high cutting rates. Higher cutting rates are always safer.

Aspiration Systems

Rapid response to a foot pedal command to decrease vacuum is far more important from a safety perspective than a command to increase vacuum. Response time is driven by many factors: size of the vacuum chamber in the cassette, proportional valve(s) response time, embedded controller, and use of a deterministic, real-time operating system. The Alcon Accurus had the first real-time operating system, and distributed embedded processing resulted in a 25-ms response time compared to the closest competitor, which was ten times slower [6]. The Constellation Vision System has true flow control using flow sensing and closed loop feedback control for phaco procedures and is twice as fast as the Accurus. This technology produces rapid, nonpulsatile control unlike the pulsatile, slow response time flow control produced by peristaltic pump systems. In addition to flow control, there is a flow limiting mode available. Port-based flow limiting produced by high cutting rates (7,500 cuts/min), smaller lumens (23, 25, and 27 gauge), and variable duty cycle control is instantaneous, while console-based flow control must interact through two-way transmission of the fluidic signal and system fluidic response through 84 inches of compliant tubing [6].

The surgeon reaction time from seeing a retina approach the port to moving a foot pedal is at least 400 ms because of visual and cognitive processing, brain calculation of a motor response, propagation through the spinal cord and leg, and contraction of the lower leg muscles. The surgeon reaction time is more than an order of magnitude longer than the 25 ms it takes an advanced venturi-based system like the Constellation to respond to a foot pedal command. The author has shown that approximately 30 times the volume of fluid contained between the tip and the port pass through the port in the time that occurs between when the surgeon decides to lift the pedal and when the vacuum is actually reduced at the cutter port [6].

Small Incision Techniques and Advantages

Small-diameter, high cutting rate cutters are especially advantageous for segmentation/delamination of ERM associated with diabetic traction retinal detachment. Small-diameter cutters limit surge produced by sudden elastic deformation of dense ERM through the cutter port. In addition, small-diameter cutters with the port close to the tip facilitate access to ERM in the context of diabetic traction retinal detachment [18–21].

Cutters can be used for segmentation of ERM as well as delamination of ERM. There are two types of cutter delamination defined by the author: (1) conformal cutter delamination and (2) fold-back delamination. Conformal cutter delamination is utilized for dense ERM and accomplished by applying the cutter port to the leading edge of the ERM, and not pushing or using excessive vacuum. The term 'conformal' was coined by the author to emphasize the need to rotate the cutter around the probe axis to adjust the angle of attack so the port is rotated somewhat away from the retina. The angle must be adjusted as the cutter traverses the convexities and concavities of the retinal surface. Fold-back delamination is used for more flexible ERM and accomplished by positioning the cutter port on top of the ERM just behind the leading edge, allowing the ERM to fold back into the port when vacuum is applied [12, 17, 22, 23].

Small-diameter, high cutting rate cutters are also advantageous for removing vitreoretinal traction on peripheral retinal breaks because they reduce pulsatile vitreoretinal traction. Small-diameter cutters are ideal for internal drainage of subretinal fluid, often eliminating the need for soft-tip cannulas and facilitating the removal of residual vitreoretinal traction during the internal drainage/fluid-air exchange sequence [10, 14].

Small-diameter cutters with high cutting rates are ideal for retinectomy – a technique which is more efficacious than relaxing retinotomy. Retinectomy is defined as removing all retina/vitreous/ERM anterior to a circumferential cut used primarily for proliferative vitreoretinopathy cases.

The author utilizes 25-gauge vitrectomy for silicone oil reoperation cases without removing oil; a two-port, sequential oil replacement method is utilized. The silicone subtype of interface vitrectomy allows retinectomy, removal of residual vitreoretinal traction, removal of subretinal fluid, and cutter delamination 'under' oil.

References

1 Wang CC, Charles S: Microsurgical instrumentation for vitrectomy, part 1. J Clin Eng 1983;8:321–328.
2 Machemer R: A new concept for vitreous surgery: two instrument techniques in pars plana vitrectomy. Arch Ophthalmol 1974;92:407–412.
3 O'Malley C, Heintz RM: Vitrectomy via the pars plana – a new instrument system. Trans Pac Coast Otoophthalmol Soc Annu Meet 1972;53:121–137.
4 O'Malley C, Heintz RM: Vitrectomy with an alternative instrument system. Ann Ophthalmol 1975;7:585–588.
5 Charles S, et al: Vitreous Microsurgery, ed 5. Baltimore, Lippincott, Williams and Wilkins, 2010.
6 Charles S: Fluidics and cutter dynamics. Retina Physician 2012;9:58–60.
7 Abulon DJ, Buboltz DC: Porcine vitreous flow behavior during high speed vitrectomy up to 7,500 cuts per minute. Invest Ophthalmol Vis Sci 2012; 53:ARVO E-Abstract 369.
8 Ray A, Abulon D, Dimalanta R, Buboltz D: Intraocular pressure and BSS flow rates at high vitrectomy probe cut rates (poster). ARVO, Fort Lauderdale, 2012.
9 Rizzo S: Performance of modified vitrectomy probe in small-gauge vitrectomy. Retina Today 2011, pp 40–42.
10 Teixeira A, Chong LP, Matsuoka N, Arana L, Kerns R, Bhadri P, Humayun M: Vitreoretinal traction created by conventional cutters during vitrectomy. Ophthalmology 2010;117:1387–1392.
11 Abulon D: Cutter velocities of two vitrectomy probes: dual pneumatic drive and single pneumatic drive with spring return (poster). ARVO, Seattle, 2013.
12 Charles S: Curved scissors delamination. Retina Today 2012, pp 52–54.
13 Fujii GY, DeJuan E Jr, Humayun MS, et al: A new 25-gauge instrument system for transconjunctival sutureless vitrectomy surgery. Ophthalmology 2002;109: 1807–1812.
14 Rizzo S, Genovesi-Ebert F, Belgting C: Comparative study between a standard 25-gauge vitrectomy system and a new ultra high-speed 25-gauge system with duty cycle control in the treatment of various vitreoretinal diseases. Retina 2011;31:2007–2011.
15 Williams GA: 25-, 23-, or 20-gauge instrumentation for vitreous surgery? Eye 2008;22:1263–1266.
16 Dugel PU, Zhou J, Abulon DJ, Buboltz DC: Tissue attraction associated with 20-gauge, 23-gauge, and enhanced 25-gauge dual-pneumatic vitrectomy probes. Retina 2012;32: 1761–1766.
17 Charles S: Principles and techniques of vitreous surgery; in Ryan S, Glaser B, Michels R (eds): Retina. St. Louis, Mosby, 1989, vol 3.

18 Oshima Y, Shima C, Wakabayashi T, et al: Microincision vitrectomy surgery and intravitreal bevacizumab as a surgical adjunct to treat diabetic traction retinal detachment. Ophthalmology 2009; 116:927–938.
19 Farouk MM, Naito T, Sayed KM, et al: Outcomes of 25-gauge vitrectomy for proliferative diabetic retinopathy. Graefes Arch Clin Exp Ophthalmol 2011;249: 369–376.
20 Sato T, Emi K, Bando H, Ikeda T: Faster recovery after 25-gauge microincision vitrectomy surgery than after 20-gauge vitrectomy in patients with proliferative diabetic retinopathy. Clin Ophthalmol 2012;6:1925–1930.
21 Wakabayashi T, Oshima Y: Microincision vitrectomy surgery for diabetic retinopathy. Retina Physician 2011;8:66–70.
22 Charles S: Techniques and tools for dissection of epiretinal membranes. Graefes Arch Clin Exp Ophthalmol 2003;241: 347–352.
23 Shimada H, et al: Expanded indications for 25-gauge transconjunctival vitrectomy. Jpn J Ophthalmol 2005;5:397–401.

Steve Charles, MD, FACS, FICS
Clinical Professor of Ophthalmology
University of Tennessee, Hamilton Eye Institute
6401 Poplar Avenue, Suite 190
Memphis, TN 38119 (USA)
E-Mail scharles@att.net

Oh H, Oshima Y (eds): Microincision Vitrectomy Surgery. Emerging Techniques and Technology.
Dev Ophthalmol. Basel, Karger, 2014, vol 54, pp 38–44 (DOI: 10.1159/000360447)

23-Gauge Vitrectomy

Peter Stalmans

Department of Ophthalmology, University Hospitals Leuven, Leuven, Belgium

Abstract

Smaller-gauge surgery enables greater precision and offers advantages in decreased surgical time, less tissue manipulation, reduced inflammation, postoperative pain, and more rapid visual recovery. While smaller instruments create smaller incisions that violate the eye less, it can be more difficult to fit the instruments required to accomplish tasks through the port. For many surgeons, 23-gauge techniques and instruments offer an ideal compromise between the cumbersome, suture-requiring 20-gauge procedures and the smaller, but more limited, 25- and 27-gauge surgeries.

Many specialists choose sutureless, small-incision surgery to ensure quieter eyes in the vitreoretinal patient. The biggest advantage over larger-gauge procedures is reduced postoperative inflammation at the sclerotomy site, enabling speedier recovery and improving postoperative patient morbidity. In addition, operating time is reduced, which cuts costs, and the small incisions are especially appropriate for working on children's eyes. 23-gauge surgery was developed to offer an alternative to 20-gauge surgery and solve many of the early issues of too much instrument flexibility and limited light options associated with smaller 25-gauge techniques. It has become the approach-of-choice for most vitreoretinal procedures today.

Development of 23-Gauge Vitrectomy

17-gauge pars plana vitrectomy was first introduced more than 40 years ago. The use of 20-gauge instrumentation became standard in the 1980s and 1990s. Sutureless procedures for 20-gauge instruments were first introduced in 1996. At the time, introducing instruments through a self-sealing, scleral-tunnel sclerotomy was a novel approach that presented many challenges. Complications such as wound leakage, vitreous incarceration, and retinal tears were common hazards, and conjunctival dissection and suturing were often required.

The introduction of small trocar-cannulas paved the way for greater advances in vitreoretinal surgery. 25-gauge instruments were developed in 1990, but 25-gauge transconjunctival sutureless vitrectomy was not introduced until 2002. Sharing characteristics of both its forerunners, 23-gauge vitrectomy soon followed in 2005. It was smaller than 20-gauge vitrectomy, but more rigid than 25-gauge vitrectomy, making procedures such as endolaser and removal of the peripheral vitreous gel easier for most surgeons. Although the use of 25-gauge instruments reduced surgery time, as suturing of the sclerotomies was omitted, and improved postoperative recovery, the narrow inner lumen of the instrument slowed down the removal of the vitreous. Moreover, the smaller gauge initially posed some problems for surgeons because of the increased flexibility of the instruments, which limited what procedures could be performed. In addition, the standard light source for 25-gauge surgery was initially less bright because fewer lumens could be transmitted through the smaller-gauge fiber optic light pipe. 23-gauge instruments and techniques were developed in response to the concerns over decreased rigidity and light in 25-gauge surgery. They provided more rigid instrumentation with better light transmission, allowing greater rotation of the eye, as well as a larger inner lumen, whereby the ability to perform a more complete vitrectomy was enhanced. Subsequent technological advances have lessened the impact of the initial issues and have made it possible to expand the scope of smaller-gauge surgery.

Because 23-gauge surgery has been performed since 2005, it has been possible to scientifically evaluate its benefits and limitations. Large-scale studies of postoperative comfort and reduced clinical risks in patients who have undergone vitrectomy using 23-gauge instruments and procedures have been undertaken and compared with surgical procedures using other gauges. The results have shown definitive benefits.

Uses of 23-Gauge Vitrectomy

23-gauge surgery was originally used for macular procedures, but with advances in instrumentation and techniques, it has become a favored approach for most vitreoretinal procedures. 23-gauge surgery is possible in all cases except removal of a foreign body, where a larger sclerotomy is needed, or removal of subretinal membrane, which requires angled instruments.

Advantages

23-gauge vitrectomy has many advantages over 25- and 27-gauge vitrectomy, mainly due to the larger diameter and greater rigidity of the instruments. One major advantage is that the plugs for the 23-gauge instrument allow the injection and extraction of silicone oil. When a narrow-wall polyamide 23-gauge cannula is fitted on the injection syringe, a complete 1,000-cSt oil fill can be obtained in less than 1 min. Since the sclerotomies are made with a myringovitreoretinal (MVR) blade in 23-gauge surgery, a slit-like incision is made obliquely in the sclera (although a 25-gauge MVR blade is also now available); these incisions are always self-sealing and postoperative hypotony is not an issue. Compared to 20-gauge vitrectomy, the 23-gauge procedure also has many advantages. Since no conjunctival peritomy is required, less discomfort and postoperative inflammation is noted in patients undergoing 23-gauge surgery. Moreover, the presence of self-closing valves over the instrument canulas prevent fluid leakage from the eye during surgery, stabilizing the intra-ocular pressure and reducing the fluid current in the vitreous cavity (fig. 1).

Sutureless Surgery

Smaller-gauge surgery, including 23-gauge procedures, can be performed without sutures because the incisions made are, of course, smaller and generally self-healing. Sutures can leave inflammatory nodules on the surface of the eye that can take weeks, or even longer, to resorb. Large incisions and sutures can leave patients with red eyes after surgery and can warp the eye's surface. Patients undergoing sutureless surgery can expect less postoperative astigmatism since sutur-

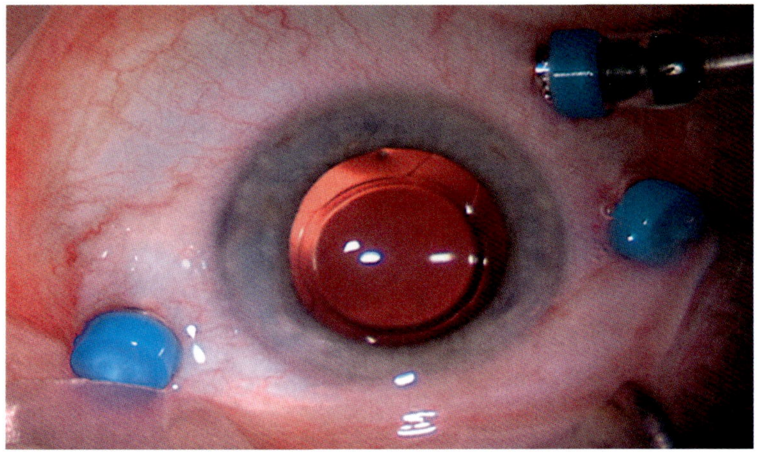

Fig. 1. Peroperative view of 23-gauge vitrectomy. All three valved cannulas are inserted in the pars plana. The infusion line is inserted into the lower temporal cannula. Since three identical cannulas are used, the surgeon can freely switch over the infusion line into another cannula if desired. The valves prevent leakage from the cannulas when no instruments are inserted.

ing of the sclerotomies is typically not required, and they can expect reduced conjunctival trauma and inflammatory response of the eye. Sutureless surgery also reduces operation time because opening and closing the sclerotomies and conjunctiva are not required.

Sclerotomies with a width of 0.72 mm are needed for 23-gauge instruments. While this would normally require closure with a suture, it can be avoided by performing a tunnel incision that achieves self-healing. Instead of a usual perpendicular incision through the sclera, as in 25-gauge surgery, a tunnel-like tangential incision is made at a 30–40° angle. Suture closure is not required because the wound borders close the incision in a valve-like manner through intraocular pressure. The transconjunctival sclera at tunnel incision created for 23-gauge instruments guarantees an almost 100% rapid self-sealing closure rate.

Increased Procedure Speed

Savings in procedure time can be achieved with 23-gauge surgery. As well as saving time in suturing, the smaller instrumentation simply enables quicker surgery. New surgical platforms, such as the Enhanced Visual Acuity System (EVA) from the Dutch Ophthalmic Research Centre (DORC) offer improved fluidic control that also contributes to enhanced procedure speed, as well as safety. In addition to improved fluidics, the system offers better control of duty cycles and cutting rates. High-speed cutting is an important option in working with smaller-gauge instrumentation, not only because it is faster, but also because it minimizes pulsatile vitreoretinal traction.

Better Efficiency

Using 23-gauge instruments, suturing the infusion and sclerotomies is no longer necessary, which not only shortens surgery time, but requires less than half as many instruments. This means that a smaller number of instruments need cleaning after surgery, saving even more time.

Reduced Risks

One of the most serious complications from vitrectomy is endophthalmitis, a serious ocular condition which can result in irreversible loss of vision. Incidence of this condition is of particular concern when evaluating any new surgical technique. Early studies indicated that incidences of endophthalmitis in 25-gauge surgery were significantly higher than 20-gauge procedures. Subsequent studies have shown that a sutureless trans-

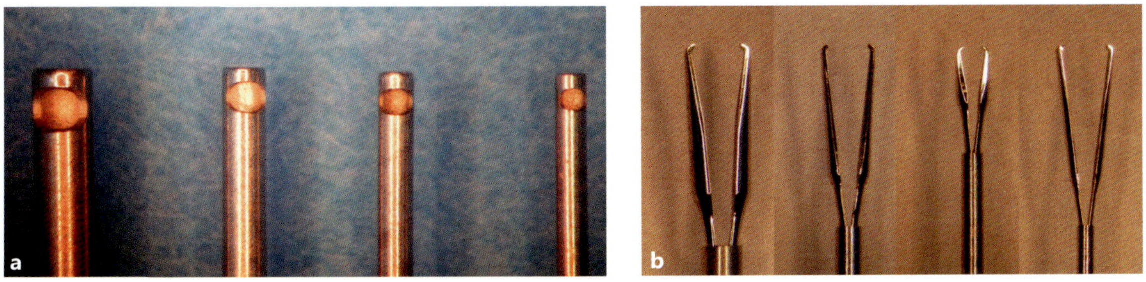

Fig. 2. Comparison of different gauges. **a** 20-, 23-, 25- and 27-gauge instruments (from left to right). The 23-gauge vitrectome offers the optimal compromise between rigidity and flow diameter. **b** 20-, 23-, 25- and 27-gauge end-gripping forceps. The tip of the 23-gauge forceps has a similar shape as the 20-gauge version, but offers markedly more grip than the 25- or 27-gauge version.

conjunctival approach using a 23-gauge procedure has a reduced risk [1] and can overcome some of the shortcomings of 25-gauge surgery with the benefits of a larger caliber, more rigid instruments, and more efficient cutters, while at the same time retaining many of the advantages of 25-gauge vitrectomy (fig. 2).

In addition, passive backflush instruments can be used in a 23-gauge system, while active aspiration is required in 25- and 27-gauge surgery. Passive aspiration is safer compared to active aspiration since no collapse of the eye can occur – a risk with active aspiration, particularly when aspiration under air infusion is performed.

Enhanced Postoperative Comfort

Postoperative pain, eye discomfort, and necessary sick leave are inevitable consequences of vitrectomy. However, studies have shown that 23-gauge pars plana vitrectomy causes significantly less postoperative pain and discomfort compared to 20-gauge pars plana vitrectomy [2]. Following 20-gauge surgery, the patients studied had a significantly increased risk of sleeping less during the first postoperative night and week, waking up due to pain during the first postoperative night and week, taking pain medication during the first postoperative night and week, and using a postoperative ointment. They also experienced a longer period of postoperative discomfort and reddish eyes. Larger incisions, longer procedures, suturing, and exposure of the bare sclera in 20-gauge surgery creates more postoperative discomfort and inflammation.

23-gauge transconjunctival sutureless techniques cause no surgical trauma to the conjunctiva, require no sclera suturing, and cause less postoperative discomfort. Compared to 20-gauge vitrectomy, both 23- and 25-gauge vitrectomy share the same advantages: little or no trauma to the conjunctiva, no suture-related inflammation or discomfort, and no postoperative astigmatism. In addition, the transconjunctival technique does not interfere with present filtration blebs or future filtration surgery. The major advantage of 23-gauge vitrectomy over 25-gauge vitrectomy is that it can be successfully performed in most complicated cases. Moreover, silicone oil can be used easily using a 23-gauge system, which is difficult in the 25-gauge variety, mainly when 5,000 cSt oil are used. The duration of sick leave in patients who had underwent 20-gauge surgery compared to 23-gauge procedures showed no significant difference [2], possibly due to the use of a fibrin sealant in conjunctival closure, which is known to reduce postoperative pain and discomfort.

Shorter Patient Hospitalization

Due to less postoperative pain and discomfort, patients undergoing 23-gauge procedures can usually be released from hospital after 1 night, providing an ambulant check-up is planned on postoperative day 2 or 3, whereas patients undergoing 20-gauge surgery tend to require 2 nights of hospitalization.

Better for Children
Smaller instruments and incisions are particularly well suited for surgery in the smaller eyes of pediatric patients, such as in cases of persistent fetal vasculature, retinopathy of prematurity, uveitis, and some instances of uncomplicated tractional or rhegmatogenous retinal detachments. Sometimes it can be necessary to use 20-gauge surgery, such as for stage 5 retinopathy of prematurity, but in most cases it makes sense to use smaller-gauge surgery in children. In really small eyes, however, the trocar can be problematic with small-gauge procedures. A 23-gauge incision can be made and the 23-gauge instrument can be used without a trocar. Using sutures after the procedure in this case, a small section of the conjunctiva can be taken down to better visualize the wound and minimize the risk of hypotony.

Limitations

Costs
The main disadvantage of 23-gauge vitrectomy is higher cost. However, requiring no sutures and fewer instruments reduces material costs, and the shorter surgery time and less postoperative treatment needed offer additional significant savings.

Training
Getting fully acquainted with performing 23-gauge surgery requires moderate adjustment, mostly with regard to the procedures. However, 23-gauge instruments nowadays are similar to 20-gauge ones in rigidity, lighting, flow, and aspiration of the vitreous cutter.

Flow Control
Smaller-gauge instruments enable greater precision in procedures and has certain advantages; however, working with smaller gauges requires a higher level of understanding of flow characteristics because all material must travel through a smaller diameter tube. Higher infusion and aspiration pressures are needed to remove the vitreous when working with 23- (25- and 27-) gauge probes. Advanced platforms offer enhanced flow control, notably EVA, which features a unique flow control system (VacuFlow VTi®) that provides a combined flow and vacuum system, enabling the surgeon to choose between vacuum and flow modes. This system overcomes the limitations of existing Venturi and peristaltic pumps and opens new possibilities in 23-gauge surgery.

Clinical Procedures
A small number of limitations in terms of the clinical procedures that can be performed exist with 23-gauge procedures. Surgery requiring curved instruments such as tractional diabetic retinal detachments and macular translocations are the only indications for 20-gauge vitrectomy.

Complications
Wound leakage and endophthalmitis are still, of course, possible complications of 23-gauge surgery; however, appropriate techniques and equipment can minimize complications.

Techniques

Techniques to minimize complications in 23-gauge surgery play a significant role in optimizing outcome.

Wound Architecture
Conjunctival displacement allows the conjunctiva to cover the wound and is an important aspect of wound construction. Additionally, construct-

ing scleral tunnels by an oblique wound is a second critical step. Angling the incision creates a flap, which pressure-closes when the instruments and trocar are pulled out. Angled incisions like these can cut leakage by half.

Fluid-Air Exchange

Another approach to minimizing postoperative wound leakage and subsequent complications is the use of fluid-air exchange at the end of a vitrectomy. Because of higher surface tension, air is less likely to leak through the incision than fluid. If leakage does occur, however, the sclerotomy site can be closed with a 7-0 or 8-0 Vicryl suture.

Antibiotics

Injection of postoperative antibiotics reduces the risk of endophthalmitis considering the 100:1 antibiotic concentration gradient between the front and back of the eye. Inject subconjunctival antibiotics under the lower lid in the inferior cul-de-sac, so if there is a subconjunctival hemorrhage, the patient will not see it and the antibiotics cannot reflux into the wounds.

High-Speed Cutting

This minimizes pulsatile vitreoretinal traction.

Instrumentation

Advances in instrumentation for 23-gauge surgery are continually expanding. Today, it is easy to find a wide range of vitreous cutters, chandeliers, curved scissors, microvitreoretinal blades, aspirating picks, and endoscopic laser probes for 23-, 25-, and 27-gauge surgery. This, in turn, has made it possible to expand the indications for these procedures.

Twin Duty Cycle Vitrectome

A new cutter type will soon be available that is equipped with an opening in the vitrectome blade (DORC's twin duty cycle cutter) for use with 23- (25- and 27-) gauge instrumentation in DORC's EVA platform. This feature offers two advantages. First, each time the cutter opens and closes, two cuts are made, which effectively produces cut rates up to 16,000 cuts/min. Secondly, even when the blade is in the closed position, the port is not occluded, which enhances the flow through the system. As a result, even at maximal cut rates and using flows around 4 ml/min, there is almost no buildup of a vacuum in the aspiration line, which provides precision control of the flow in the tubing.

With the twin duty cycle cutter, the vitreous is brought into the inner aperture and cut in a forward and backward movement, increasing the amount of vitreous that is cut in a single motion. The aperture in the inner tube results in almost constant aspiration flow into the port. The inner port on the new cutter is larger than previous designs which should enable a larger amount of material to be taken in per cut and increase the speed of surgical procedures. The twin duty cycle vitrectome removes 2–3 times more vitreous than a standard cutter.

23-Gauge Dual Light Probe

While many vitreoretinal procedures can be performed using a conventional hand-held light probe for endoillumination, more complicated cases require chandelier illumination. A new 23-gauge dual light probe (DORC) resembles a conventional 23-gauge light probe, with 27-gauge light fiber offering wide-angle viewing and a 23-gauge hand piece. However, the fiber can be moved in and out of its posterior end and features a small adjustable silicone disk which serves as a stopper. For use as a chandelier endoilluminator during vitrectomy, the silicone stopper can be positioned 4 mm from the end of the fiber and the fiber can be inserted into one of the two ports of the trocar-microcannula system with the other port accessible for instrumentation. The change from a hand-held probe to a chandelier takes only a few seconds.

Developments in the Pipeline

While a two-step cannula system with separate MVR knife was previously considered to be the best way of achieving an accurate incision with minimal insertion force, creating a self-healing wound, DORC is developing the new-generation One-Step MVR Cannula System, which has an integrated MVR blade providing all these benefits plus added convenience. The system is available for 23-, 25-, and 27-gauge instrumentation.

Implications for Industry

23-gauge techniques and instruments are ideal for many surgeons and are likely to lead to rapid further development of new instrumentation and systems that optimize this modality.

References

1 Paolini B, Romanelli F, Prigione G, Pertile G: Incidence of endophthalmitis in a large series of 23-gauge and 20-gauge transconjunctival pars plana vitrectomy. Graefes Arch Clin Exp Ophthalamol 2009;247:895–898.

2 Mentens R, Stalmans P: Comparison of postoperative comfort in 20 gauge versus 23 gauge pars plana vitrectomy. Bull Soc Belge Ophtalmol 2009;311:5–10.

Peter Stalmans, MD, PhD
University Hospitals Leuven, Campus Sint-Rafaël, Ophthalmology
Kapucijnenvoer 33
BE–3000 Leuven (Belgium)
E-Mail peter.stalmans@uzleuven.be

Oh H, Oshima Y (eds): Microincision Vitrectomy Surgery. Emerging Techniques and Technology.
Dev Ophthalmol. Basel, Karger, 2014, vol 54, pp 45–53 (DOI: 10.1159/000360448)

25-Gauge Vitrectomy

Marco Mura[a] · Francesco Barca[b]

[a]Academic Medical Center, University of Amsterdam, Amsterdam, The Netherlands;
[b]U.O. Chirurgia Oftalmica, Azienda Ospedaliero Universitaria Pisana (AOUP), Pisa, Italy

Abstract

The development of a 25-gauge vitrectomy system represents a major step forward in vitreoretinal surgery. The main advantages of small-gauge incisions are reduction of surgical time, decreased postoperative inflammation, and fast postoperative recovery time. The use of this technique requires research, training, knowledge, and experience on the part of the vitreoretinal surgeon and the personnel in the operation room. At the same time the indications for 25-gauge vitrectomy have changed a lot in the last years due to improvement in materials and technology and the advent of new instruments. Nowadays, with the development of new surgical instrumentation and the improvement of surgical skills, we can approach the whole spectrum of vitreoretinal pathology. This chapter describes the instruments used in 25-gauge vitrectomy, explains how to set the vitrectomy machine for safe surgery and what the indications for 25-gauge vitrectomy are (with particular reference to vitreoretinal interface diseases, retinal detachment, and proliferative diabetic retinopathy) as well as the complications that can occur, and provides some pearls for challenging cases.

The development of the 25-gauge vitrectomy system was an important step in vitreoretinal surgery. Introduced and developed by de Juan and colleagues in 2002 [1, 2], it is now widely used in the treatment of several vitreoretinal diseases. This technique, called 'transconjunctival sutureless vitrectomy', can achieve real sutureless surgery due to its small caliber. The main advantages of small-gauge incisions are shortening of surgical time, reduction of postoperative inflammation, and fast postoperative recovery time. The use of this technique requires research, training, knowledge, and experience on the part of the vitreoretinal surgeon and the personnel in the operation room. At the same time, the surgical tools have to be constantly updated.

Indications

The indications for 25-gauge vitrectomy have changed a great deal in the last years due to improvement in materials and technology and the advent of new instruments. Initially the 25-gauge vitrectomy system was used to treat less complicated elective vitreoretinal pathology such as macular holes and macular pucker, moderate vitreous bleedings, and uncomplicated primary retinal detachments [3]. Nowadays, with the development of new surgical instrumentation and the improvement of the individual surgical skills, we can approach the whole spectrum of the vitreoretinal pathology [4]. Many surgeons, including the authors, make use of this technology not only to treat common disease of the vitreoretinal interface, but also for more complex cases like vitreous hemorrhages, retinal detachments complicated with proliferative vitreoretinopathy (PVR) or giant retinal tear, proliferative diabetic retinopathy with or without tractional retinal detachment, and ocular trauma. The 25-gauge system can be used to perform challenging surgical procedures like macular translocation or retinal pigment epithelium (RPE)-choroid transplantation, which previously was only possible with 20-gauge instrumentation.

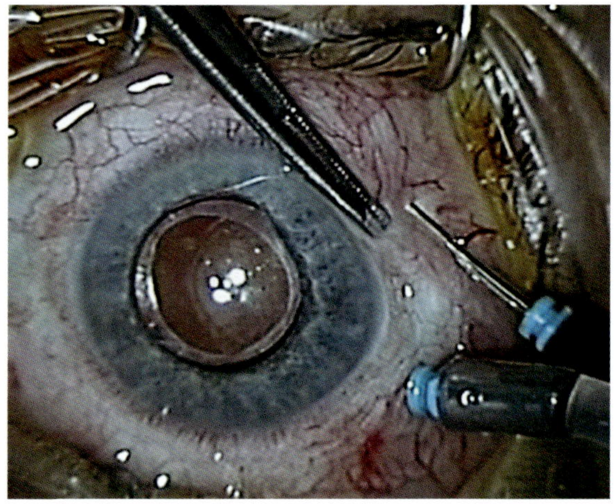

Fig. 1. 25-gauge trocar insertion. The conjunctiva is displaced superiorly with an anatomic forceps while the trocar cannula is inserted at about a 30° angle through the conjunctiva and sclera.

Instrumentation

The system consists of a specific set of microcannulas and a series of instruments specifically designed for this gauge. Standard microcannulas have a shaft 3.5 mm in length (usually polyamide or steel) with an internal and external diameter of 0.4 and 0.5 mm, respectively. On the extraocular portion, they have a little collar that can be grabbed to manipulate the cannula itself. Once introduced through the scleral wall they maintain their position without the need for suturing. In cases with a thickened eye wall (e.g. choroidal detachment), longer microcannulas (5 mm) are available to avoid suprachoroidal infusion.

Multiple surgical instruments have been designed for the 25-gauge system: vitrectomy probe, light fibers, laser probes (straight, curved, directional), microforceps [internal limiting membrane (ILM) forceps, serrated jaws, end-grasping, asymmetrical, etc.], scissors (horizontal or vertical cutting), bipolar cautery, illuminated pick, diamond-dusted scraper, etc. In combination with these instruments, several types of 25-gauge light probes for wide-angle endoillumination are currently available. These are called chandelier-style illuminators that produce homogenous and wide-angle endoillumination, making them perfect for use in combination with a panoramic-viewing system.

Wound Construction and Cannula Removal

Sclerotomy construction is fundamental in sutureless surgery because a good result is dependent on the water tightness of the sclerotomy (fig. 1). Before inserting the trocar cannula, the conjunctiva should be displaced (with blunt forceps or cotton tip) in such a way to obtain a misalignment of the sclerotomy and the conjuctival wound when the cannula is removed. The authors perform sclerotomies 3.5 mm from the limbus in pseudophakic and aphakic eyes and 4 mm in phakic patients. We introduce the microvitreoretinal blade with a 30° angle until the edge of the shaft of the microcannula is reached; the microblade is then verticalized and introduced in the vitreous cavity perpendicular to the scleral plane. This technique creates a biplanar self-sealing scleral incision at the end of the operation. The trocar cannulas are essential in modern 25-gauge vitrectomy because they allow the alignment between displaced conjunctiva and sclera, making possible an atraumatic insertion and removal of the different types of instruments in and out the eye protecting the vitreous base from possible iatrogenic damage. The trocar cannulas can be with or without valves. In the authors' experience, a valved system offers major stability for the vitreous cavity, which avoids leakage of vitreous and fluid. This reduces the risk of vitreoretinal incarceration in the scleral wound and helps to keep intraocular pressure stable during surgery. The cannulas have to be removed tangentially to facilitate the apposition of the internal and external aspects of the sclerotomy with the pressure exerted by the intraocular pressure. In case of sclerotomy leakage, it is usually sufficient to massage the sclerotomy itself in a gentle and accurate way to allow the closure of the wound. In those cases where a tamponade agent (gas or silicone oil) is not required, the authors perform a complete fluid-air exchange. In fact, the higher superficial tension of the air bubble compared to the irrigation fluid allows a better closure of the scleral wound.

High-Speed Vitrectomy and Machine Set

All the vitrectomy machines that are currently available can simultaneously cut and aspirate the vitreous, which generates pulsatile traction on the retinal surface. An ideal vitrectomy machine would not exert such traction. Today, with the new small-gauge instruments and high cut rate (high-speed vitrectomy), it is possible to reduce the amount of pulsatile traction generated during a vitrectomy procedure. Thanks to this technology, the new vitrectomy platforms are able to drastically reduce the traction applied to the retina because the vitreous can be fragmented in very small pieces before been aspirated by the vitrectomy probe. This has also made it possible to return to a proportional aspiration system (proportional vacuum). Until a few years ago, the majority of the vitreoretinal surgeons performed 25-gauge vitrectomy with a 3D modality to partially compensate for the reduced aspiration flow rate at the highest cut rate and the increased traction at high vacuum levels. The new generation of vitrectomy systems have cutters and aspiration pumps which are able to ensure an optimal flow rate at a very high cut rate, minimizing vitreoretinal traction. The high-speed vitrectomy probe is able to cut the vitreous in very small fragments, which reduces the viscosity of the vitreous and the resistance inside the probe lumen and tubing, which substantially increases the flow rate and reduces indirectly the traction from the vitreous on the retina. The machine is set with an initial aspiration of 0 mm Hg and moves linearly to 650 mm Hg when the foot pedal is fully depressed, maintaining a fixed cut rate of 5,000, 6,000, or 7,500 cuts/min depending on the platform used. In this way, we have a maximum aspiration flow and cut rate during core vitrectomy, and, vice versa, a minimum aspiration flow during vitreous shaving when lower traction on the vitreoretinal surface is required.

Vitrectomy

25-gauge vitrectomy consists of three main steps: core vitrectomy, posterior hyaloid separation (if uncompleted), and peripheral vitrectomy ('vitreous shaving'). Core vitrectomy is the first step, and has the goal of making an opening in the anterior vitreous cortex and creating a cavity in the central vitreous. In this phase it is possible to use the maximum vacuum (650 mm Hg) with the highest cut rate (5,000, 6,000, or 7,500 cuts/min). Once the central vitreous is removed, the second step is the induction or the completion of posterior vitreous detachment. Posterior vitreous detachment is induced approximating the port of the vitreous probe (with the cutter off) to the optic disc and increasing progressively the aspiration until reaching the maximum level (range: 500–650 mm Hg). The maneuver needs to be repeated several times until the posterior hyaloid becomes visibly engaged in the vitrectomy port, after which the separation from the optic disc is completed along the whole disc circumference. At this stage, the hyaloid is slowly pulled anteriorly towards the lens, keeping a constant aspiration of about 300–400 mm Hg. We suggest performing this maneuver only until reaching the midperiphery to avoid retina traction at the level of the vitreous base with consequent iatrogenic retinal breaks. During this procedure it is mandatory to pay attention to the presence of abnormal vitreoretinal adhesion, such as in cases of diabetic patients who have undergone panretinal photocoagulation or in cases or lattice degeneration areas. In these cases, the adherence between vitreous and retina is stronger than normal and the risk of an iatrogenic break is very high. We believe that the induction of posterior vitreous detachment is the most important surgical moment. Leaving the hyaloid in place could in fact work as a scaffold for cell proliferation, creating tangential traction that could result in macular puckers and/or PVR. Vitreous shaving is the last step of the vitrectomy. If accessory illumination is present, the shaving can be performed by the surgeon himself; otherwise, the assistant will be the one performing the scleral depression (fig. 2).

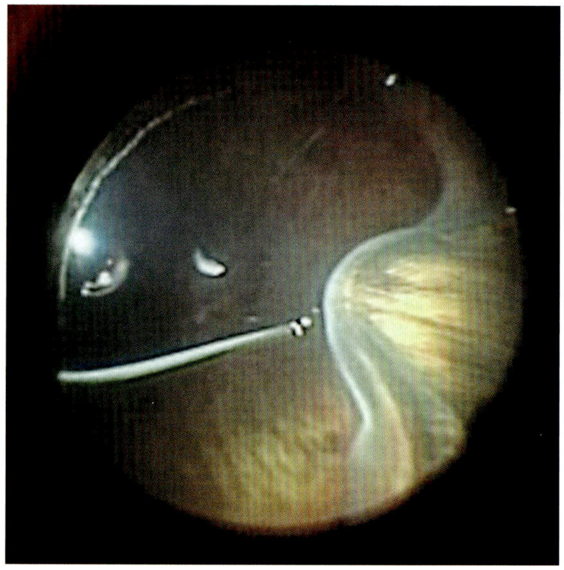

Fig. 2. 25-gauge cannula location during retinal detachment surgery with the chandelier in the inferonasal quadrant.

Macular Surgery

In macular surgery, removal of all macular epiretinal membranes is essential for a good surgical outcome. For the removal of these membranes we have several types of 25-gauge forceps, for example the Tano or Eckardt ILM forceps and end-grasping or asymmetrical forceps. We usually start the peeling from the center of the membrane (inside-out peeling technique [5]), which can be identified by the orientation of the retinal folds, or we start from the thicker part of the epiretinal membrane, usually recognizable as the most opaque area. Once the membrane is pinched and peeling is started, it is essential to proceed tangentially to the retinal plane and with circular movements around the foveal area to avoid inadvertent retinal touches. It is also very important to observe the fovea throughout the entire procedure to avoid iatrogenic foveal decapitation or breaks. ILM peeling is also achievable with the same technique, and adjuvant staining solutions even make it easier by providing better visualization of the ILM itself as well as enhancing the cleavage plane between the retina and ILM.

Retinal Detachment

The small caliber of the 25-gauge probe and the high cut rate are of extreme importance in the treatment of a retinal detachment because they have the advantage of reducing the number of intraoperative retinal breaks, thus minimizing vitreous turbulence and reducing dynamic vitreoretinal traction. This is a very important aspect considering that a recently detached retina is usually very mobile. For this reason, having technology that can reduce the vitreous traction on a mobile retina makes the procedure much safer. We use the 25-gauge vitrectomy system [4, 6] in all types of retinal detachment, and in those complicated by PVR [7], giant retinal tears, choroidal detachment, etc. To ensure a good surgical outcome, posterior vitreous detachment induction (when not present) represents for us the key to the surgical procedure because the traction exerted by the hyaloid left in place is the primary cause of development of new retinal breaks and PVR.

Another key point is the removal of the traction at the level of the anterior edge of the retinal breaks; sometimes the amputation of the anterior flap of the retinal break is necessary to be sure all vitreoretinal tractions have been removed. We do not believe it is necessary to perform a complete vitrectomy (vitreous shaving with deep sclera depression) in every case. In fact, we routinely perform vitreous base shaving in cases with posterior attachment of the vitreous base, in myopic cases with peripheral retinal degeneration, in diabetics and sickle cell cases with fibrovascular proliferation, and in cases with PVR grade C and higher (fig. 3). We always make sure that the subretinal fluid is thoroughly aspirated to facilitate retina RPE adhesion and avoid the formation of undesirable retinal folds at the macular level. The fluid is removed from the preexisting retinal break when this is accessible; otherwise, a new retinotomy is performed peripherally (nasal better than temporal, and superior better than inferior quadrant). Perfluorocarbon liquid (PFCL) helps make the procedure simpler. Another technique we use is to first drain the subretinal fluid during fluid-air exchange as routinely done; if subretinal fluid is still present in macular area, it can be pushed away towards the primary break using PFCL under air. PFCL is then removed making sure to aspirate the little amount of water from the PFCL-air interface. The breaks are then treated with endolaser or cryotherapy. We use cryotherapy to treat breaks when a single small break (≤1 o'clock) is present as well as with multiple (2–3 max.) and superior breaks. Endolaser is performed for larger (>1 o'clock) and/or inferior breaks, multiple breaks (>3), and for giant retinal breaks, retinectomies, and PVR cases.

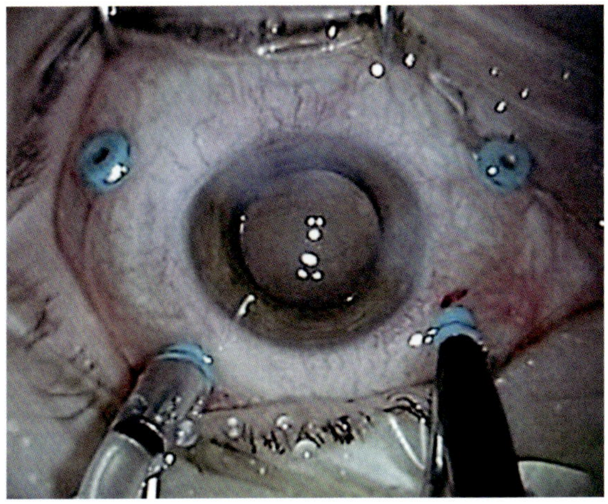

Fig. 3. 25-gauge vitreous base dissection using the bimanual technique with scleral depression and chandelier light system.

Giant Break

The surgical treatment of the giant retinal breaks [8], both associated or not associated with retinal detachment, is a challenge even for experienced retinal surgeons. The biggest improvement in the treatment of this disease has probably been the introduction of PFCL, which has improved the prognosis of this disease. We perform a complete vitrectomy with vitreous base shaving. The edge of the giant tear is then unrolled with the help of gentle suction (vitrectomy probe or soft-tipped extrusion needle) when PVR is not present or with the bimanual technique with the use of an illuminated spatula or chandelier light and a serrated jaws-type forceps when PVR has already developed. With a soft-tipped cannula, the disinserted edge of the retina is then lifted and PFCL is injected towards the optic disc until the edge of the giant break is adherent to the underlying RPE. Endolaser photocoagulation is now applied to the posterior edge of the tear making sure to seal it up to the ora serrata on both sides. The choice of the tamponade agent depends on the retinal conditions and the location of the giant break. A superior giant retinal break without PVR can be tamponaded with a long-acting gas such as perfluoropropane (C_3F_8 12%). Silicone oil is still the best option for giant retinal breaks with PVR that are not superiorly located.

Management of Proliferative Vitreoretinopathy

PVR is an excessive healing reaction of the retina to damage (e.g. retinal detachment, trauma). We routinely perform 25-gauge vitrectomy in every retinal detachment with PVR. In planning the surgery, it is extremely important to localize the PVR (anterior and/or posterior; epiretinal and/or subretinal) and its extension (number of quadrants involved). PFCL is very useful because it has a very low viscosity (2–3 cSt) and is easily injected through small-caliber cannulas (e.g. 25 gauge). In fact, PFCL has modified the surgical approach to PVR. The traditional approach before its introduction was first the management of the anterior PVR and then the posterior PVR. The use of PFCL has reversed this strategy, leading to management from the posterior pole to the ora serrata [9]. Nowadays, we first address the posterior PVR; once it is completely removed we stabilize the posterior retina with PFCL and can address the anterior PVR safely. If the retina is not flattened with a PFCL bubble, it means that there is residual epiretinal traction that needs further peeling, sometimes associated with retinectomy. In case of epiretinal proliferation, we stain the membranes with a mixture of trypan blue and brilliant peel to better identify the tissue and make sure with a second staining the tissue has been removed.

Subretinal proliferation needs to be addressed in a different way. It is not always necessary to remove cases in which the membranes are flat and very localized. In such cases, it is possible to test the elasticity of the retina by performing fluid-air exchange and drainage of the subretinal fluid; if the retina goes flat, it means that the elasticity is well preserved and the focal membrane does not need to be removed. If the retina does not flatten, removal of the subretinal membrane is then necessary. Subretinal dendritic PVR needs to be removed and can be done with end-grasping or serrated jaws forceps via a small retinotomy. When the PVR is very extensive, it is usually necessary to perform a retinectomy and access the subretinal space by flipping the retina outside-in. Also in this case, serrated jaws and/or end-grasping forceps are the preferred choice in our center.

Proliferative Diabetic Retinopathy

The improvement of medical care, new laser technology, and advent of the intravitreal injection of different sorts of drugs has reduced the need for a surgical approach to diabetic retinopathy. Vitrectomy, however, plays a crucial role in the management and treatment of the complications of diabetic retinopathy [10]. Surgical indications for 25-gauge vitrectomy are tractional retinal detachment threatening or involving the macula, neovascular glaucoma, anterior vitreous cortex fibrovascular proliferation, and vitreous or preretinal hemorrhage. The first surgical step when approaching an eye with proliferative diabetic retinopathy is to evaluate the condition of the posterior vitreous cortex (PVC) and its relation with the retinal surface; in fact, the PVC can be totally or partially detached from the retina or completely adherent. The cases in which the PVC is totally detached from the retinal surface are generally the less complex to treat. In these cases there is no trac-

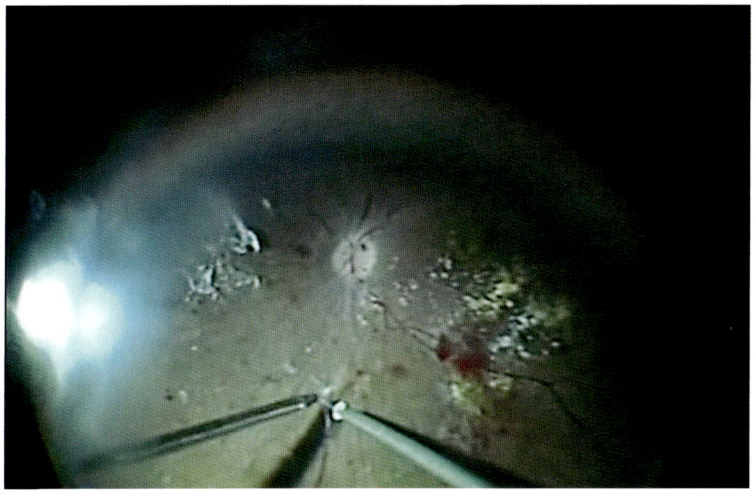

Fig. 4. Bimanual cutter delamination in proliferative diabetic retinopathy. Chandelier light provides illumination while the surgeon lifts the fibrovascular tissue with end-grasping forceps and cuts the tissue with the cutter.

tion on the retina, and once the vitreous and the PVC have been removed, the surgery can be completed with panretinal endolaser photocoagulation if necessary. When the PVC is adherent, the complexity of the surgery varies proportionally to the degree of adherence of the cortex to the retina. In such cases, there are several possible techniques.

We do not use the segmentation technique anymore, but we still employ delamination because we think that leaving residual fibrovascular tissue on the retinal surface may result in chronically elevated retinal areas that may also lead to rhegmatogenous retinal detachment in case of atrophic hole formation, or to a recurrent vitreous hemorrhage. However, the segmentation technique can be helpful as a first step of delamination when very broad and long fibrovascular adhesion is present; segmenting these broad areas before delaminating them can reduce traction on adjacent retinal tissue, with consequent reduction of iatrogenic breaks. Vitreoretinal proliferation usually arises at the level of the optic disc and the major retinal vessels. As a first step, we advise removing or circumscribing the PVC and to isolate every fibrovascular attachment point to avoid anteroposterior traction and iatrogenic retinal tears during delamination. This step is achieved using the highest cut rate and the lowest vacuum possible. Afterwards, we proceed to the delamination of the fibrovascular pegs. In cases of focal and/or weak adhesion, delamination is possible using simple end-grasping forceps (fig. 4). However, if the adhesion is broad and/or strong, it is better to use a bimanual technique that requires the use of an additional chandelier light, end-grasping forceps, and the vitrectomy probe or curved scissors. Delamination is then performed lifting the fibrovascular pegs with the forceps and cutting with the blade of the scissors or the port of the vitrectomy probe at the root of the fibrovascular peg, removing the tissue completely. The advantage of 25-gauge vitrectomy is evident; in fact, the small caliber of the probe and the position of the port located on the distal end of the shaft makes it possible to insert it in narrow spaces such as between the retina and the fibrovascular tissue.

Challenging and Other Cases

The old concept that 25-gauge vitrectomy is not suitable for the most challenging cases was revised many years ago. Excessive flexibility, reduced caliber and poor efficiency of the pumps, and being unable to reach usable aspiration flow with reduced gauge were the reasons many surgeons gave for not using this system for difficult cases. Technology has evolved and today we have vitrectomy machines able to reach high vacuum levels and a high cut rate without compromising aspiration flow. According to Poiseuille's law, the resistance to flow in a capillary tube is inversely proportional to the fourth power of the radius, i.e. to overcome this limit and reach acceptable flows, it was necessary develop vitrectomy machines able to reach high vacuum levels as well as very high cut rates to cut the vitreous fibers in pieces small enough to be aspirated without blocking the lumen of the vitrectomy probe. Evolution in the materials has also made possible the production of stiffer probes comparable to a bigger gauge possible. In our clinical practice, we perform 25-gauge vitrectomy in every case: ocular trauma (open or closed), intraocular foreign body removal, removal of dense subretinal blood, macular translocation, and RPE-choroid transplantation [11–13].

Complications

Minimally invasive surgery has become more popular since it became available on a large scale in 2004. A 2012 survey presented at the American Society of Retina Specialists showed that in 2005 only 20% of the surgeons were using small-gauge surgery as a first technique, while 90% of surgeons were using it in 2012. We feel this data can be explained by the fact that complications during a vitreoretinal procedure are not related to the gauge used. Some years ago Kunimoto and Kaiser [14] and Scott et al. [15] reported a higher incidence of endophthalmitis using small-gauge sutureless instruments. Other studies have shown that the higher risk was only due to wrong construction of the sclerotomy ports. Changing from a straight to oblique incision reduced the incidence of endophthalmitis and postoperative hypotony to values comparable to the 20-gauge sutured technique [16].

A high cut rate [17, 18], small gauges, and the use of trocar cannulas have also reduced the incidence of iatrogenic retinal breaks and consequent retinal detachment.

Conclusions

A new technique must be shown to be safe and efficient at least as much as the standard technique before it can be introduced to the market. 25-gauge vitrectomy was immediately shown to be safe and efficient, ensuring a faster and painless postoperative recovery for the patient. Initially considered as a possibility for less complex surgical cases (e.g. macular surgery), this technology, due to continuous research and the improvement in materials, is now used to treat every type of pathology in vitreoretinal surgery. The majority of the complications are independent from the gauge used. Surgery without risks is a utopian dream. Endophthalmitis, iatrogenic retinal breaks, and retinal detachment are just some examples of complications possible with any technique used. In our experience, and supported by clinical studies, having a technique that generates less vitreoretinal traction [19] represents undoubtedly a great advantage in terms of safety and efficacy [17].

References

1 Fujii GY, de Juan E Jr, Humayun MS, Pieramici DJ, Chang TS, Awh C, Ng E, Barnes A, Wu SL, Sommerville DN: A new 25-gauge instrument system for transconjunctival sutureless vitrectomy surgery. Ophthalmology 2002;109: 1807–1812.

2 de Juan E Jr, Hickingbotham D: Refinements in microinstrumentation for vitreous surgery. Am J Ophthalmol 1990; 109:218–220.

3 Ibarra MS, Hermel M, Prenner JL, Hassan TS: Longer-term outcomes of transconjunctival sutureless 25-gauge vitrectomy. Am J Ophthalmol 2005;139: 831–836.

4 Mura M, Tan SH, de Smet MD: Use of 25-gauge vitrectomy in the management of primary rhegmatogenous retinal detachment. Retina 2009;29:1299–1304.
5 Charles S, Calzada J, Wood B: Vitreous Microsurgery, ed 5. Philadelphia, Wolters Kluwer/Lippincott Williams & Wilkins, 2011, p 62.
6 Dell'Omo R, Barca F, Tan HS, Bijl HM, Oberstein SY, Mura M: Pars plana vitrectomy for the repair of primary, inferior rhegmatogenous retinal detachment associated to inferior breaks. A comparison of a 25-gauge versus a 20-gauge system. Graefes Arch Clin Exp Ophthalmol 2013;251:485–490.
7 Iwahashi-Shima C, Sato T, Bando H, Ikeda T, Emi K: Anatomic and functional outcomes of 25-gauge vitrectomy for repair of eyes with rhegmatogenous retinal detachment complicated by proliferative vitreoretinopathy. Clin Ophthalmol 2013;7:2043–2049.
8 Kunikata H, Abe T, Nishida K: Successful outcomes of 25- and 23-gauge vitrectomies for giant retinal tear detachments. Ophthalmic Surg Lasers Imaging 2011;42:487–492.
9 Ryan JS: Perfluorocarbon liquids in vitreoretinal surgery; in: Retina, ed 4. Amsterdam, Elsevier Mosby, 2005, vol 3, p 2179.
10 Farouk MM, Naito T, Sayed KM, Nagasawa T, Katome T, Radwan G, Abdallah A, Elagouz M: Outcomes of 25-gauge vitrectomy for proliferative diabetic retinopathy. Graefes Arch Clin Exp Ophthalmol 2011;249:369–376.
11 Kunikata H, Uematsu M, Nakazawa T, Fuse N: Successful removal of large intraocular foreign body by 25-gauge microincision vitrectomy surgery. J Ophthalmol 2011;2011:940323.
12 Kunikata H, Fuse N, Abe T: Fixating dislocated intraocular lens by 25-gauge vitrectomy. Ophthalmic Surg Lasers Imaging 2011;42:297–301.
13 Ho LY, Walsh MK, Hassan TS: 25-gauge pars plana vitrectomy for retained lens fragments. Retina 2010;30:843–849.
14 Kunimoto DY, Kaiser RS: Incidence of endophthalmitis after 20- and 25-gauge vitrectomy. Ophthalmology 2007;114:2133–2137.
15 Scott IU, Flynn HW Jr, Dev S, Shaikh S, Mittra RA, Arevalo JF, Kychenthal A, Acar N: Endophthalmitis after 25-gauge and 20-gauge pars plana vitrectomy: incidence and outcomes. Retina 2008;28:138–142.
16 Oshima Y, Kadonosono K, Yamaji H, Inoue M, Yoshida M, Kimura H, Ohji M, Shiraga F, Hamasaki T, Japan Microincision Vitrectomy Surgery Study Group: Multicenter survey with a systematic overview of acute-onset endophthalmitis after transconjunctival microincision vitrectomy surgery. Am J Ophthalmol 2010;150:716–725.
17 Rizzo S, Genovesi-Ebert F, Belting C: Comparative study between a standard 25-gauge vitrectomy system and a new ultrahigh-speed 25-gauge system with duty-cycle control in the management treatment of various vitreoretinal pathologies. Retina 2011;31:2007–2013.
18 Rizzo S, Belting C, Genovesi-Ebert F, di Bartolo E: Incidence of retinal detachment after small-incision, sutureless pars plana vitrectomy compared with conventional 20-gauge vitrectomy in macular hole and epiretinal membrane surgery. Retina 2010;30:1065–1071.
19 Teixeira A, Chong LP, Matsuoka N, Arana L, Kerns R, Bhadri P, Humayun M: Vitreoretinal traction created by conventional cutters during vitrectomy. Ophthalmology 2010;117:1387–1392.

Marco Mura
Academic Medical Center, University of Amsterdam
Meibergdreef 9
NL–1105AZ Amsterdam (The Netherlands)
E-Mail m.mura@amc.uva.nl

Oh H, Oshima Y (eds): Microincision Vitrectomy Surgery. Emerging Techniques and Technology.
Dev Ophthalmol. Basel, Karger, 2014, vol 54, pp 54–62 (DOI: 10.1159/000360449)

27-Gauge Vitrectomy

Shunsuke Osawa[a] · Yusuke Oshima[b]

[a]Department of Ophthalmology, Okanami General Hospital, Mie, and
[b]Vitreoretina & Cataract Surgery Center, Oshima Eye Clinic, Osaka, Japan

Abstract

Ten years or more have passed since the current concept of 25-gauge transconjunctival sutureless vitrectomy with a trocar-cannula system emerged. There is no doubt that current microincision vitrectomy surgery with 25- or 23-gauge instrumentation has simplified the vitrectomy procedure and has provided numerous potential advantages over traditional 20-gauge surgery. The established theory regarding surgical wounds is that 'much smaller is better'. Along with the development of new-generation vitrectomy machines with ergonomic instruments, surgeons have been shifting dramatically from 20-gauge systems to 23- and 25-gauge systems over the last years. Thanks to recent innovations and improvements in high-end multifunctional vitrectomy machines and ultrahigh-speed cutters, the development of powerful light sources, and wide-angle viewing systems, several new techniques have also encouraged us to launch the development of a 27-gauge vitrectomy system over the past several years. Similar to the recent evolution in 23- and 25-gauge systems, further development and refinement of the functionality of instruments with a gauge of 27 or more are under way and will continue over the coming years, which in the future will allow us to establish this system for ultra-minimally invasive surgery for the full spectrum of vitreoretinal pathologies.

Ten years or more have passed since Eugene de Juan and colleagues [1, 2] first brought out the current concept of transconjunctival sutureless vitrectomy with a trocar-cannula system and 25-gauge instrumentation. Afterwards in 2005, Eckardt [3] introduced a 23-gauge system. There is no doubt that current microincision vitrectomy surgery (MIVS) with 25- or 23-gauge instrumentation has simplified the vitrectomy procedure and has provided numerous potential advantages over traditional 20-gauge surgery, including faster wound healing, decreased conjunctival scarring, shorter operating time, less postoperative inflammation, reduced corneal astigmatism, and improved patient comfort with earlier visual recovery [4–9]. In 25- and 23-g systems, stiffer instruments and wide-angle viewing systems have ended the frustration with small-gauge tool fragility. More powerful light sources like xenon, mercury vapor, and LED combined with a chandelier system have improved the endoillumination brightness through a smaller-gauge optic fiber. Thanks to recent innovations and improvements in high-end multifunctional vitrectomy machines and ultrahigh-speed cutters, several new techniques have also encouraged us to launch the development of a 27-gauge vitrectomy system over the past several years. In this chapter, we describe the evolution of 27-gauge vitrectomy systems.

Criticisms of Microincision Vitrectomy Surgery

The most serious and common criticisms regarding the current 23- and 25-gauge vitrectomy systems have focused on complications related to wound sealing, such as hypotony due to leakage, choroidal detachment, and an increasingly higher incidence of bacterial contamination or postoperative endophthalmitis. Although the recent refinement of trocar-cannula systems has improved their self-sealing architectures, special techniques (2-step oblique insertion, 1-step extremely oblique insertion, etc.) are still required. Complete self-sealing wounds are not yet achievable in every case, even with 25-gauge systems. The established theory regarding surgical wounds is that 'much smaller is much better'. On the basis of the above-mentioned facts of modern MIVS, the gauge size for MIVS will likely decrease in the future. In fact, before the introduction of 25- and 23-gauge MIVS, much smaller-gauge instrumentation had been used for postoperative management. For example, we performed transconjunctival fluid-fluid exchange and fluid-air exchange in vitrectomized eyes through a 27-gauge needle for many years. There have been no previous reports on complications related to wound integrity with a 27-gauge (0.40-mm) needles, which some have proposed as the optimal size for easy self-sealing of scleral wounds.

Development of the 27-Gauge System

In the beginning, a crucial concern in developing the 27-gauge system was a reduced endoillumination light source. Fortunately, the introduction of powerful sources using xenon light and mercury vapor light enabled us to develop more smaller-gauge illumination tools [10]. Nowadays, we can use a more powerful, safe, and efficient light source using a light-emitting diode (LED) source (fig. 1). Development of a practical 27-gauge vitreous cutter was the most crucial step for establishing the 27-gauge vitrectomy system. We developed a prototype pneumatic 27-gauge cutter in collaboration with DORC (Zuidland, the Netherlands). Surprisingly, the duty cycle of the 27-gauge cutter was equal to or slightly better than that of a 25-gauge cutter at 1,000 or 1,500 cuts/min [Y. Oshima, unpubl. data, 2008]. In 2008, we were very excited to first report preliminary results using a first-generation 27-gauge system. Although at that time it was used only in selected cases, mainly macular disease and simple vitreous hemorrhage, both the anatomical and visual results were promising [11]. 27-gauge vitrectomy could be started immediately after the sclerotomies at the pars plana by simple vertical insertion. After simple removal of all instruments, surgery was finished at once and all sclerotomies self-sealed completely without the required suturing. Outstandingly, no hypotony was observed, and there was no need to convert to a larger-gauge system in any of the study cases. Encouraged by the promising pilot study results, we succeeded in collaborating with two companies (DORC and Synergetics Inc., St. Charles, Mo., USA) to launch a 27-gauge system pack including a 2,500-cuts/min high-speed pneumatic cutter for macular surgery. And now, DORC has developed a pneumatic high-speed 6,000-cuts/min 27-gauge vitrectomy system available for most vitrectomy systems (fig. 2). More recently, we worked with Alcon Laboratories Inc. (Fort Worth, Tex., USA) to launch the 27+-gauge UltraVit probe system with a Constellation vision system, featuring dual-pneumatic-driven technology, capable of 7,500 cuts/min with duty cycle control in 2012 [12–14].

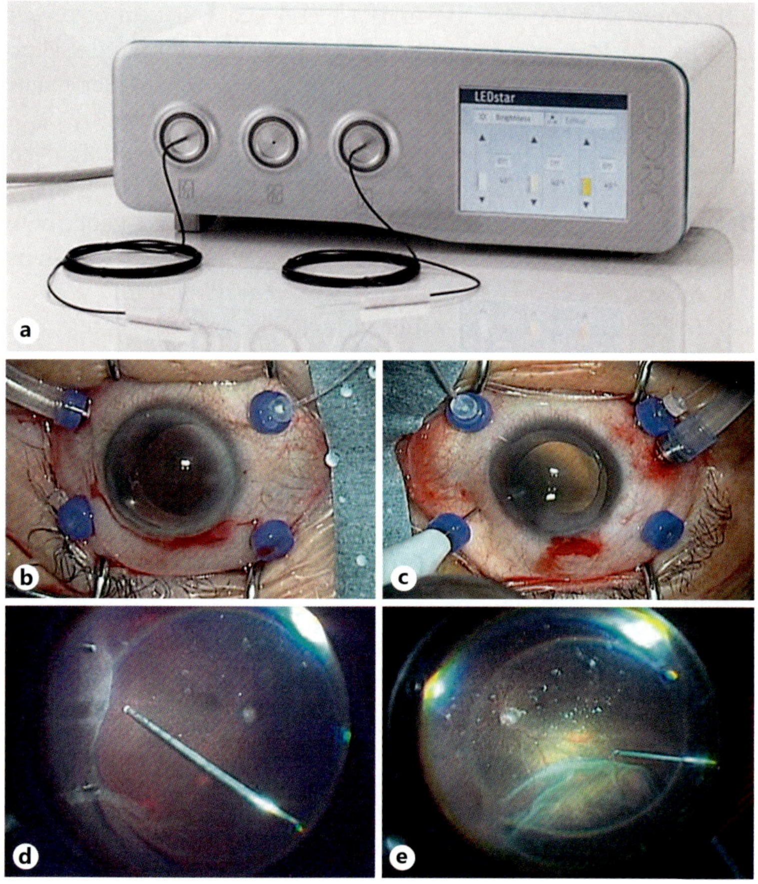

Fig. 1. The more powerful, safe, and efficient light source using LED.
a LED Star (DORC). **b, d** Peripheral shaving under 27-gauge single chandelier illumination.
c, e Releasing the vitreous traction around the retinal break under dual (twin) chandelier illumination.

Efficiency of 27-Gauge Ultrahigh-Speed Vitrectomy

Efficiency of the vitrectomy system is measured by various parameters, but the most important is flow rate. The flow rate of viscous fluid, such as vitreous, is modulated by the Hagen-Poiseuille law, which states that flow through the vitreous cutter is proportional to the aspiration force, the fourth power of the radius, and operating time, and on the other hand inversely proportional to the length of the cutter and the coefficient of viscosity. In a 27-gauge system, a decrease of the inner lumen radius by 20% theoretically results in a decrease of flow rate by about 60%. In our experience, there is the recognition that flow rate decreases, but an actual decrease is not felt with 60%. Therefore, we compared the practical performance of the 27+-gauge ultrahigh-speed vitreous cutter and that of the 25+ ultrahigh-speed cutter using porcine eyes with Constellation. As a result,

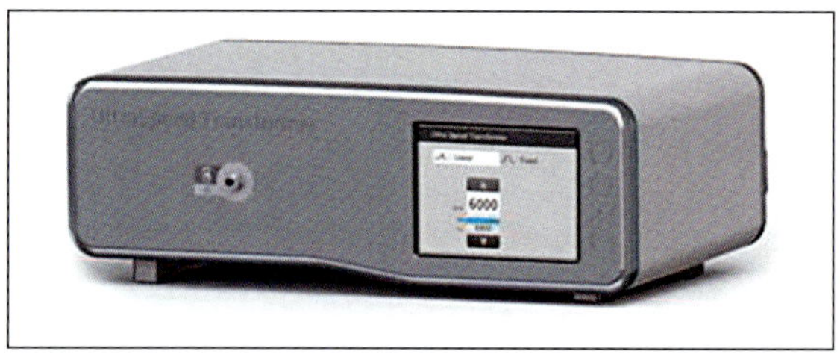

Fig. 2. Pneumatic high-speed 6,000-cuts/min vitrectomy system; Ultra Speed Transformer (DORC).

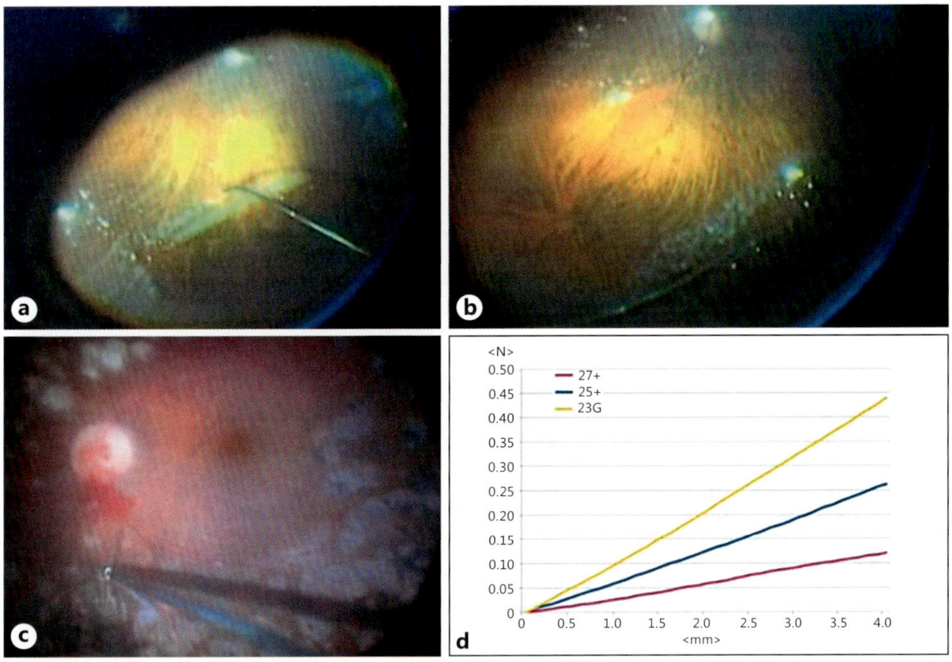

Fig. 3. Rigidity of 27-guage instruments. **a, b** Stretch out the rolled-up retina with 27-gauge cutter like a soft-tip needle. **c** 27-gauge cutter used like a membrane pick. **d** Rigidity test, 27+-gauge vs. 25+- and 23-gauge.

the 27+-gauge cutter showed approximately 60% of efficiency of the 25+-gauge [Y. Oshima, unpubl. data, 2013]. As a matter of fact, by using an ultrahigh-speed vitreous cutter with duty cycle control, the vitreous is cut into very fine fragments, and an efficient vitreous flow rate can be achieved because the vitreous viscosity decreases. Furthermore, the rise in vitreous flow rate is accompanied by a rise in cut rate. In vitreous cutting flow rate, the efficiency of the 27+-gauge ultrahigh-speed vitreous cutter (7,500 cuts/min) is approximately twice that of the 25+-gauge cutter (2,500 cuts/min) [Y. Oshima, unpubl. data, 2013].

Actual Fragility

The 27-gauge instrumentation, for which fragility was one of the major concerns, has been made stiffer by featuring a stiffness sleeve. We tested the 27+-gauge cutter for actual rigidity, comparing it to the 23- and 25+-gauge cutter. The rigidity of the 27+-gauge cutter was approximately half that of the 25+-gauge cutter. Therefore, it is considerably more fragile than the 25+-gauge cutter. On the other hand, we often use the 27-gauge cutter like a membrane pick and a soft-tip needle by taking advantage of bending (fig. 3). Surgeons must consider the fragility of the 27+-gauge instrumentation, but our experience with the 27+-gauge instrumentation has shown that there is only a slight difference in rigidity compared to the 25+-gauge instrumentation. One reason for this is that the tapered stiffening sleeve, designed by Alcon, enters the valve-cannula well and provides maximum stiffness by using the cannula as a stiffening sleeve (fig. 4). In this way, the 27+-gauge instrumentation achieved a higher degree of stiffness than the standard 25-gauge instrumentation.

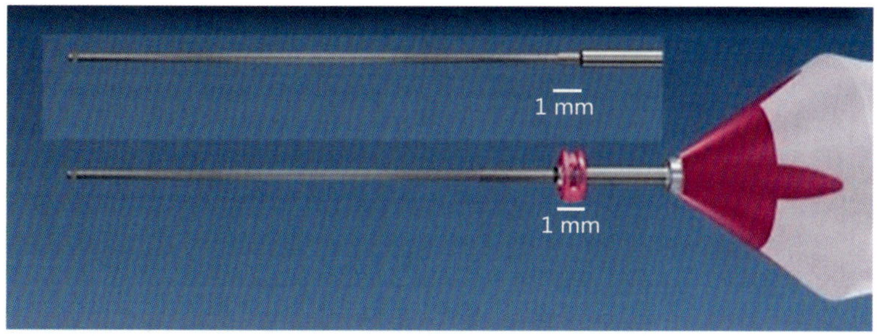

Fig. 4. Tapered stiffening sleeve of the 27+-gauge cutter.

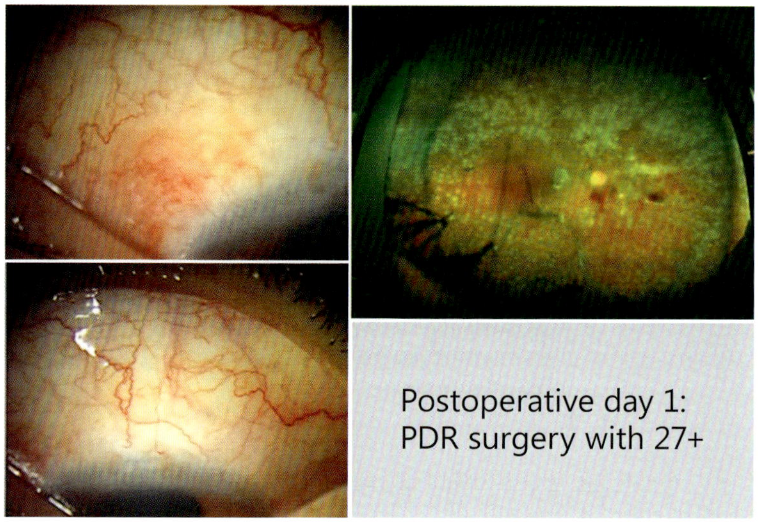

Fig. 5. Postoperative day 1 findings of proliferative diabetic retinopathy surgery with the 27+-gauge system.

Techniques, Indications, and Clinical Experiences with 27- and 27+-Gauge Systems

The surgeon can begin 27-gauge vitrectomy immediately after creating sclerotomies at the pars plana by one-step vertical insertion. Complex techniques for creating a self-sealing wound are no longer required. The postoperative findings, including the anterior segment, are in most cases perfect, even on the first day after surgery (fig. 5). Thanks to the improvement of the cutting efficiency described above, the current indications for the 27-gauge vitrectomy have expanded (table 1; fig. 6). More recently, it has been useful for treating severe retinal detachment and moderately severe-to-challenging proliferative diabetic cases, along with the very efficient and safe ultrahigh-speed vitreous cutter and the development of a variety of accessories in the 27+-gauge instrumentation (fig. 7). With wide-angle fundus viewing, it is also easy to perform bimanual membrane segmentation and dissection with a 27-gauge system. Nevertheless, overall we had fewer chances to perform bimanual manipulation in the 27+-gauge diabetic series than we did in the past with the 25-gauge systems because the 27-gauge cutter can be more easily inserted into the tiny space between the membrane and the retina. This also explains why the 27+-gauge cutter with shave mode, '3D vertical scissors mode', is sufficient for several roles (fig. 8a–c). In this 3D 'shave' sub-mode, we can use the 27+-gauge cutter safely and efficiently

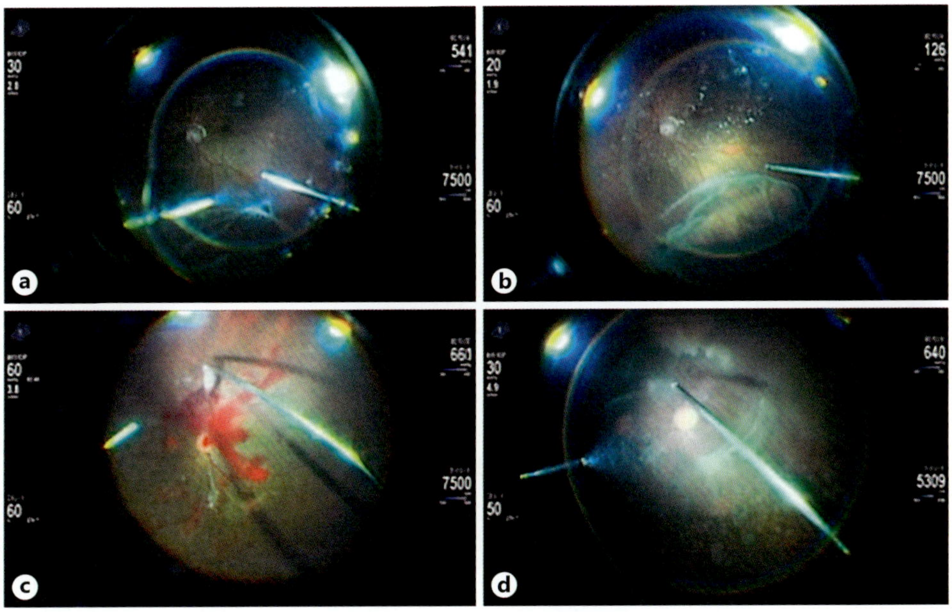

Fig. 6. The current indications for 27-gauge vitrectomy have expanded. **a**, **b** Core vitrectomy and peripheral shaving under scleral indentation with the 27-gauge cutter for rhegmatogenous retinal detachment. **c** Fibrovascular membranes were cut and removed using the 27-gauge cutter. **d** Ultrahigh-speed cutting with the 27+-gauge cutter for a massive old vitreous hemorrhage.

Table 1. Current indications for 27-gauge vitrectomy

Macular diseases
    Epiretinal membrane proliferation
    Idiopathic or secondary macular hole
    Macular traction syndrome
    Macular edema associated with
        Diabetic retinopathy
        Retinal vein occlusion
        Uveitis
    Persistent pseudophakic cystoid macular edema
    Subinternal limiting membrane hemorrhage

Simple vitreous hemorrhage
Vitreous biopsy
Primary rhegmatogenous retinal detachment
Moderate proliferative diabetic retinopathy with or without focal tractional retinal detachment
Subretinal hemorrhage

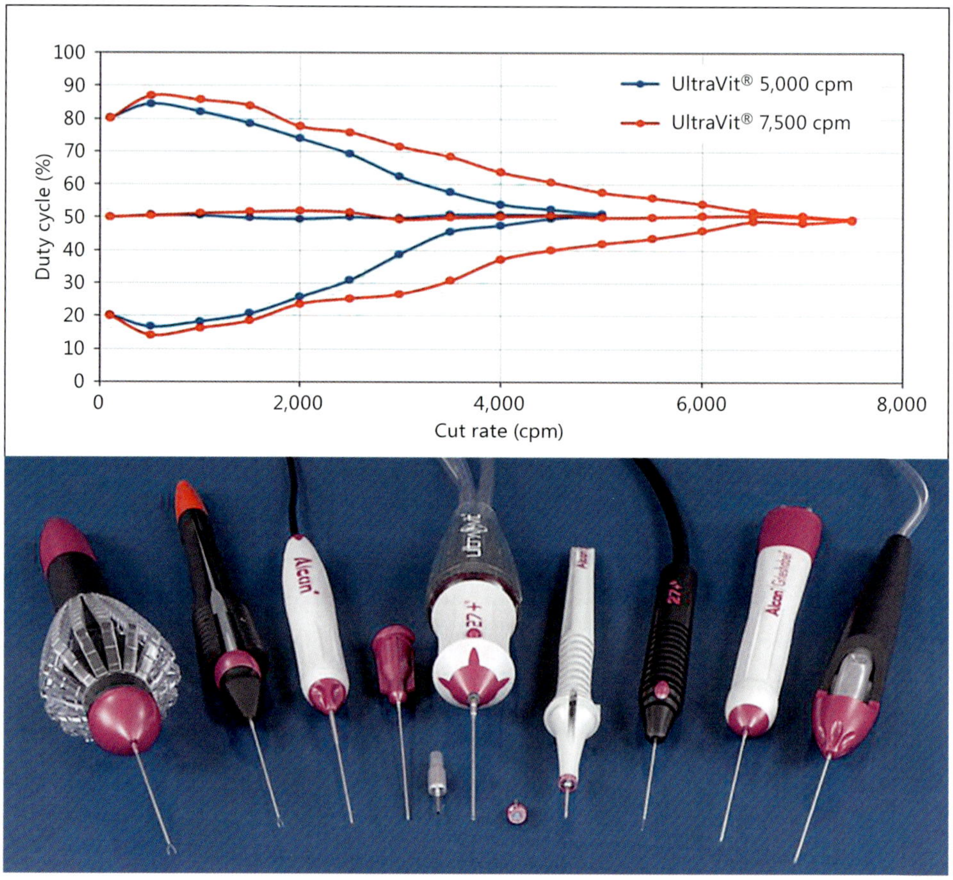

Fig. 7. The 27+-gauge system with Constellation. Comparison of duty cycle changes of dual-pneumatic driven cutters (5,000 vs. 7,500 cuts/min). The three settings of Constellation: 'core' (port biased open), 'shave' (port biased closed), and 50/50. The open biased setting renders the port mostly open in the cutting cycle, maximizing the flow for the given cut rate and vacuum. The closed biased setting renders the port mostly closed in the cutting cycle, minimizing the flow and traction force for the given cutting rate and vacuum.

like vertical scissors. Because of an initial cut rate of 100 cuts/min and end limit of 1,000–1,500 cuts/min, it can move very slow and linearly to 100 mm Hg when the treadle ramping is 70% depressed; after membrane segmentation has been completed, aspiration and cut rate gradually increase until the treadle is fully depressed (fig. 8d).

Constellation's new program 'CR3' can change the treadle setting for each surgeon like a racing car. For example, 'tuned proportional mode by 3D' (fig. 9), we have a delicate adjustment vitreous flow during peripheral shaving and powerful vitreous flow during core vitrectomy. Using the 27+-gauge system will simplify opening and closing procedures, which may save total operating time. Also, because of the small size, safety, efficiency, and multifunctionality of the 27+-gauge cutter, reducing the use of various instruments for manipulation in complex and challenging cases will minimize the time wasted in instrument exchanges and, as a result, also contribute to the reduction of total operating time.

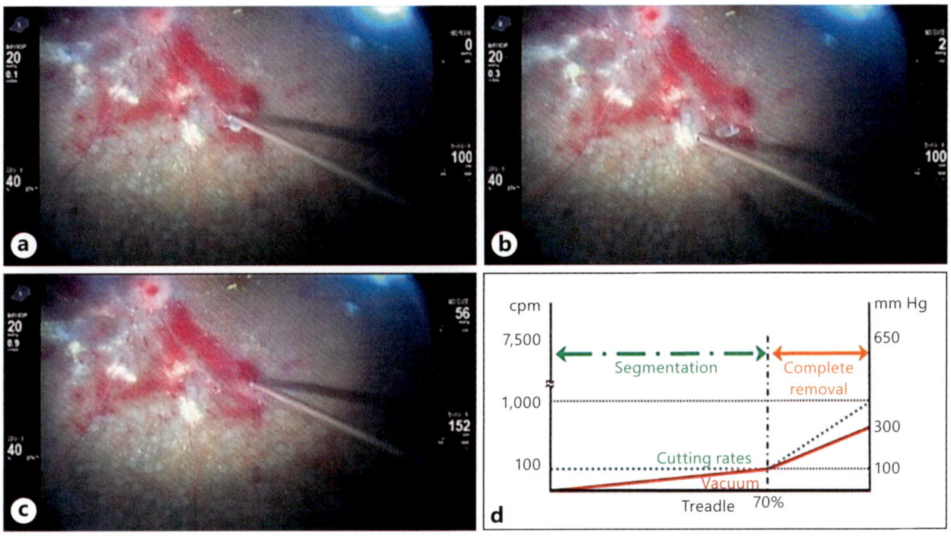

Fig. 8. The 27+-gauge cutter allows safe, efficient, and elegant removal in proliferative cases. **a** The small probe can act like a pick and allow one to lift up abnormal tissue and get into the space between the proliferative membrane and the retina. **b** The 27+-gauge cutter can also act like vertical scissors by cutting the proliferative membrane safely with efficient segmentation. **c** The treadle is fully depressed, the proliferative membrane is removed safely and quickly by fold-back delamination. **d** '3D vertical scissors mode' of the 27+-gauge cutter with shave mode.

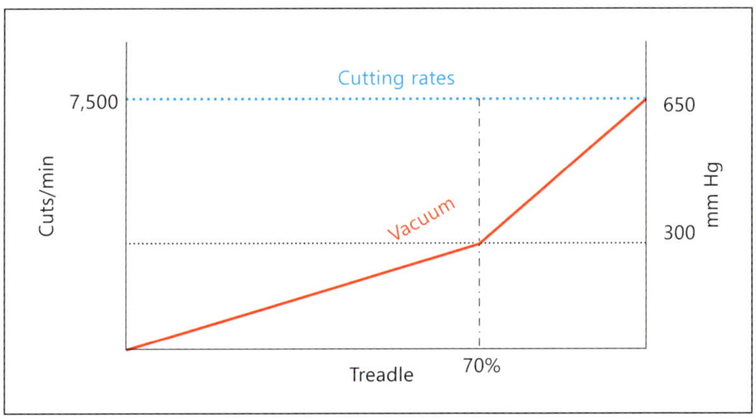

Fig. 9. 'Tuned proportional mode by 3D': we can perform a comfortable and efficient vitrectomy during peripheral shaving with a gentle slope of 0–70% and during core vitrectomy with a steep slope 70% to the treadle when it is fully depressed.

A Promising Outlook

The ultimate goal of vitrectomy is to achieve favorable anatomic success and early vision restoration, with an acceptable operating time and minimal complications, perfect self-sealing wounds, and only slight changes on the ocular surface. The 27-gauge system may have brought us one step closer to these goals. Although the development 27-gauge vitrectomy is an ongoing project, and it has not yet been established as a widely accepted system, its feasibility and safety in selected cases have been demonstrated and confirmed. The 27-gauge ultrahigh-speed vitrectomy has the theoretical advantage of high efficiency and safety. These new technologies, however, must achieve much higher performance rates. Similar to the recent evolution in 23- and 25-gauge systems, further development and refinement of the functionality of the 27-gauge instruments are under way and will continue over the coming years, allowing us in the future to establish this system for ultra-minimally invasive surgery for the full spectrum of vitreoretinal pathologies.

References

1 Fujii GY, De Juan E Jr, Humayun MS, et al: A new 25-gauge instrument system for transconjunctival sutureless vitrectomy surgery. Ophthalmology 2002;109:1807–1812.

2 Fujii GY, De Juan E Jr, Humayun MS, et al: Initial experience using the transconjunctival sutureless vitrectomy system for vitreoretinal surgery. Ophthalmology 2002;109:1814–1820.

3 Eckardt C: Transconjunctival sutureless 23-gauge vitrectomy. Retina 2005;25:208–211.

4 Recchia FM, Scott IU, Brown GC, et al: Small-gauge pars plana vitrectomy: a report by the American Academy of Ophthalmology. Ophthalmology 2010;117:1851–1857.

5 Fine HF, Iranmanesh R, Iturralde D, Spaide RF: Outcomes of 77 consecutive cases of 23-gauge transconjunctival vitrectomy surgery for posterior segment disease. Ophthalmology 2007;114:1197–1200.

6 Kadonosono K, Yamakawa T, Uchio E, et al: Comparison of visual function after epiretinal membrane removal by 20-gauge and 25-gauge vitrectomy. Am J Ophthalmol 2006;142:513–515.

7 Rizzo S, Genovesi-Evert F, Murri S, et al: 25-gauge, sutureless vitrectomy and standard 20-gauge pars plana vitrectomy in idiopathic epiretinal membrane surgery: a comparative pilot study. Graefes Arch Clin Exp Ophthalmol 2006;244:472–479.

8 Okamoto F, Okamoto C, Sakata N, et al: Changes in corneal topography after 25-gauge transconjunctival sutureless vitrectomy versus after 20-gauge standard vitrectomy. Ophthalmology 2007;114:2138–2141.

9 Shinoda H, Shinoda K, Satofuka S, et al: Visual recovery after vitrectomy for macular hole using 25-gauge instruments. Acta Ophthalmol 2008;86:151–155.

10 Oshima Y, Awh C, Tano Y: Self-retaining 27-gauge transconjunctival chandelier endoillumination for panoramic viewing during vitreous surgery. Am J Ophthalmolol 2007;143:166–167.

11 Oshima Y, Wakabayashi T, Sato T, et al: A 27-gauge instrument system for transconjunctival sutureless microincision vitrectomy surgery. Ophthalmology 2010;117:93–102.

12 Rizzo S, Genovesi-Ebert F, Belting C: Comparative study between a standard 25-gauge vitrectomy system and a new ultrahigh-speed 25-gauge system with duty cycle control in the treatment of various vitreoretinal diseases. Retina 2011;31:2007–2013.

13 Oshima Y: Continuing development of 27-gauge vitrectomy systems: where are we now? Retinal Physician 2012, pp 20–25.

14 Rizzo S, Barca F: Twenty-seven-gauge sutureless microincision vitrectomy surgery: a new frontier? Retina Today 2013, pp 37–40.

Yusuke Oshima, MD, PhD
Founder and Director
Vitreoretina & Cataract Surgery Center, Oshima Eye Clinic
1-12-8 Nishikanmuri, Takatsuki-city
Osaka 569-0055 (Japan)
E-Mail yusukeoshima@gmail.com

Oh H, Oshima Y (eds): Microincision Vitrectomy Surgery. Emerging Techniques and Technology.
Dev Ophthalmol. Basel, Karger, 2014, vol 54, pp 63–70 (DOI: 10.1159/000360450)

Basic Setup and Disinfection

Hiroyuki Shimada

Department of Ophthalmology, Surugadai Hospital of Nihon University, Tokyo, Japan

Abstract

Vitrectomy is one of the ophthalmic surgeries that require a large number of instruments. Despite a growing array of single-use disposable instruments, vitrectomies for refractory diseases still involve complicated procedures and many surgical devices. As to the arrangement of materials and instruments on the surgical table, fluids that must not be introduced intraocularly, infusion fluid for washing the ocular surface, fluids for intraocular injection, and fluids for periocular injection are classified and marked to avoid using the wrong fluid. Since bacteria are present in the fluid retained in the fluid catch bag, the accumulated infusion fluid should be removed by aspiration.

Povidone-iodine exhibits a broad range of microbicidal activities against multidrug resistant bacteria, *Candida* species, viruses, and *Acanthamoeba* species, as well as the capability of destroying biofilms, and no resistance is known. Studies on the oculotoxicity of povidone-iodine have shown that the concentrations that are safe for ocular tissues and provide high bactericidal effect range from 0.05 to 0.5%. Upon applying 10% povidone-iodine on the skin, the conjunctival sac should be disinfected using 0.25% povidone-iodine. Even with thorough disinfection of the eyelid and conjunctiva with povidone-iodine and proper draping, bacteria may still gain access to the surgical field after the speculum is placed. Therefore, during vitreous surgery, bacteria may enter the eye easily via the ocular surface fluid. To prevent endophthalmitis, it is necessary to make efforts to achieve 'transient sterilization' of the surgical field by repeated irrigation with 0.25% povidone-iodine.

Basic Setup

Vitrectomy is one of the ophthalmic surgical procedures that require a large number of instruments. Despite a growing array of single-use disposable instruments, vitrectomies for refractory diseases still involve complicated procedures and many surgical devices.

Figure 1 shows the basic setup of a university hospital that treats many refractory diseases. A general surgical table is used. The vitrectomy machine is placed on the left of the patient, and the operating microscope stand is placed posterior to the surgeon. The operating microscope has two side scopes, one for the first and the other for the second assistant. A large-sized instrument table is

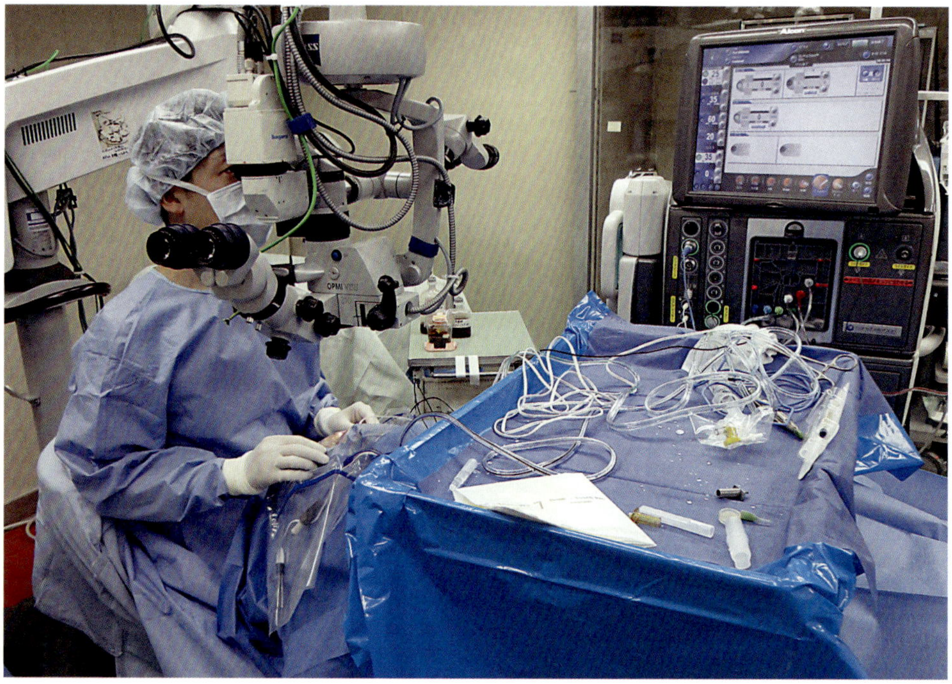

Fig. 1. Basic setup of a university hospital that treats many refractory diseases. A general surgical table and a large-sized instrument table are used.

set at a fixed height and positioned above the trunk of the patient.

Figure 2 shows the basic setup used in a clinic that treats mostly mild diseases. An electric ophthalmic operating table is used. The operating microscope is placed on the left of the patient and the vitrectomy machine is positioned on the right of the surgeon. The operating microscope has only one side scope for the first assistant. The small instrument table provided with the vitrectomy is positioned above the trunk of the patient.

Regardless of facility, instruments such as the aspirator, guide light, and vitreous cutters should be placed securely on the instrument table to prevent them from falling from the table. To avoid obstruction to surgical procedures, the vitreous cutter and other devices should be placed orienting from the inferior side of the patient's trunk toward the surgical field. The intraocular infusion line should be positioned perpendicular to the eyeball and stabilized by tape or forceps. In the past, a hand rest was placed at the patient's head for holding instruments. However, bacteria-containing infusion fluid would accumulate in the space between the hand rest and the patient's head, causing contamination of the instruments. The hand rest is therefore no longer used. Without the hand rest, the infusion fluid flows more easily into the fluid catch bag. Since bacteria are present in the fluid retained in the fluid catch bag [1], the accumulated infusion fluid should be removed by aspiration.

As to the arrangement of materials and instruments on the surgical table, fluids that must not be introduced intraocularly, infusion fluid for washing the ocular surface, fluids for intraocular injection, and fluids for periocular injection are classified and marked to avoid using the wrong

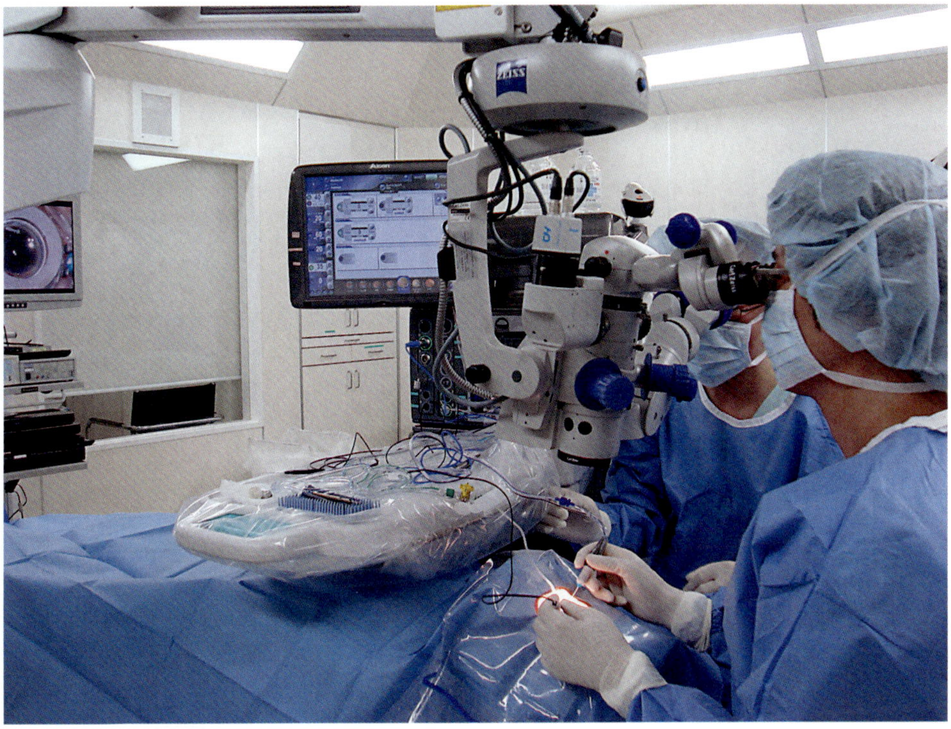

Fig. 2. Basic setup of a clinic that treats mostly mild diseases. An electric ophthalmic operating table and a small-sized instrument table provided with the vitrectomy machine are used.

fluid (fig. 3). Fluids that must not be introduced intraocularly, i.e. 4% xylocaine [1] and 0.25% povidone-iodine for ocular surface irrigation during surgery [2], are filled into syringes and not fitted with needles. Balanced salt solution for irrigating the ocular surface [3] is filled into a 20-ml syringe fitted with a blunt 25-gauge needle. Fluids for intraocular injection, comprising balanced salt solution [4] and vitreous body visualization agent [5], are filled into 2.5-ml syringes and fitted with blunt 25-gauge needles. Brilliant blue G [6] is filled into a 2.5-ml syringe and fitted with a 25-gauge soft-tapered needle. Xylocaine 2% for sub-Tenon injection [7] is filled into a 2.5-ml syringe labeled with a red tape, antibiotic [8] with a white label bearing the name, and steroid [9] also with a white label bearing the name, and fitted with 27-gauge needles.

Disinfection

Povidone-iodine exhibits a broad range of microbicidal activities against multidrug-resistant bacteria, *Candida* species, viruses, and *Acanthamoeba* species, and has the capability of destroying biofilms; no resistance to it is known. The microbicidal activities of povidone-iodine are observed over a wide concentration range from 0.005% [2] to 10% (fig. 4). Povidone-iodine is an intriguing agent; the microbicidal effect is not more powerful at higher concentrations. There is a misunderstanding that the neat solution, 10% povidone-iodine, has the most potent microbicidal effect and requires the shortest time to kill microorganisms. The truth is that the bactericidal effect of povidone-iodine peaks at 0.1% [3] (fig. 5). The exposure time necessary to

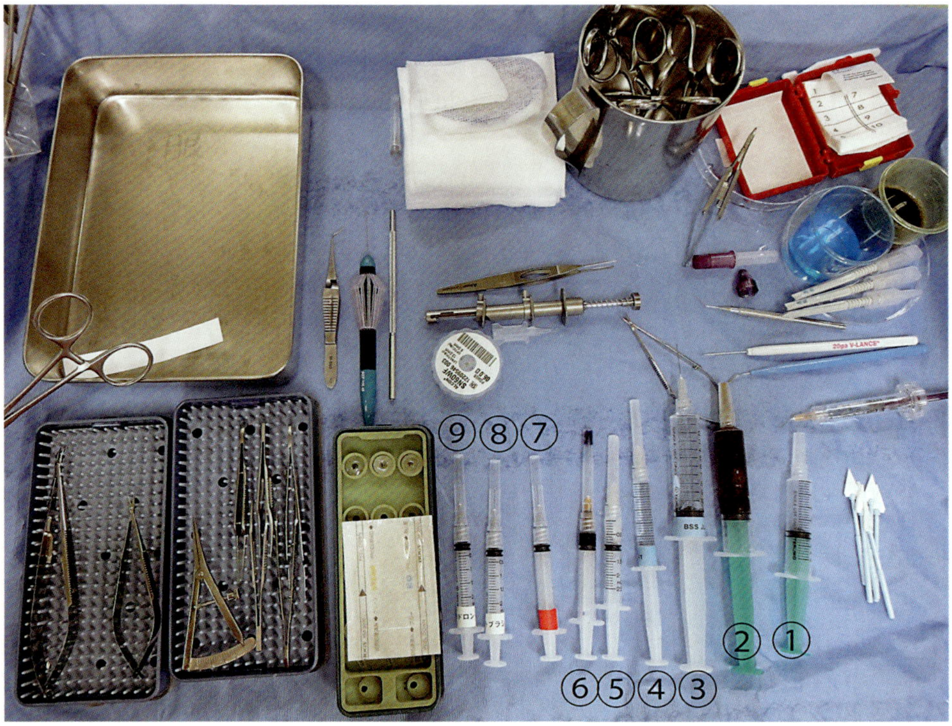

Fig. 3. Arrangement of materials on the surgical table. Fluids that must not be introduced intraocularly (1 and 2), infusion fluid for washing the ocular surface fluids for intraocular injection (4, 5, and 6), and fluids for periocular injection (7, 8, and 9) are classified and marked to avoid using the wrong fluid.

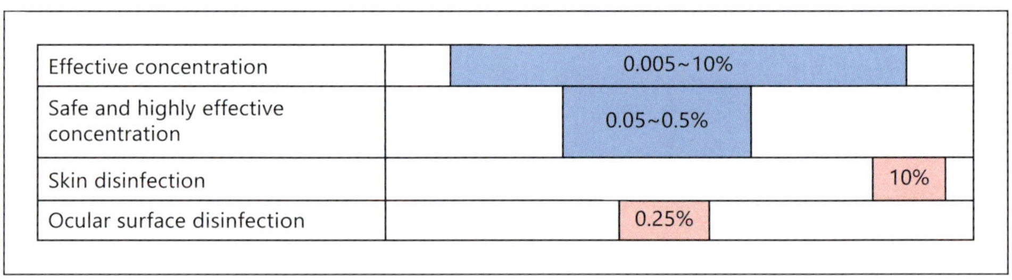

Fig. 4. Safe and effective concentrations of povidone-iodine reported in the literature and concentrations used in intraocular surgeries. The diagram shows the effective bactericidal concentrations against bacteria in vitro (0.005–10%) and the safe and highly effective concentrations in vivo (0.05–0.5%) compared with the concentration used for skin disinfection (10%: mildly effective and oculotoxic) and that for repeated ocular surface irrigation during intraocular surgeries (0.25%: highly effective and nontoxic).

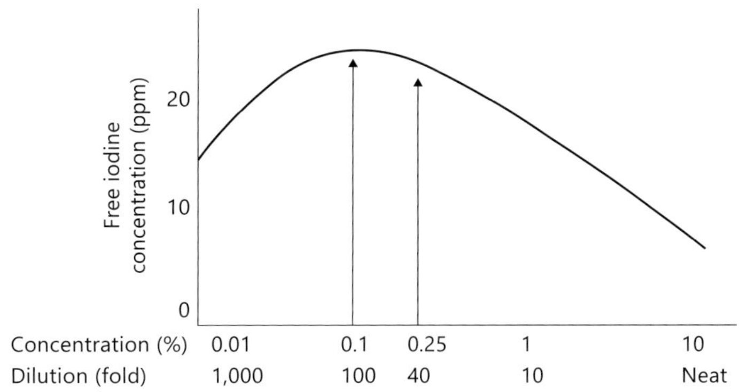

Fig. 5. Free iodine concentration at various dilutions of povidone-iodine. As the available free iodine concentration is highest at 0.1%, the bactericidal effect is most potent at this concentration. The reason for this phenomenon is that free iodine is released more easily at higher dilutions.

Table 1. Comparison between 0.25 and 10% povidone-iodine

	0.25% povidone-iodine	10% povidone-iodine
Free iodine concentration	25 ppm high bactericidal effect	10 ppm low bactericidal effect
Time required for bactericidal effect	15–30 s	2–3 min
Bactericidal duration	short	long
Ocular toxicity	nontoxic	toxic
Washing method	repeated washing (to replenish iodine)	applying once (no need to replenish iodine)
Usage	ocular surface disinfection (low bacterial load)	skin disinfection (high bacterial load)

kill bacteria is shorter at 0.1–1.0% (15 s) than at 2.5–10% (30–120 s) [4]. The reason is that more free iodine is available at higher dilutions, consequently providing higher bactericidal effect (table 1). Studies on the oculotoxicity of povidone-iodine have shown that the concentrations that are safe for ocular tissues and provide high bactericidal effect range from 0.05 to 0.5% [5]. The midpoint of this range, 0.25%, is recommended for use in ocular surface disinfection [6].

Preoperative Disinfection of Eyelid Skin

Use a sponge soaked in 10% povidone-iodine to disinfect the eyelid skin. Do not use a cotton ball because cotton fibers (lint) adhere to surgical instruments and may be introduced inside the eye [7]. Since 10% povidone-iodine is a concentration that may cause corneal damage, care has to be exercised not to allow the solution to flow inside the eyelids. To disinfect the eyelid skin, use a sponge soaked in povidone-iodine and apply it in a concentric circular movement gradually

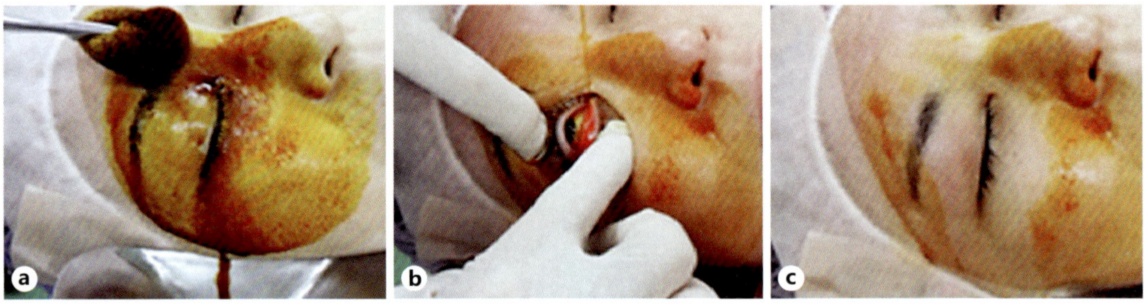

Fig. 6. Procedures of preoperative disinfection. **a** Disinfection of eyelid skin: use a cotton sponge soaked with 10% povidone-iodine and apply for 2–3 min to obtain the bactericidal effect. **b** Disinfection of conjunctival sac: with the 10% solution remaining on the skin, apply 0.25% povidone-iodine to the conjunctival sac. **c** Wiping of 0.25% solution: using a piece of gauze, press lightly to wipe off the excess 0.25% solution. Do not wipe off the 10% solution around the eye, as it serves to provide a continuous bactericidal effect and to identify the eye being operated on.

spreading toward the periphery (fig. 6a). Repeat the procedure 3–4 times. The area of disinfection extends superiorly to slightly above the eyebrow, medially to slightly exceeding the nose bridge, laterally to the midpoint between the lateral canthus and the ear, and inferiorly to around the ala of nose. There is also a misunderstanding when using 10% povidone-iodine that sufficient bactericidal effect cannot be obtained without drying. This only means that to obtain sufficient bactericidal activity, an exposure time long enough for the solution to dry (2–3 min) is required. After applying the solution, do not rinse with physiological saline, but leave the agent on the skin so that continuous bactericidal effect can be expected.

Preoperative Disinfection of the Conjunctival Sac

Upon applying the 10% povidone-iodine on the skin, disinfect the conjunctival sac using 0.25% povidone-iodine (fig. 6b). Leaving the 0.25% povidone-iodine in the conjunctival sac without rinsing off with physiological saline will ensure continuous bactericidal activity. The yellow coloration from applying 10% povidone-iodine on the skin around the eye also serves to identify the eye to be operated on when the eye is draped (fig. 6c).

Intraoperative Disinfection of the Surgical Field

Even with thorough disinfection of the eyelid and conjunctiva with povidone-iodine and proper draping, bacteria may still gain access to the surgical field after the speculum is placed. During operation, despite physically washing the surgical field with infusion fluid, bacteria are detected from the ocular surface in 10–20% of the cases [8]. Therefore, during cataract surgery [6], vitreous surgery [9], and intravitreal injection [10], bacteria may enter the eye easily via the ocular surface fluid. To prevent endophthalmitis, it is necessary to make efforts to achieve 'transient sterilization' of the surgical field by repeated irrigation with 0.25% povidone-iodine instead of the conventional 'bacteria reduction' by physically washing out the normal flora on the ocular surface with infusion fluid.

For this purpose, after placing the speculum, wash the surgical field again with 0.25% povidone-iodine and wait 30 s before inserting the trocar (fig. 7a). During procedures such as placing

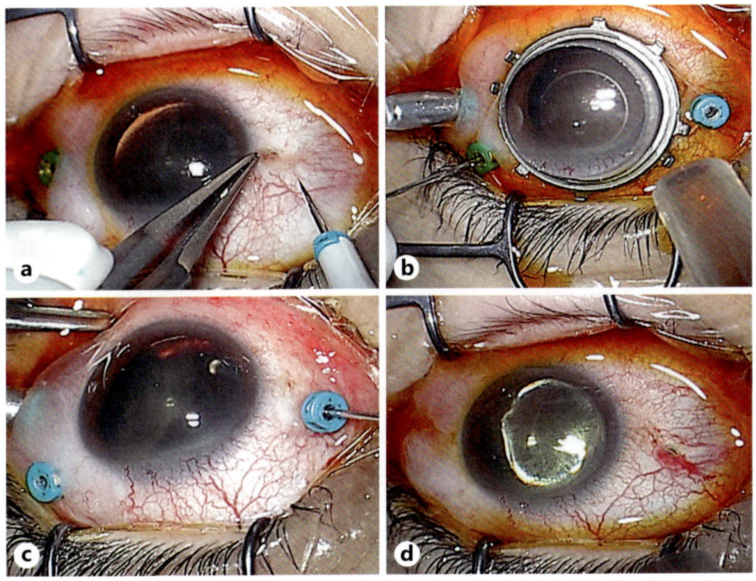

Fig. 7. Intraoperative disinfection. **a** After placing the speculum, irrigate the surgical field with 0.25% povidone-iodine and wait 30 s before inserting the trocar into the sclera. During intraoperative procedures such as placement of contact lens (**b**) and depression of the sclera (**c**), irrigate with 0.25% povidone-iodine every 20–30 s so that the solution is retained in the conjunctival sac. **d** Finally, wash the operative field again with povidone-iodine before surgery is completed.

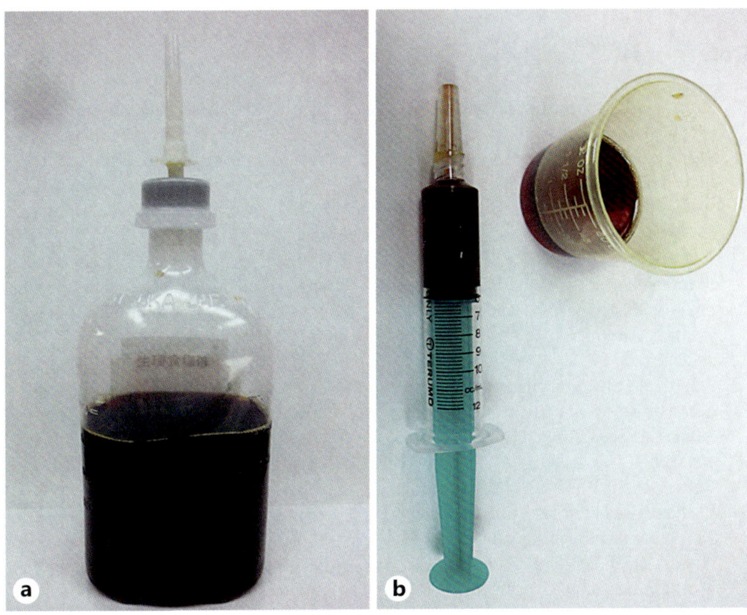

Fig. 8. Preparation and use of 0.25% povidone-iodine. **a** In the operating room, prepare a 0.25% solution by adding 10% povidone-iodine into a bottle of physiological saline. Storing in a bottle reduces decoloration of iodine. **b** For use, transfer the solution into a container and fill a syringe with the required amount.

the contact lens (fig. 7b) and depressing the sclera (fig. 7c), irrigate with 0.25% povidone-iodine so that the solution is retained in the conjunctival sac. During surgery, irrigate repeatedly with 0.25% povidone-iodine every 20–30 s in the same manner as washing the ocular surface with infusion fluid. No corneal damage has been experienced with a povidone-iodine concentration of 0.25%, even with repeated application to the ocular surface. Even if introduced into the anterior chamber or vitreous body, it will be diluted by the infusion fluid, and the intraocular concentration of povidone-iodine is negligible at the end of surgery. Procedures such as simultaneous cataract surgery, buckling for retinal detachment [11], and insertion of a chandelier light fiber should be performed in the presence of iodine solution. At the end of surgery, wash the surgical field again with 0.25% povidone-iodine to complete the surgery (fig. 7d).

Even with careful irrigation of the surgical field, surgeons should always assume a scenario that bacteria have gained access into the vitreous cavity [12]. Precautions such as shaving the peripheral vitreous to remove any foothold for bacteria, sufficient perfusion of the vitreous body to remove bacteria that may have entered, and securely closing the scleral wound are necessary [13].

Preparation of 0.25% Povidone-Iodine Solution

Use physiological saline to dilute povidone-iodine. If distilled water were to be used for diluting, the low osmolality would cause corneal epithelial damage. Povidone-iodine becomes unstable once diluted, with gradual attenuation of the bactericidal effect. Therefore, when used at room temperature, preparing a fresh solution twice daily is recommended. The diluted solution is prepared in the operating room by adding 10% povidone-iodine to a bottle of physiological saline. Attaching a sterilized nozzle to the bottle makes it more convenient to use and reduces attenuation of the bactericidal effect (fig. 8a). For use, dispense the prepared solution into a container and fill a syringe with the required amount (fig. 8b).

References

1 Shimada H, Nakashizuka H, Hattori T, et al: Reducing bacterial contamination inside fluid catch bag in 25-gauge vitrectomy by 0.25% povidone-iodine ocular surface irrigation. Int Ophthalmol 2013;33:35–38.

2 Van den Broek PJ, Buys LF, Van Furth R: Interaction of povidone-iodine compounds, phagocytic cells, and microorganisms. Antimicrob Agents Chemother 1982;22:593–597.

3 Zamora JL: Chemical and microbiologic characteristics and toxicity of povidone-iodine solutions. Am J Surg 1986;151:400–406.

4 Berkelman RL, Holland BW, Anderson RL: Increased bactericidal activity of dilute preparations of povidone-iodine solutions. J Clin Microbiol 1982;15:635–639.

5 Trost LW, Kivilcim M, Peyman GA, et al: The effect of intravitreally injected povidone-iodine on *Staphylococcus epidermidis* in rabbit eyes. J Ocul Pharmacol Ther 2007;23:70–77.

6 Shimada H, Nakashizuka H, Hattori T, et al: Reduction of anterior chamber contamination rate after cataract surgery by intraoperative irrigation with 0.25% povidone-iodine. Am J Ophthalmol 2011;151:11–17.

7 Shimada H, Nakashizuka H, Hattori T, et al: Frequency, source and prevention of cotton fibers in the anterior chamber during cataract surgery. J Cataract Refract Surg 2008;34:1389–1392.

8 Miño de Kaspar H, Kreutzer TC, Aguirre-Romo I, et al: A prospective randomized study to determine the efficacy of preoperative topical levofloxacin in reducing conjunctival bacterial flora. Am J Ophthalmol 2008;145:136–142.

9 Shimada H, Nakashizuka H, Hattori T, et al: Reduction of vitreous contamination rate after 25-gauge vitrectomy by surface irrigation with 0.25% povidone-iodine. Retina 2013;33:143–151.

10 Shimada H, Hattori T, Mori R, et al: Minimizing the endophthalmitis rate following intravitreal injections using 0.25% povidone-iodine irrigation and surgical mask. Graefes Arch Clin Exp Ophthalmol 2013;251:1185–1189.

11 Shimada H, Nakashizuka H, Hattori T, et al: Prophylaxis for acute scleral buckle infection using 0.25% povidone-iodine ocular surface irrigation during surgery. Int Ophthalmol 2014;34:211–216.

12 Tominaga A, Oshima Y, Wakabayashi T, et al: Bacterial contamination of the vitreous cavity associated with transconjunctival 25-gauge microincision vitrectomy surgery. Ophthalmology 2010;117:811–817.

13 Shimada H, Nakashizuka H, Hattori T, et al: Incidence of endophthalmitis following 20- and 25-gauge vitrectomy causes and prevention. Ophthalmology 2008;115:2215–2220.

Hiroyuki Shimada, MD, PhD
Department of Ophthalmology, Surugadai Hospital of Nihon University
1-8-13 Surugadai, Kanda, Chiyodaku
Tokyo 101-8309 (Japan)
E-Mail sshimada@olive.ocn.ne.jp

Oh H, Oshima Y (eds): Microincision Vitrectomy Surgery. Emerging Techniques and Technology.
Dev Ophthalmol. Basel, Karger, 2014, vol 54, pp 71–76 (DOI: 10.1159/000360451)

Wound Construction

George Trichonas · Peter K. Kaiser
Cole Eye Institute, Cleveland Clinic, Cleveland, Ohio, USA

Abstract

Wound construction is critical in microincision vitrectomy surgery. The three main steps in constructing a proper wound include displacing the conjunctiva away from the sclera, flattening the sclera on insertion, and angling the incision. Each one of these steps helps create wounds that will not leak. Misaligning the conjunctiva from the scleral hole prevents a vitreous wick from extending external to the conjunctiva. Flattening the sclera on trocar insertion provides a longer wound cord length, which is less likely to leak, and angling the incision has been proven to seal better in both anterior and posterior segment incisions. When you make an angled incision, you initially insert the blade at a 30° angle (at least). This will make the wound more stable because it is less likely to cause internal disruption of the wound edges. These three basic steps are simple, but very important to follow when constructing a microincision wound in order to limit postoperative complications including wound leakage, gas leak, hypotony, and endophthalmitis.

While there have been reports of scissors to cut the vitreous in the past, the history of modern pars plana vitrectomy dates back to Dr. Robert Machemer, who in 1971 used a 17-gauge sclerotomy port for his first pars plana vitrectomy in a diabetic nonclearing vitreous hemorrhage [1]. Since then the field has changed dramatically and we have moved from 17-gauge to 20-gauge vitrectomy and more recently in 2002 to microincision vitrectomy surgery (MIVS) with gauges as small as 27 gauge [2]. MIVS has become very popular among retina surgeons over the past 11 years [3]. Advances in technology, biomedical engineering, and instrumentation have made it possible to consistently shrink the size of the entry cannula from 23- to 25-gauge and more recently to 27-gauge vitrectomy. Smaller incisions are less traumatic to the eye and do not require sutures. The absence of sutures helps with patient comfort, decreases surgical time, decreases postoperative inflammation, and speeds up recovery. However, the sutureless nature of MIVS poses risks related to postoperative hypotony, choroidal hemorrhage, gas or silicon oil leakage, and even endophthalmitis. Initial studies comparing endophthalmitis rates between microincision surgeries and 20-gauge vitrectomy revealed higher rates of endophthalmitis with microincision surgery [4, 5]. This was alarming to all retina surgeons. A careful analysis of the data, however, showed that different wound construction techniques had different endophthalmitis rates [6–8].

While other factors like the intraoperative use of corticosteroids, subconjunctival injection of antibiotics, and incomplete removal of the peripheral vitreous skirt have been hypothesized to result in bacterial in-growth predisposing the patient to endophthalmitis, the most critical part remains wound construction. The principal of wound construction is similar to a self-sealing limbal incision for phacoemulsification. The idea is to create a multiplanar wound that is stable and prevents bacterial migration in the eye. Herein, we will discuss the different techniques to successfully produce good wound construction in microincision surgery.

Instrumentation

Microincision surgery is predicated on introducing either flexible or rigid cannulas into the eye that allow the insertion of the microsurgical instruments without disrupting the sclera. The insertion of a cannula in the eye during vitrectomy is currently a single-step technique, although dual-step systems have been used in the past with success. The cannula fits over a sharp trocar, which allows simultaneous opening of the sclera and insertion of the microincision cannula. This creates an entry system that provides the vitrectomy instruments unobstructed access to the eye. Other components of the instrumentation include cannula plugs and an infusion line. Early-generation microvitreoretinal blades were stiletto-like. Beveled blades that created linear incisions replaced these because linear incisions tend to close easier. The newer EdgePlus microvitreoretinal blades (Alcon Laboratories Inc., Fort Worth, Tex., USA) have a hump perpendicular to the horizontal plane of the blade, which stretches the tissue and ensures a slit-like incision with minimal insertion force.

Globe Fixation and Site Preparation

The first step in wound construction is displacing the conjunctiva. Many surgeons will mark the entry site first with calipers (approx. 3–4 mm from the limbus depending on phakic status) and then hold the conjunctiva with nontoothed forceps in order to displace it away from the incision site. Care must be taken not to tear the conjunctiva. Others use a cotton swab or another instrument to displace the conjunctiva before entering with the trocar. The main benefit of misaligning the scleral and conjunctival incisions is to prevent any vitreous wick from extending beyond the sclera and through the conjunctiva.

Flattening the sclera is another critical step before inserting the trocar. The globe is a curved structure and by flattening it you will end up with a longer chord length within the sclera. This creates a better sealing wound. Thus, by not following the natural curve of the eye and by flattening the sclera you can create a wound with a longer cord length that is less likely to leak.

Some surgeons prefer the use of a fixation plate to fixate the globe, displace the conjunctiva, and flatten the sclera in one step. The pressure plate has caliper marks incorporated within the plate to measure the distance from the limbus, and on the undersurface it has serrations that allow displacement and holding of the conjunctiva. There are several different types of fixation plates on the market. Alternatively, one can even use a cotton tip applicator to fixate the globe.

Different Types of Incisions

Stab or Straight Incision

With the stab or straight incision, the direction of the trocar is kept perpendicular to the globe and enters without any angulation. Direct entry is made after conjunctival displacement at the pars plana. The advantage of this wound construction is that it is very simple to perform and fast. The disadvantage, as seen histologically, is that it is often not self-sealing and creates a gap that tends to leak, especially with larger-gauge vitrectomy, increasing the chances of postoperative endophthalmitis [9, 10] (fig. 1). In smaller-gauge surgery (>25

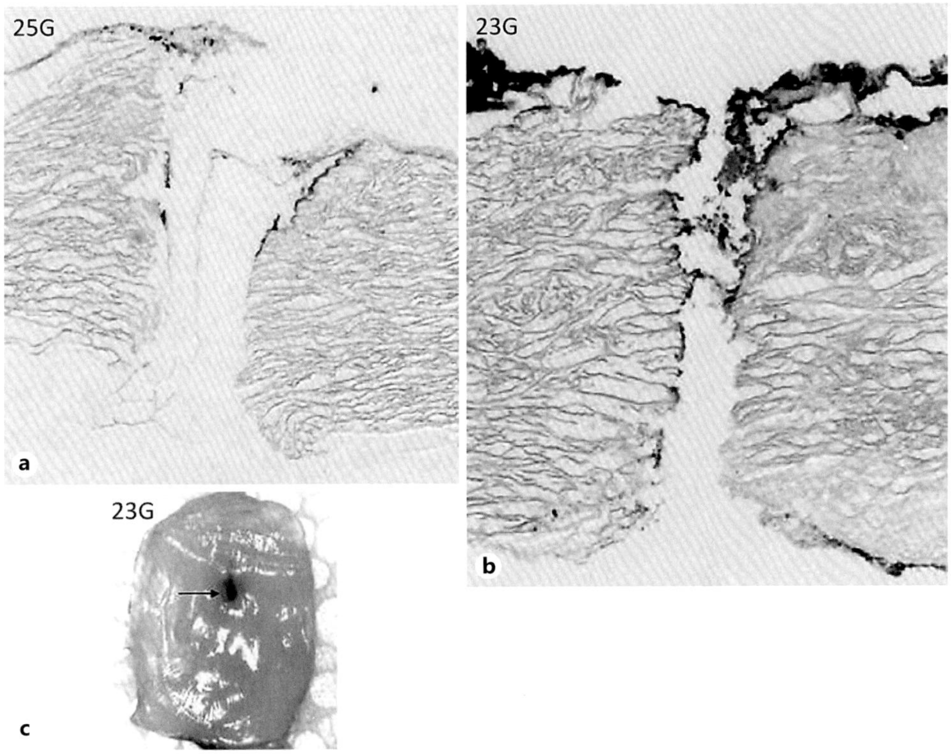

Fig. 1. Histopathology slide demonstrates gaping of straight 25-gauge (25G) (**a**) and straight 23-gauge (23G) (**b**) incisions and India ink (that mimics the size of bacteria) visible on and within straight incisions. **c** India ink is grossly visible at the internal hole (arrow) of the sclera of straight sutureless 23-gauge incision.

gauge), a stab incision is not ideal but often does not leak, whereas in larger gauges (<23 gauge) it is very likely to leak and is not recommended.

Oblique or Angled Incision

An oblique or angled incision is when the direction of the trocar is at least 30° to the sclera. The length of the incision inside the sclera is variable depending on the exact angle of insertion of the trocar. The angled incision has been proven by histology and anterior segment optical coherence tomography to be more stable and less likely to leak regardless of the pressure in the eye as compared to stab incisions [11]. When evaluated with spectral domain anterior segment optical coherence tomography, all 23- or 25-gauge stab incisions were open and readily visible immediately after removing the cannulas, whereas angled incisions had better apposition and were often very difficult to find. Experiments using India ink, which mimics the size of bacteria, placed on the surface of cadaver eyes after removing cannulas showed India ink inside the wound and often inside the eye in all 23- or 25-gauge stab incisions with penetration across the whole incision in some wounds, whereas no ink particles were observed in the wound or eye with angled incisions (fig. 2). This indicates the potential for surface fluid and bacterial inflow through stab incisions before the occurrence of any wound healing. This risk, however, is very low with angled incisions. Therefore, it has been speculated that angled inci-

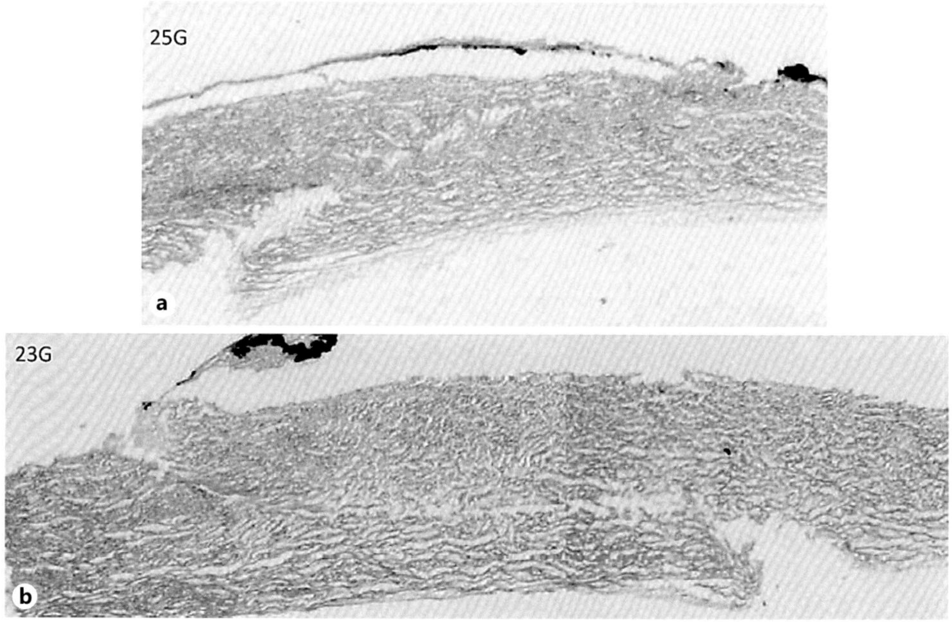

Fig. 2. Histopathology slide demonstrates good approximation and closure of angled 25-gauge (25G) (**a**) and angled 23-gauge (23G) (**b**) incisions. India ink is not visible on or within the angled incisions.

sions are safer postoperatively, leading to lower rates of endophthalmitis and infection. The main disadvantages of angled incisions are that the inner tissues when you enter obliquely in the vitreous may be disrupted as seen on histology, and it takes more time [9]. However, the advantages appear to far outweigh the disadvantages for this type of incision.

Regardless of incision type, it is important not to rotate the trocar as you enter the sclera. Many beginning surgeons mistakenly perform this maneuver when entering the globe thinking it helps with entry. In fact, this rotation of the trocar tears scleral fibers, thus creating a very unstable wound.

Wound Closure

Wound closure is critical after completing the vitrectomy. Careful inspection of the wound after removal of the cannula will help determine the stability of the wound and prevent postoperative leaks and hypotony. The formation of a conjunctival bleb is a sign of wound leakage. There are several tips to insure that this does not happen. When you remove the cannula, it is very important to place a solid instrument into the cannula as you are removing it to prevent suction from the removal of the hollow cannula from producing a vitreous wick through the wound. A light pipe or a plug can be used for this purpose.

Performing a partial or complete air-fluid exchange is also suggested before removing the cannulas. The air/gas bubble inside the eye will help close the internal lip of the wound by increasing the surface tension. Postoperative hypotony rates are less in eyes left with some degree of air fill compared to fluid-filled eyes [12, 13]. A small air bubble also makes it easier to visualize small wound leaks since small bubbles appear around leaks. In contrast, small leaks in a fluid-filled eye may be difficult to see as no bleb forms. Moreover, when leaks of air occur, they are easy to displace to allow the surgeon to place a suture. In many cases, patience and pressure with a blunt-tipped instrument is enough to cause cessation of most instances of leakage.

It is important to note that if any incision is leaking or appears unusual at the end of the case, the threshold for placing a suture should be low. Other parameters that should make the surgeon consider placing a suture are prolonged time of surgery, excessive manipulation of instruments, monocular patients, highly myopic or uveitic patients with thin sclera, and active external infection such as conjunctivitis or severe blepharitis. Prolonged surgery times and excessive manipulation disrupts the wound architecture and causes swelling and subsequent gaping between the inner and outer wound leafs. If wound leaks are detected, placing a suture, preferably an absorbable 7-0 or 8-0 suture, is the best option given the increased risk of complications. Patients with blepharitis have increased secretions and bacterial load on the eyelids that can potentially enter the eye when the surgical wounds are unstable. Overall, the surgeon should be very cautious during wound closure even when a proper wound was constructed, evaluating carefully the wound at the end of the case and having low threshold for placing a suture.

Complications

Hypotony

Leakage through the sclerotomy is the main cause of hypotony, especially in the early postoperative period. Even a small amount of pressure on the eye while removing the speculum or patching the eye can cause a significant amount of leakage if the wound is unstable. Persistent hypotony can lead to potentially sight-threatening complications such as choroidal effusions and endophthalmitis. Early postoperative hypotony can create a siphon effect drawing bacteria into the vitreous cavity. Thus, all ports should be carefully observed for leakage, which usually manifests as a subconjunctival bleb. In this case, placement of a suture is indicated.

Endophthalmitis

There have been several reports of increased incidence of endophthalmitis associated with MIVS. This has been attributed to wound construction and straight or stab incisions. In the largest study to date, Kunimoto and Kaiser [4] reported an 11-fold increase in the rate of endophthalmitis from 0.018% after 20-gauge to 0.23% after 25-gauge sutureless vitrectomy. Similarly, Scott et al. [5] reported 0.03% with 20-gauge and 0.84% with 25-gauge sutureless vitrectomy, and Shaikh et al. [14] in a small case series noted 0.0% with 20-gauge and 1.6% with 25-gauge sutureless vitrectomy. In addition, Eifrig et al. [8] reported similar endophthalmitis rates after 20-gauge vitrectomy, approximately 0.03–0.05% [15–18]. Therefore, the increased incidence of endophthalmitis with MIVS was of great concern. However, a careful analysis of the studies mentioned above showed that the highest incidence of endophthalmitis was related to those cases that used a stab incision. Angled incisions had similar rates of endophthalmitis as 20-gauge incisions.

Conclusions

Wound construction is critical in microincision surgery and angled incisions are superior to straight incisions regardless of the gauge. Postoperative endophthalmitis is the major concern; however, after analyzing the data, we are comfortable that angled incisions are safe for patients. Linear incisions heal better compared to chevron-shaped incisions, and this observation led to the development of new trocars that make slit incisions. Wound closure is as important as wound construction. Partial or complete air-fluid exchange will help close the internal lip of the wound. However, since the surgery is sutureless, the surgeon should be very meticulous and observant at the end of the case for wound leakage. As surgeons become more comfortable with MIVS, their threshold to place a suture at the end of the case should be low, especially in the beginning of their career given the detrimental complications that open wounds can cause.

Disclosure Statement

Financial support was received from Research to Prevent Blindness (P.K.K.). P.K.K. is a consultant for Alcon, Bausch and Lomb, and Novartis.

References

1 Machemer R, Buettner H, Norton EW, Parel JM: Vitrectomy: a pars plana approach. Trans Am Acad Ophthalmol Otolaryngol 1971;75:813–820.
2 Fujii GY, De Juan E Jr, Humayun MS, et al: A new 25-gauge instrument system for transconjunctival sutureless vitrectomy surgery. Ophthalmology 2002;109:1807–1812.
3 American Society of Retina Specialists Annual Preferences and Trends Survey. 2010. http://www.asrs.org.
4 Kunimoto DY, Kaiser RS: Incidence of endophthalmitis after 20- and 25-gauge vitrectomy. Ophthalmology 2007;114:2133–2137.
5 Scott IU, Flynn HW Jr, Dev S, Shaikh S, Mittra RA, Arevalo JF, et al: Endophthalmitis after 25-gauge and 20-gauge pars plana vitrectomy: incidence and outcomes. Retina 2008;28:138–142.
6 Mason JO 3rd, Yunker JJ, Vail RS, White MF Jr, Feist RM, Thomley ML, et al: Incidence of endophthalmitis following 20-gauge and 25-gauge vitrectomy. Retina 2008;28:1352–1354.
7 Chen JK, Khurana RN, Nguyen QD, Do DV: The incidence of endophthalmitis following transconjunctival sutureless 25- vs 20-gauge vitrectomy. Eye (Lond) 2009;23:780–784.
8 Eifrig CW, Scott IU, Flynn HW Jr, Smiddy WE, Newton J: Endophthalmitis after pars plana vitrectomy: incidence, causative organisms, and visual acuity outcomes. Am J Ophthalmol 2004;138:799–802.
9 Singh A, Stewart JM: 25-gauge sutureless vitrectomy: variations in incision architecture. Retina 2009;29:451–455.
10 Singh RP, Bando H, Brasil OF, Williams DR, Kaiser PK: Evaluation of wound closure using different incision techniques with 23-gauge and 25-gauge microincision vitrectomy systems. Retina 2008;28:242–248.
11 Taban M, Ventura AA, Sharma S, Kaiser PK: Dynamic evaluation of sutureless vitrectomy wounds: an optical coherence tomography and histopathology study. Ophthalmology 2008;115:2221–2228.
12 Shimada H, Nakashizuka H, Hattori T, Mori R, et al: Incidence of endophthalmitis after 20- and 25-gauge vitrectomy: causes and prevention. Ophthalmology 2008;15:2215–2220.
13 Bamonte G, Mura M, Tan HS: Hypotony after 25-gauge vitrectomy. Am J Ophthalmol 2011;151:156–160.
14 Shaikh S, Ho S, Richmond PP, et al: Untoward outcomes in 25-gauge versus 20-gauge vitreoretinal surgery. Retina 2007;27:1048–1053.
15 Mollan SP, Mollan AJ, Konstantinos C, et al: Incidence of endophthalmitis following vitreoretinal surgery. Int Ophthalmol 2009;29:203–205.
16 Eifrig CW, Flynn HW Jr, Scott IU, Newton J: Acute-onset postoperative endophthalmitis: review of incidence and visual outcomes (1995–2001). Ophthalmic Surg Lasers 2002;33:373–378.
17 Eifrig CW, Scott IU, Flynn HW Jr, et al: Endophthalmitis after pars plana vitrectomy: incidence, causative organisms, and visual acuity outcomes. Am J Ophthalmol 2004;138:799–802.
18 Aaberg TM Jr, Flynn HW Jr, Schiffman J, Newton J: Nosocomial acute-onset postoperative endophthalmitis survey: a 10-year review of incidence and outcomes. Ophthalmology 1998;105:1004–1010.

Peter K. Kaiser, MD
Cole Eye Institute, Cleveland Clinic
9500 Euclid Avenue, Desk i3
Cleveland, OH 44195 (USA)
E-Mail pkkaiser@gmail.com

Oh H, Oshima Y (eds): Microincision Vitrectomy Surgery. Emerging Techniques and Technology.
Dev Ophthalmol. Basel, Karger, 2014, vol 54, pp 77–86 (DOI: 10.1159/000360452)

The Evolution of Endoillumination

David R. Chow

Assistant Professor University of Toronto, St. Michaels Hospital, Director Toronto Retina Institute, Toronto, Ont., Canada

Abstract

Advances in endoillumination over the last decade have been numerous and were necessary to allow transition to smaller-gauge vitrectomy systems. Advances in light sources and their associated filters have resulted in safer, more powerful light sources that provide enough output to drive small fibers for 27-gauge surgery, chandeliers, and lighted instrumentation. Filtered light can also be used to enhance tissue visualization. This chapter will review the history and advances in light sources.

There have been some major advances in endoillumination over the past decade. Historically, retina surgeons have relied on light sources integrated into their vitrectomy systems for their endoillumination requirements. Prior to the mid-2000s this meant a halogen light source for Alcon Accurus users and a metal halide light source for Bausch and Lomb Millennium users. Clinically, these older sources of illumination have provided a safe viewing environment with adequate illumination for most tasks using a standard 20-gauge light probe. Unfortunately, these illumination sources lacked the power to provide adequate viewing for lighted instrumentation, wide-angle probes, and chandelier systems, which is why these secondary illumination options failed to develop during this era. Of even greater importance at the time was the inadequate illumination these sources provided for smaller-gauge vitrectomy which was gaining momentum. The output of 25-gauge light probes on these light sources provided roughly 40% of the typical output of 20-gauge light probes. As a result, many of the early 'adopters' of 25-gauge instrumentation frequently complained that their view was inadequate. The inadequacies of the halogen and metal halide light sources were recognized by many companies, leading to the release of stand-alone xenon light sources (Synergetics Photon 1, Alcon AHBI, DORC) that addressed the power problem. This enabled a whole new range of lighted instrumentation to gain popular acceptance, including chandeliers which allow 'true' bimanual surgery. In addition, the power of the xenon light sources allowed the integration of different light filters to be explored to improve safety, allow greater brightness, and possibly enhance tissue visualization. The Synergetics Photon 1 was the first light source to integrate a strong yellow filter to improve safety and allow surgeons the ability to turn up the brightness when necessary. As the product cycle of the older platforms came to an end, newer vitrectomy systems were released (Alcon Constellation, Bausch and Lomb

Stellaris PC), all of which incorporated stronger xenon light sources and even the addition of various light filters in some. Most recently, DORC has introduced a new vitrectomy platform, the EVA, which integrates the first LED light source with a tunable filter option.

As retina surgeons, we need to ask ourselves what we want in a light source. Almost every surgical lighting study has shown the key to visualization is maximizing brightness. The problem for us as retina surgeons is that unlike all the other surgical subspecialties, the tissue we operate on is prone to light damage or phototoxicity which can be blinding. As a result, most would agree that the most important factor in choosing a light source is safety. The interchange between improving the brightness of our viewing environment and the effect that it has on safety is one we need to understand at all times. The other factors to consider in a light source are its color and the effect it has on tissue visualization. There are also differences in the quality of illumination provided by focal, wide-angle, and chandelier lighting systems. This chapter will review some of these basic concepts in endoillumination.

Safety

There are two major forms of phototoxicity: thermal and photochemical. Thermal phototoxicity is a risk for endoscopes, but not really an issue to us as retinal surgeons. Photochemical or UV/blue light toxicity is our major concern. The understanding of risk associated with UV/blue light exposure was determined by Ham et al. [1] in his work on rhesus monkeys. To this day, his aphakic hazard curve is used to determine the risk of inducing UV/blue light toxicity with a light source. This curve shows that the risk of inducing phototoxicity increases with exposure to lower UV/blue light wavelengths. As such, to calculate the safety of a light source, the first thing you need to do is obtain the spectral output of a given light source. This is obtained with an instrument called a spectrophotometer. When a light probe is shined into a spectrophotometer, the components of that light source are displayed as a function of wavelength and intensity of output at that wavelength (fig. 1). The aphakic hazard sum is the calculation of the output of a light source and its intersection with the aphakic hazard curve defined by Ham et al. [1]. It is essentially an area under the curve function. This aphakic hazard sum, which is essentially the standard measure of light source safety, can be inversed to determine the number of lumens that are necessary to create a watt of hazard (lumens/hazard watt).

Over the last decade I have performed a number of studies on clinically available light sources to determine their safety calculations. The two largest being in 2004 and 2010. Figure 2 shows the output curves obtained with the 2010 testing of clinically available light sources. The first thing to note is that the spectral output of each light source has a characteristic curve that is independent of the manufacturer and purely a function of the type of light bulb used. The only variable that can be really altered by the manufacturer is the addition of a cutoff UV/blue light filter to the light source they have chosen. As a result, there are some generalities of safety which can be made by knowing just the type of light source and the filter used. The study I performed in 2010 showed that mercury vapor light sources (Synergetics Photon 2, Bausch and Lomb Stellaris PC) had the best safety calculations, followed by xenon light sources with a 435-nm UV filter and halogen light sources (Alcon Constellation, Bausch and Lomb Stellaris, Alcon Accurus, Synergetics Photon 1), and finally the xenon lights sources with a 420-nm filter and metal halide light sources (DORC Bright Star Xenon, Bausch and Lomb Millennium Metal Halide, Alcon AHBI Xenon; fig. 3). It is important to understand, however, that these safety calculations, which were measured in lumens/hazard watt, are

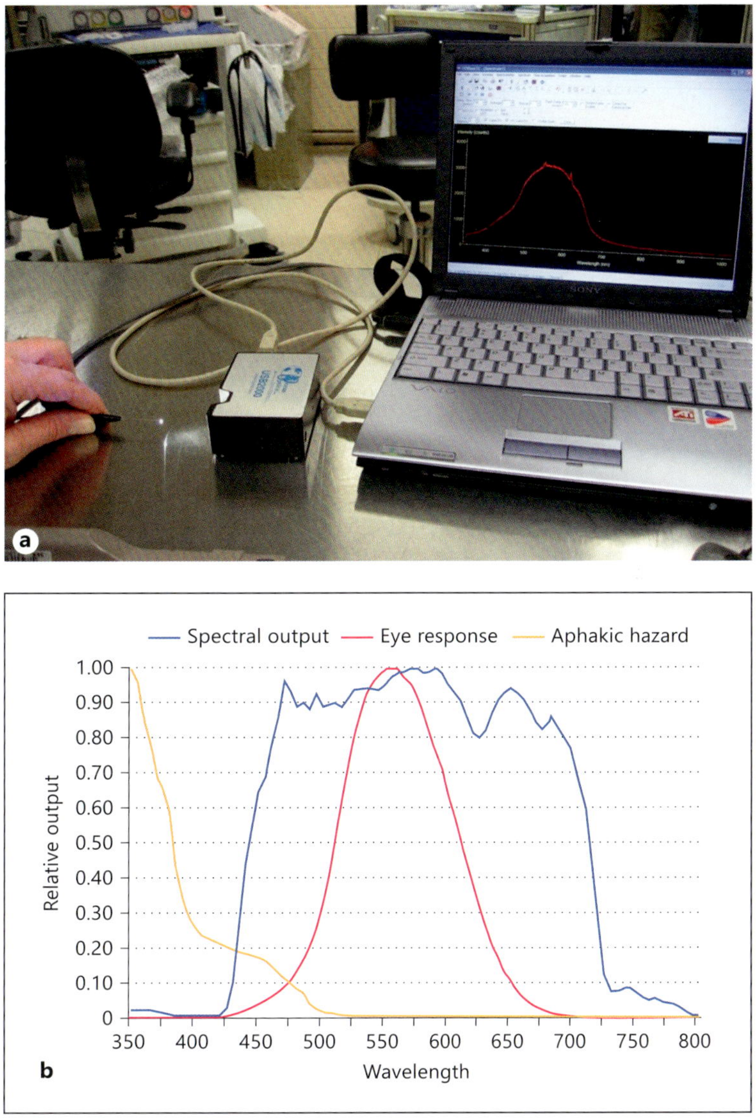

Fig. 1. a Light probe shined into a spectrophotometer with a computer screen showing output of the light source as a function of wavelength and intensity of output. **b** Output of a xenon light source (blue), shown against an aphakic hazard curve (yellow) and photopic response curve (purple).

a measure of the baseline safety of light sources and only allow direct comparative assessments if the brightness, working distance, and cone of illumination are all kept constant between the comparers.

For most clinicians, the calculation that is relevant to them surgically is referred to as the retinal threshold time, a calculation that incorporates the brightness of the light source, its inherent safety calculation (aphakic hazard sum or lumens/hazard watt), the working distance, the numerical aperture of the fiber, and the industry standard hazard threshold of 25 J/cm^2. This calculation provides a theoretical safe working time for the variables used in the calculation. These calculations also allow surgeons to compare the effect of varying the working distance and brightness on clinically available light

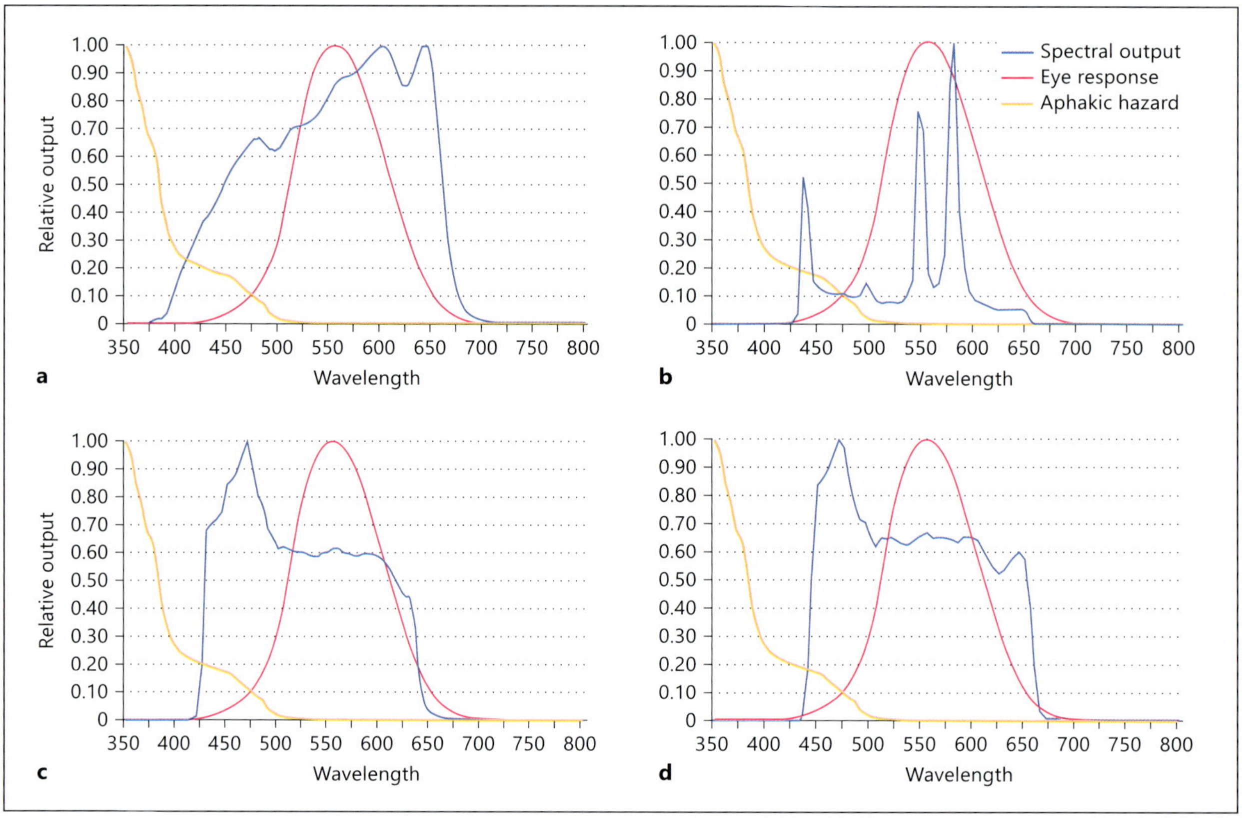

Fig. 2. a Alcon Accurus halogen. **b** Bausch and Lomb Millennium metal halide. **c** Alcon AHBI xenon. **d** Synergetics Photon 1 xenon.

sources with respect to safety (table 1). From these calculations an obvious clinical pearl is that the greatest increase in surgical safety can be obtained by increasing the working distance. For example, with the Alcon Constellation the retinal threshold time when a 23-gauge light pipe is used at 8 lumens and a working distance of 4 mm is kept is 12 min 25 s; however, this increases to 41 min 29 s when the working distance is increased to 8 mm! When you look at the differences between light sources you can see that a mercury vapor light source (Bausch and Lomb Stellaris PC/Synergetics Photon 2) used at 8 lumens and a working distance of 4 mm has a retinal threshold time of 15 min 16 s which is greater than a xenon light source used at the same brightness and working distance, like the Alcon Constellation which had a threshold time of 12 min 25 s.

For years when I would discuss the safety of light sources, many surgeons found the topic of minimal importance since they had no experience with phototoxicity. Over the last few years, however, interest in the topic has increased. The FDA has a database of over 16 cases of phototoxicity that were associated with the use of a xenon light source with a 420-nm filter between 2006 and 2009. In addition, a poll of the graduating retina fellows from North American fellowships over the last few years (Retina Fellow Forum) has shown a steady number of cases still occurring. In 2011, 30% of fellows reported having seen at least 1 case,

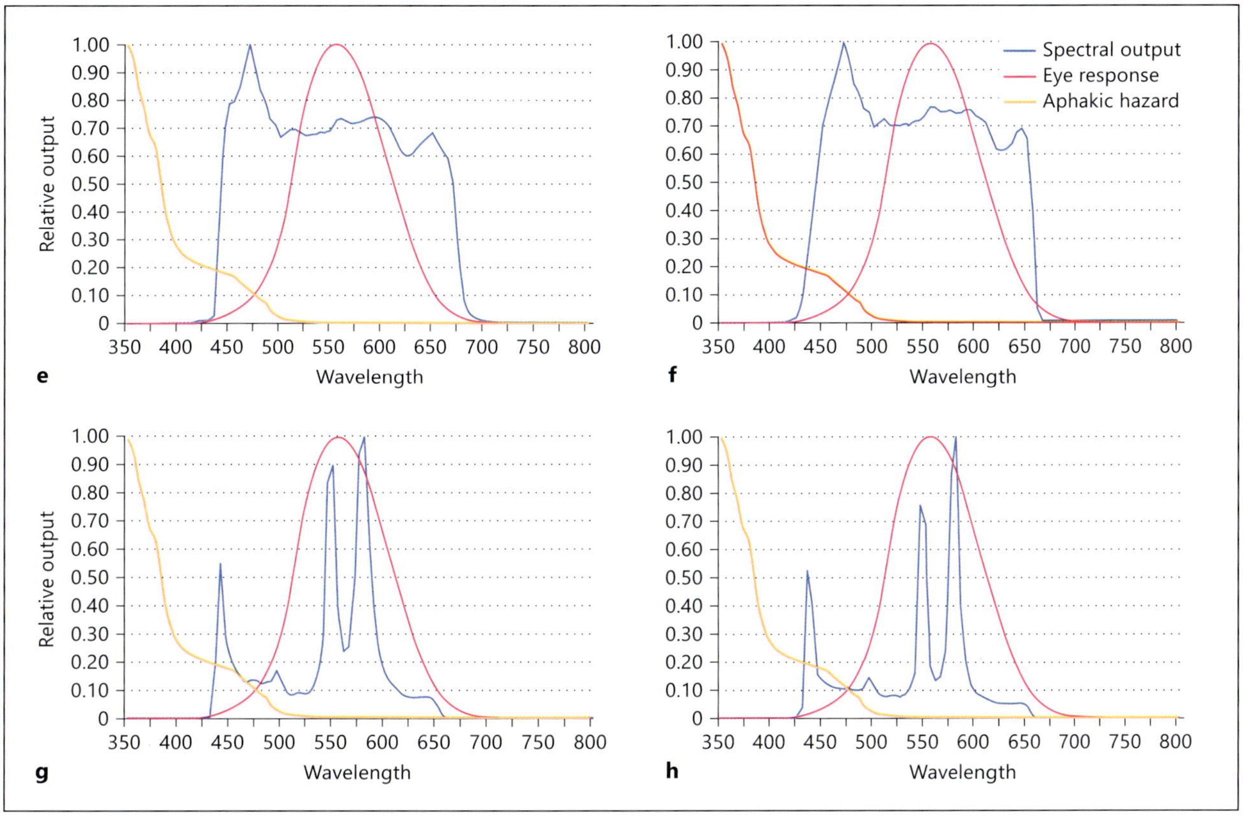

Fig. 2. e Alcon Constellation xenon. **f** Bausch and Lomb Stellaris PC xenon. **g** Synergetics Photon 2 mercury vapor. **h** Bausch and Lomb Stellaris PC mercury vapor.

Chow; Vail Vitrectomy meeting Feb 2010	Lumens/hazard watt (aphakic hazard sum)
Synergetics Photon 2 Mercury Vapor	1,980
B&L Stellaris PC Mercury Vapor	1,965
B&L Stellaris PC Xenon (435)	1,622
Alcon Constellation Xenon	1,608
Alcon Accurus Halogen	1,533
Synergetics Photon 1 Xenon	1,503
DORC Bright Star Xenon (420)	1,292
Bausch and Lomb Metal Halide	1,144
Alcon AHBI Xenon	1,000

↑ Safety

Fig. 3. Safety calculations of light sources expressed in lumens/hazard watt (aphakic hazard sum).

Table 1. Retinal threshold times

	4-mm working distance	8-mm working distance
Alcon Accurus halogen 20-gauge light pipe; high 3 = 8 lumens	10 min 7 s	33 min 48 s
Alcon Xenon AHBI 20-gauge light pipe = 8 lumens	7 min 43 s	25 min 49 s
Alcon Xenon AHBI 20-gauge light pipe; max. = 21.58 lumens	2 min 51 s	9 min 34 s
Alcon Constellation xenon 20-gauge light pipe = 8 lumens	12 min 25 s	41 min 29 s
Synergetics Photon 1 xenon 20-gauge light pipe; max. = 12.03 lumens	7 min 43 s	25 min 49 s
B&L Stellaris PC/Synergetics Photon 2 mercury vapor 20-gauge light pipe = 8 lumens	15 min 16 s	50 min 59 s
B&L Stellaris PC/Synergetics Photon 2 mercury vapor 20-gauge light pipe = 16 lumens	7 min 38 s	25 min 29 s

a number that dropped to 18% in 2013 and 17% in 2014.

Another strategy that can be used to improve light source safety is the incorporation of light filters. In a 2005 study, I integrated many different filters into the Synergetics Photon 1 to see what effect they had on safety calculations and by extension a surgeon's ability to use more brightness. Another potential advantage of using light filters, i.e. tissue visualization, was preliminarily explored in this study. The data from this study showed that a strong yellow filter (amber with a cutoff around 480 nm) improved the safety calculation of the Photon 1 with its baseline UV 435-nm filter from 1,922 lumens/hazard watt up to 20,543 lumens/hazard watt, an over 10-fold increase in safety. With the amber filter in place, there was no loss of brightness and the retinal threshold time increased to 1 h 58 min 15 s. The overall viewing environment was felt to be comfortable for all situations. The value of this increase in safety can most readily be seen by turning up the brightness to 30 lumens (3 times the normal brightness) and repeating the safety calculations which show a retinal threshold time of 42 min 8 s, which is still a 4.5-fold longer safety time than that of a 435-nm filter. As a result, using an amber light filter provides a significant increase in safety to the point where surgeons can then turn up the brightness on their light source if they need to while still operating in a safer environment! Since this study, a number of light sources have released yellow filters to aid in safety, allow the use of brighter light, and possibly improve tissue visualization. Synergetics released an add-on yellow filter that can be used on the Photon 1 or 2, which improved their safety calculations 26- and 30-fold, respectively. DORC released two yellow filters on the Bright Star (475 and 515 nm) that increased its safety by 5- and 33-fold, respectively. Bausch and Lomb released three filters on the Stellaris PC: a yellow tint with a 16% increase in safety, a green tint that offered no safety advantage but potential tissue visualization advantages, and an amber filter that improved safety 118-fold.

Brightness

The second most important variable to understand about endoillumination and light sources is their brightness. Most nonophthalmic surgical studies have shown that the single greatest improvement in visualization is obtained through increasing the brightness on the operating field. For most surgical specialties, turning up the brightness can be done without risk; however, retina surgeons always need to be cognizant of the risk of phototoxicity. The calculation of the brightness of a light source involves measuring the output of the light source, which can be done with a power meter, and then modulating this power output by the photopic response curve that we as surgeons have to obtain the brightness perceived by us when we are operating (expressed in lumens).

The perfect way to understand this concept is to consider the brightness of a red light source. Although it has a lot of power, because its output does not intersect with our photopic response curve, it looks very dark to us versus a green or yellow light source that has moderate power but an output curve that overlaps the photopic response curve which looks very bright to us. This can be articulated in a calculation referred to as a light source's luminous efficacy. The calculations that I performed in 2004 and then again in 2011 revealed that the light sources on the Alcon Accurus and Bausch and Lomb Millennium both had an output of around 6–8 lumens with a standard 20-gauge light pipe. At the time this was felt to be an adequate amount of light by most surgeons, but the 6–8 lumens was not scientifically based but empiric. When 25-gauge technology was originally introduced, many surgeons complained that the light was inadequate and visualization was difficult. The calculations on these same light sources with standard 25-gauge light pipes confirmed their complaints with only 3–4 lumens available on halogen/metal halide light sources. This was one of the driving forces behind the creation of the xenon light sources which addressed the inadequate power available on the older light sources. Calculations on the newer xenon light sources revealed power outputs as high as 40–60 lumens with 20-gauge light pipes. Although this power was not necessary for a 20-gauge light pipe, it became clinically useful for driving enough light down the smaller fibers inherent to 23-, 25-, and now 27-gauge light pipes and still have enough left over to provide a good clinical view. It also became critical in the development of clinically useful chandeliers and lighted instrumentation.

How Much Light Do We Really Need?

Many surgeons have commented that they do not need more than 8 lumens of light on their light source. The problem with this perception is that the lighting requirements vary from case to case and from operating room to operating room. I think most of us would inherently agree that the amount of light we need to peel the internal limiting membrane in a high myope with a pale fundus, a nuclear sclerotic cataract, a microscope with an active laser filter, an assistant scope with a 50:50 beam splitter, a surgeon with early nuclear sclerosis who is older is very different from the amount of light we would need to remove a vitreous hemorrhage in a pseudophake with a pigmented fundus, a passive laser filter, a modern microscope with no loss of light to the assistant eyepieces, and a young surgeon. The newer xenon and mercury vapor light sources provide that power capability if it is necessary.

In 2005, I performed another study at the Zeiss research facility in Switzerland where we systematically evaluated the amount of light loss along the visual pathway coming up to the eyepieces. As you can imagine, the effect of a newer microscope without a beam splitter and the removal of a laser filter made huge differences in the amount of light loss along the visual pathway. Of interest, the non-contact wide-angle viewing systems resulted in less light loss than the contact wide-angle viewing systems, a concept not appreciated at the time.

Chandeliers

One of the true clinical advances that has come out of the new generation of light sources has been the creation of useful chandeliers. The concept of chandeliers is not new, as they existed prior to the creation of the newer xenon/mercury vapor light sources, but were limited at the time by the power capabilities of the light sources present and by the large multiple fibers that were necessary to create an adequate view. Modern chandeliers offer a significant advantage of allowing ‘true’ bimanual surgery. This is extremely useful when trimming the vitreous base where the surgeon can depress for himself or when trying to perform complex diabetic dissections. It has taken a while, but the usage of chandeliers has gradually increased over the last 10 years. At the Retina Fellow Forum in 2014, 73% of the graduating retina fellows in North America reported that they would routinely use a chandelier for complex retinal detachment or diabetic tractional retinal detachment. This is a significant jump from 49% in 2010. On the other hand 17% of the fellows reported that they have never used a chandelier. Another major advantage of chandeliers is the safety obtained through a maximized working distance. When the retinal threshold time of a chandelier is calculated, the safety calculations are orders of magnitude higher than those obtained with standard light pipes held at 4 or 8 mm from the retinal surface. Instead of minutes, the calculations are all in the order of hours and this is with the chandelier being used at full output, reinforcing the value of maximizing working distance on the risk of phototoxicity!

There have been multiple chandelier designs over the last decade since the release of the newer generation light sources. There are one- and two-step designs for insertion of the fiber. Generally, most recent designs have moved to a one-step concept and there is a gradual move towards housing the chandelier fiber in another cannula so as to allow the possibility of moving the fiber to a different cannula during the operation as necessary. There are single- and dual-fiber chandeliers. Proponents of dual-fiber chandeliers were concerned with the positioning of single-fiber chandeliers and with the shadowing created 180° away from the fiber insertion site. As a single-fiber chandelier user, I think the advantage of a single additional wound outweighs the positioning and shadowing issues. The positioning of a single-fiber chandelier is an issue I have often been asked about. Generally, I place the chandelier at the 6-o’clock position and pay a great deal of attention to bending the distal tubing and the angulation of the fiber tip to obtain an optimal view. At this point, I will loosely secure the tubing in place and commence with the case. Sometimes during the operation the movement of the eye results in the chandelier losing its placement. In those situations I think it is important to not get frustrated but to angle the fiber to illuminate the hemiretina you are working on and then to flip it over to illuminate the other hemiretina when you are ready. As for the shadowing complaints, this will only be relevant in my setup when I am operating at the 12-o’clock position. Through depression and rotation of the eye I have found this not to be an issue clinically.

Tissue Visualization

The idea of changing the color of a light source to enhance tissue visualization is a relatively novel concept. The only work in this area was done over 15 years ago with green light to enhance visualization of the nerve fiber layer and inner retinal surface for macular surgery. Although the authors felt the green light did enhance the contrast on the macular surface, the reduced light output or brightness with the green filter in place was felt to be limiting.

With the introduction of the Synergetics Photon 1 xenon light source, I performed a study in 2005 to evaluate the effect of various filters on the basic parameters of safety and brightness, and initially explored the concept of enhanced tissue visualization. As previously alluded to, the yellow filters were found in this study to incrementally and dramatically improve the safety calculations, allowing surgeons the option to increase the power or brightness of their light source without compromising the retinal threshold times. The overall viewing environment with the yellow filter in place was found to be quite satisfactory. The green filter, although providing only a small improvement in safety, did appear to have enhanced contrast for macular work and unlike the previous studies, the power or brightness was adequate due to the more powerful underlying xenon light source. The blue filter, to no surprise, did not provide any tissue visualization enhancements and had a detrimental effect on the safety calculations to a great degree. The red filter, although providing an extremely safe working environment, had very poor brightness and as a result a viewing environment that was unacceptable. Following this work, yellow filters were integrated as an option into multiple light sources.

The Synergetics Photon 2 was the first mercury vapor light source to enter the retina market and it had a distinctly greenish hue associated with its base spectral curve. This greenish hue was received by the community with a decidedly mixed reaction – some loved the view it provided, others hated it. The Bausch and Lomb Stellaris PC integrated three filters into its light source: a green tint, a yellow tint, and an amber filter. Although the yellow tint and amber filter provided an undeniable improvement in safety, the unknown question was whether these filters provided any real improvement in tissue visualization.

To try and properly address this, a multicenter trial was organized with 26 surgeons worldwide who systematically evaluated the baseline xenon and mercury vapor light sources and the three filters in all stages of a vitrectomy, across all pathologies. The surgeons were asked to record their impressions of the view obtained and to comparatively assess the views across all the options. The results in 348 cases over a 4-month period in 2013 were intriguing. To no surprise the baseline xenon light source was well accepted by the surgeons in almost all situations. The green filter was the preferred choice of most surgeons for macular surgery with no dye, with intravitreal Kenalog for visualization, and with indocyanine green dye. The one exception was macular surgery with brilliant blue dye where the preferred filter, particularly for European surgeons, was the amber filter. The most controversial of the filters was the amber filter. This filter was poorly accepted in most situations; however, there were two notable exceptions. The first and strongest exception was during air-fluid exchange where the amber filter was found to provide a superior view by the majority of surgeons. In this situation the amber filter was felt to significantly reduce glare. The other exception was, as mentioned above, for surgeons using brilliant blue dye for macular surgery who felt the amber filter improved contrast.

Future Directions

The most recent changes in the field of endoillumination involve the creation of LED light sources. The obvious advantage of these light sources is the significant increase in bulb life up to 10,000 h. In addition, DORC has added the capability of titrating the color of their LED light source on the EVA platform along a fixed pathway to a more yellow hue. The concept of a titratable light source with respect to hue is certainly an advance in the concept of giving surgeons the ability to choose the ideal 'color' of illumination for a given patient or procedure. There are some novel light sources being explored as well which may also provide surgeons more choice in their illumination options.

Reference

1 Ham WT, Mueller HA, Ruffolo JJ, Guerry D, Geurry RK: Action spectrum for retinal injury from near-ultraviolet radiation in the aphakic monkey. Am J Ophth 1982;93:299–306.

Disclosure Statement

The author has been a consultant/speaker for Bausch and Lomb, Allergan, Alcon, DORC, Synergetics, Katalyst, OptoVue, Lumenis, Arctic Dx, Novartis, Thrombogenics.

David R. Chow, MD, FRCSC
23 Ivor Rd
North York, ON M4N 2H3 (Canada)
E-Mail davidrchow@me.com

Oh H, Oshima Y (eds): Microincision Vitrectomy Surgery. Emerging Techniques and Technology.
Dev Ophthalmol. Basel, Karger, 2014, vol 54, pp 87–91 (DOI: 10.1159/000360453)

Wide-Angle Viewing System

Makoto Inoue

Kyorin Eye Center, Kyorin University School of Medicine, Tokyo, Japan

Abstract

A wide-angle viewing system offers a panoramic view of the surgical field and also improves the safety and efficacy of the vitreoretinal surgical procedure. Surgeons can easily observe the fundus in almost the whole area and evaluate the retinal pathologies through the panoramic view even in eyes with small pupils, corneal opacity, or eyes implanted with multifocal intraocular lens or toric intraocular lens. Recent wide-angle viewing systems consist of two types: contact lens and non-contact lens. The benefit of the contact lens type is better resolution and contrast of the fundus image compared to the non-contact lens type. The contact lens is directly attached to the cornea and the aberration and the reflection from the corneal surface are canceled. However, the eye position needs to be fixed and surgical procedures that rotate the eye should be avoided because incomplete attachment of the contact lens causes decreased visibility of the fundus image. The benefit of the non-contact lens type is that the viewing angle can be changed by moving the front lens up and down to adjust the distance between the cornea and the front lens. The surgical procedures are more flexible and the eye can be rotated. Dehydration of the corneal surface decreases the visibility of the fundus image and the corneal surface needs to be covered with viscoelastic material to avoid dehydration. Condensation of the front lens also decreases the visibility of fundus. Understanding the optical characteristics of the wide-angle viewing system is the key to a successful vitreoretinal surgery.

A wide-angle viewing system offers a panoramic view of the surgical field and also improves the safety and efficacy of vitreoretinal surgical procedures [1]. Surgeons can easily observe the fundus in almost the whole area and evaluate the retinal pathologies through the panoramic view even in eyes with small pupils, corneal opacity, or eyes implanted with multifocal intraocular lens or toric intraocular lens [2, 3]. The peripheral retina can be observed at a glance without rotating the eye excessively and depressing the sclera as with conventional floating prism contact lenses. This wide-angle viewing system is extremely useful especially for retinal detachment associated with giant breaks because the edges of the retinal break can be seen in one view (fig. 1). In conjunction with chandelier illumination, a bimanual technique allows a wide area, including the peripheral retina, to be observed without rotating the eye, and thus creation of peripheral retinal breaks can be avoided (fig. 2). Chandelier illumination or slit-lamp illumination built in the microscope in conjunction with a wide-angle viewing system provides wide, excellent visibility of the funduscopic images for scleral buckling procedures without wearing indirect binocular ophthalmoscopy [4]. Adjusting the viewing focus and magnification under the surgical microscope may be more helpful for identifying small tears during surgery which were unrecognized preoperatively. A wide-angle viewing system and chandelier illumination also contributes to expanded use of small-gauge vitrectomy for various vitreoretinal pathologies. Understanding recent developments and optical characteristics of a wide-angle viewing system are essential for achieving successful vitreoretinal surgery.

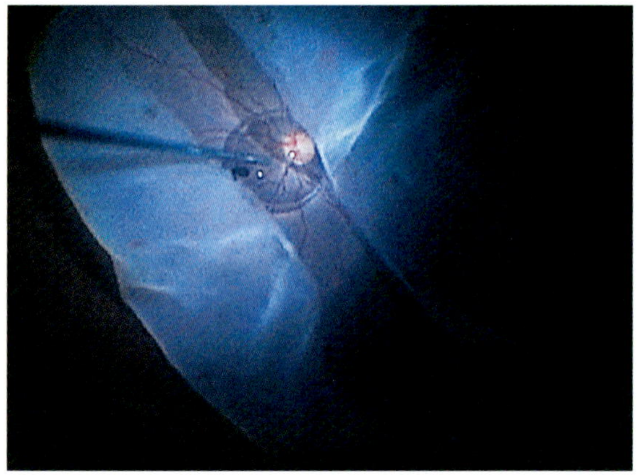

Fig. 1. Intraoperative wide-angle view of an eye with giant break retinal detachment. Wide-angle viewing with the RESIGHT system enables the visualization of the detached retina to the edge of the retinal break with a conventional light pipe when the perfluorocarbon liquid is injected.

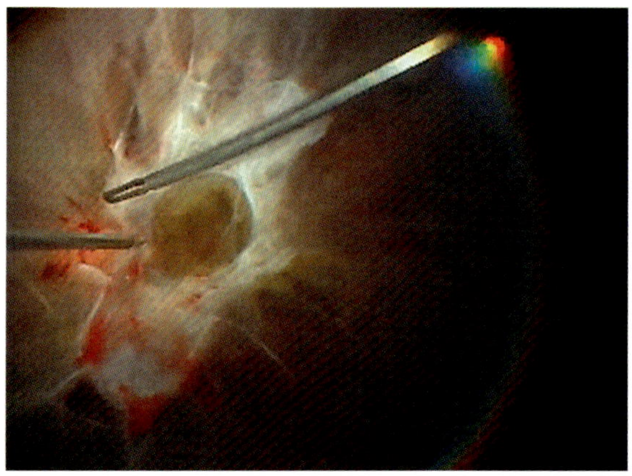

Fig. 2. Bimanual technique with a wide-angle viewing system for proliferative diabetic retinopathy. The peripheral retina is avoided tracting when the fibrovascular membrane is held by forceps and dissected with scissors.

History of the Wide-Angle Viewing System

Dominguez [5] introduced an observation system in which a front lens was used with slit-lamp examination to observe the fundus in the operating microscope in 1981; however, the image was inverted and not widely used. Spitznas and Reiner [6] invented the stereoscopic diagonal inverter, which is attached to a microscope and converts the inverted image through the front lens for wide-angle viewing. Spitznas [7] also introduced a non-contact wide-angle viewing system, the Binocular Indirect Ophthalmo Microscope (BIOM), which consists of a non-contact front lens, reduction lens, and stereoscopic inverter.

EIBOS was introduced in 1993 and this system was integrated with a stereoscopic inverter and front lens with manual focusing. The Peyman-Wessels-Landers 132D upright vitrectomy lens was introduced in 1990, and is also an integrated system of a front lens and stereoscopic inverter. The contact lens-type wide-angle viewing system, which enables better resolution of fundus images, was also introduced during this period [8, 9].

An optical fiber-free intravitreal surgery system (OFFISS), which was initially introduced for

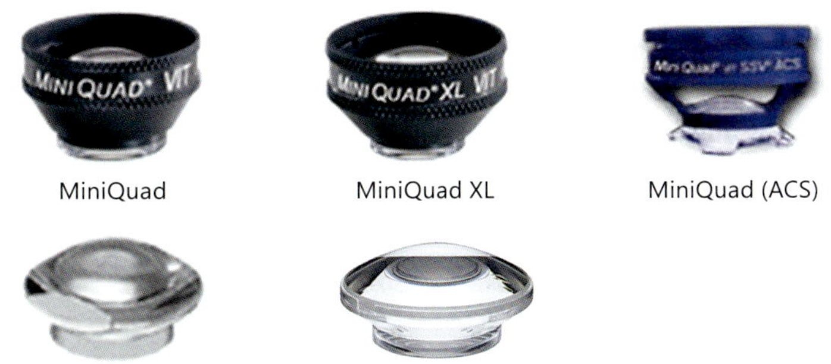

Fig. 3. Contact lens-type wide-angle viewing system. MiniQuad (ACS) has a stabilizer to stand on the cornea without holding. The height of the Panora View lens is designed to be lower for better stabilization. ACS = Autoclave sterilization lens.

Table 1. Catalog data of contact lens-type wide-angle viewing systems

	Refractive powers, D	Magnification	Viewing angle[1] (straight/tilting)	Diameter of the lens (up/bottom), mm	Height, mm
MiniQuad	156	0.39×	106/127	18.4/11.45	11.9
MiniQuad XL	156	0.39×	112/134	21.4/11.45	13.3
ClariVit wide angle	156	0.39×	110/132	0.19/10	10.6
Panora View	128	0.47×	110/132	16.6/11.2	8.2

[1] The parameters differ in a measuring condition.

vitreous surgery without endoillumination for complicated bimanual surgery, provided a wide-angle front lens [10]. This system enables electric control of focusing, magnifying, and the observation angle, and X-Y moving is automatically reversed when the front lens is used. The front lens of OFFISS was attached to the frame of the microscope, not to the main body, to enable focusing with the foot pedal by moving the main body of the microscope up and down and maintaining the distance between the front lens and the cornea. The RESIGHT system has an inner focusing system by moving the reduction lens up and down. This system does not require moving the main body of the microscope upward to make it focused for wide-angle viewing, and the surgery can be seamlessly switched between conventional viewing through the contact lens and wide-angle viewing.

Contact Lens-Type Wide-Angle Viewing System

The benefit of a contact lens-type wide-angle viewing system is the ability to achieve better resolution and contrast of the fundus image compared to the non-contact lens-type wide-angle viewing system (fig. 3, table 1). The contact lens is directly attached to the cornea and the aberration of the cornea and the reflection from the corneal surface are canceled. The surgeons do not have to worry excessively about dehydration of the corneal surface. However, the eye position needs to be fixed and the surgical procedures for the peripheral retina involving rotating the eye should be avoided because incomplete attachment of the contact lens causes decreased visibility of the fundus image. The contact lens needs to be held by a skilled assis-

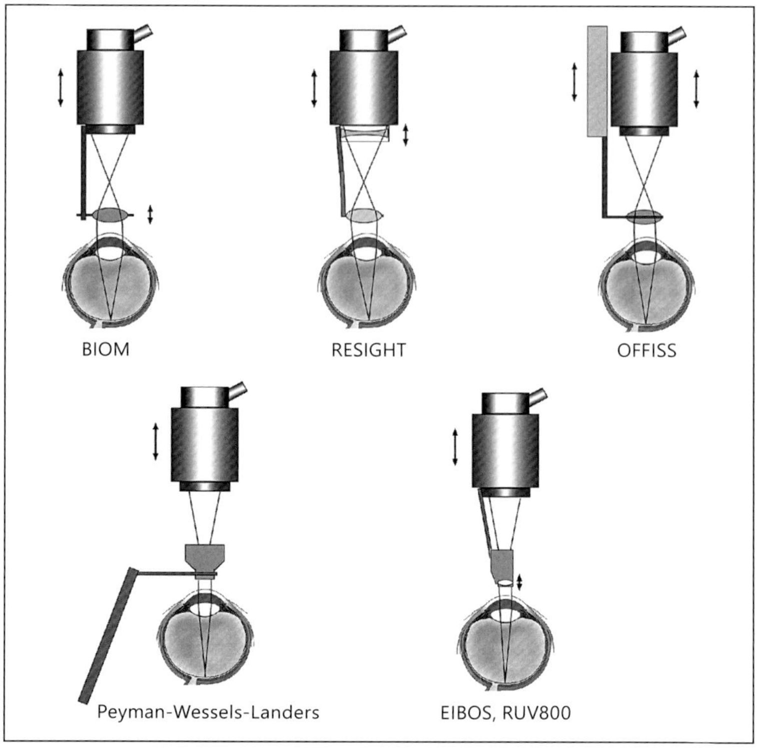

Fig. 4. Non-contact lens-type wide-angle viewing system. The field of view and the focus can be adjusted by moving the front lens and the cornea or the reduction lens.

tant to keep the contact lens stable and perfectly upright. When using chandelier illumination, the surgeon can hold the contact lens instead of a light guide. The surgeon performs the operation with one hand, and can use the other hand to switch the chandelier light to another sclerotomy port.

Another benefit of the contact lens-type wide-angle viewing system is less cost compared to the non-contact lens-type wide-angle viewing system. A stereo-converter is required for the surgery, but the cost is almost reduced by half.

Non-Contact Lens-Type Wide-Angle Viewing System

The benefit of non-contact lens is the ability to change the viewing angle by moving the front lens up and down and adjusting the distance between the cornea and the front lens (fig. 4, table 2). When the eye is rotated to view the more peripheral areas of the retina, better visibility of the fundus can be achieved with the non-contact lens-type wide-angle viewing system than with the contact lens type. The surgical procedures are more flexible and a skilled assistant to hold the front lens is not required. This is why the non-contact lens-type wide-angle viewing system requires less training time and has a smaller learning curve.

Dehydration of the corneal surface decreases the visibility of the fundus image and the corneal surface needs to be covered with viscoelastic material or a hard contact lens should be applied to avoid dehydration. The condensation on the front lens is also a factor that decreases visibility. Draping around the eye must be completely isolated from the breath of the patient to avoid condensation on the front lens.

Table 2. Catalog data of non-contact-type wide-angle viewing systems

	Diameter of front lens, mm	Refractive power of front lens, D	Viewing angle
BIOM	19	132	102.9
RESIGHT	17	128	94.9
OFFISS	21	120	130.2
MERLIN	14	140	88.9
Landers	18	132	99.9
EIBOS	20	132	105.8
RUV800	20	132	105.8

Landers = Peyman-Wessels-Landers lens.

Ohji et al. [11] described that a meniscus contact lens combined with a non-contact lens Peyman-Wessels-Landers wide-angle system increased the intraoperative field of view and improved the sharpness of the peripheral images. Ohtsuki et al. [12] described a modified technique to enhance the visual field through the RESIGHT wide-angle viewing system by applying a magnifying prism meniscus contact lens when the eye is rotated. This technique can eliminate the aberration so as to observe the peripheral retina when rotating the eye.

References

1 Chalam KV, Shah VA: Optics of wide-angle panoramic viewing system-assisted vitreous surgery. Surv Ophthalmol 2004;49:437–445.
2 Inoue M, Noda T, Mihashi T, et al: Quality of image of grating target placed in model of human eye with corneal aberrations as observed through multifocal intraocular lenses. Am J Ophthalmol 2011;151:644–652.
3 Inoue M, Noda T, Ohnuma K, et al: Quality of image of grating target placed in model eye and observed through toric intraocular lenses. Am J Ophthalmol 2013;155:243–252.
4 Aras C, Ucar D, Koytak A, Yetik H: Scleral buckling with a non-contact wide-angle viewing system. Ophthalmologica 2012;227:107–110.
5 Dominguez A: Oftalmoscopia cinematografica de imagen invertida. Arch Soc Espan Ophthal 1981;41:701–702.
6 Spitznas M, Reiner J: A stereoscopic diagonal inverter (SDI) for wide-angle vitreous surgery. Graefes Arch Clin Exp Ophthalmol 1987;225:9–12.
7 Spitznas M: A binocular indirect ophthalmo microscope (BIOM) for non-contact wide-angle vitreous surgery. Graefes Arch Clin Exp Ophthalmol 1987;225:13–15.
8 Shah VA, Chalam KV: Self-stabilizing wide-angle contact lens for vitreous surgery. Retina 2003;23:667–669.
9 Nakata K, Ohji M, Ikuno Y, et al: Wide-angle viewing lens for vitrectomy. Am J Ophthalmol 2004;137:760–762.
10 Horiguchi M, Kojima Y, Shimada Y: New system for fiberoptic-free bimanual vitreous surgery. Arch Ophthalmol 2002;120:491–494.
11 Ohji M, Tada E, Futamura H: Combining a contact lens and wide-angle viewing system for a wider fundus view. Retina 2011;31:1958–1960.
12 Ohtsuki M, Inoue M, Uda S, et al: Combining magnifying prismatic lens with a wide-angle viewing system to enhance view of peripheral retina during vitreous surgery. Retina 2012;32:1983–1987.

Makoto Inoue
Kyorin Eye Center, Kyorin University School of Medicine
6-20-2 Shinkawa
Mitaka, Tokyo, 181-8611 (Japan)
E-Mail inoue@eye-center.org

Oh H, Oshima Y (eds): Microincision Vitrectomy Surgery. Emerging Techniques and Technology.
Dev Ophthalmol. Basel, Karger, 2014, vol 54, pp 92–101 (DOI: 10.1159/000360454)

Vitreous Substitute and Tamponade Substances for Microincision Vitreoretinal Surgery

Stanislao Rizzo · Francesco Barca
U.O. Chirurgia Oftalmica, Azienda Ospedaliero Universitaria Pisana (AOUP), Pisa, Italy

Abstract
Intraocular tamponades are important tools in vitreoretinal surgery and their introduction has represented a pivotal moment in the management of ophthalmic surgery as they are equipped with a combination of chemical and physical properties that have propelled their surgical use. There are two ophthalmic tamponades, liquid and gas, both of which are currently used in microincision vitreoretinal surgery (MIVS). ***Methods:*** Perfluorocarbon liquids (PFCLs) are effective in a wide range of situations, not only for repair of complex retinal detachment, but also for a variety of intraocular surgical maneuvers since they have physical properties that render them very useful for vitreoretinal surgeons. These include transparency, high specific gravity, and immiscibility with water. Thanks to their low viscosity, PFCLs are easy to use with MIVS. The intraocular gases are important tools used primarily for the ability to provide internal tamponade for retinal tears or holes. Performing oblique sclerotomy has overtaken the risk of postoperative hypotony. Silicon oil (SO) describes a group of hydrophobic polymeric and monomeric compounds made up of silicon-oxygen bonds, which have the capability to be lighter or heavier than water (heavy SO). In MIVS there is an increase in the use of SO with lower viscosity. ***Conclusions:*** Intraocular tamponades are very useful surgical tools because they have simplified the surgical management of many vitreoretinal diseases. With modern vitrectomy systems, the possibility to use different tamponade substances has improved the prognosis of several diseases.

Intraocular tamponades are important tools in vitreoretinal surgery and their introduction has represented a pivotal moment in the management of ophthalmic diseases. There are two types of tamponades for ophthalmic surgical use: liquid and gas. An ideal vitreous substitute should have the following: tamponade every break in every quadrant (both superior and inferior), block or minimize fluid circulation around breaks, protect against proliferative vitreoretinopathies, and be inert and compatible for ocular tissues. The safe and effective use of tamponade substances requires knowledge of their physical and chemical properties because it is on the basis of this knowledge that surgeons have to decide what kind of tamponade to use. In this chapter we focus on the use of these tamponades in microincision vitreoretinal surgery (MIVS).

Physical Properties of Tamponades and Clinical Consequences

To be effective as an internal tamponade, a substance has to have the ability to displace aqueous substances from the retinal surface. The following four physical parameters influence this function:

(1) Specific gravity: substances with a specific gravity of 1 are neutrally buoyant in water, those with a specific gravity >1 are denser than water, and so will sink in it, and those with a specific gravity of <1 are less dense than water, and so will float.

(2) Buoyancy: an intraocular bubble of tamponade agent is acted upon by two opposing forces, buoyancy (upward force) and the gravity on the bubble (downward force). Regarding the vitreous cavity, the result is the force with which the bubble presses against the retina. The force is greatest with air or gas, as the specific gravity is very low at 0.001.

(3) Interfacial tension: defined as a physical rating of the difference between the intermolecular force of the two liquids, it is responsible for the shape of liquid bubbles. Therefore, a substance with a high interfacial tension will have a greater tendency to stay as one large bubble without dispersion into small bubbles. Gas or air has the highest interfacial tension against water (around 80 mN/m), whereas perfluorocarbon liquids (PFCLs) and silicone oil (SO) are lower, around 40–45 mN/m and 35 mN/m, respectively.

(4) Viscosity: physical property of a fluid which measures its resistance to gradual deformation by shear stress. The tendency of a substance to emulsify and disperse into droplets over time is also dependent on its viscosity. The less viscous a substance, the lower the energy that is required to disperse a large bubble of the substance into small droplets.

Here we review the major indications and complications regarding the use of some current types of intraocular tamponades used during MIVS.

Perfluorocarbon Liquids

PFCLs are synthetic fluorinated liquids which contain carbon-fluorine bonds [1] and are particularly effective in a wide range of situations since they have physical properties that render them very useful for a vitreoretinal surgeon as an intraoperative tool. Their specific gravity has a range of 1.76–2.03, whereby they sink and flatten the retina with a force 10 times higher than an equivalent volume of SO and only slightly lower than that exerted by intraocular gases. Due to their high superficial tension (range: 14–21.6 din/cm at 25°C) PFCLs tend to stay as a whole bubble without blending in water and have a poor tendency to go in the subretinal space through a retinal break.

Uses in Microincision Vitreoretinal Surgery

Unlike SO, PFCLs have a low viscosity (2–3 cSt), allowing injection and removal with small-gauge instruments. As with all fluids, PFCLs are incompressible, whereby if injected into a closed system such as a vitreous cavity they will induce an increase of the intraocular pressure (IOP). Independently of surgical techniques, it is therefore necessary to allow a way out of the irrigation solution when PFCL is injected. If a second illumination is present, PFCL can be injected leaving one cannula open or using an extrusion cannula through which the saline solution can exit (fig. 1). If there is not a second illumination, we usually keep the infusion pressure down until 10–15 mm Hg and open a way out in the valve that is connected to the infusion line in order to allow a retrograde flux of the saline solution. In this way, surgeons can keep the IOP under a correct control during the entire procedure and avoid dan-

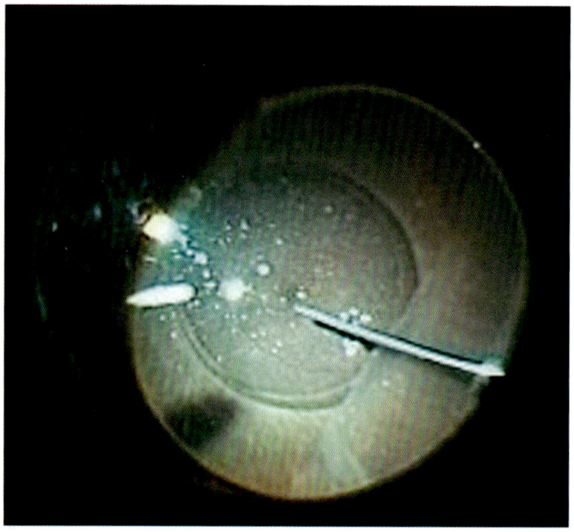

Fig. 1. PFCL injection with secondary illumination in rhegmatogenous retinal detachment with giant retinal tear repair. While PFCL is injected into the vitreous cavity (right hand), the irrigation solution is actively aspirated using the probe (cutter off) (left hand).

gerous increases in pressure. Alternatively, a dual-bore needle like Charles et al. [2] may be used. We, however, do not use this technique because, due to the smaller caliber, it easily induces an increase IOP with the formation of many droplets of PFCL that can migrate under the detached retina through a retinal break.

Regarding the surgical indications, however, there is no difference with the old 20-gauge system. The main indication for PFCL use is still retinal detachment (both uncomplicated and complicated) in those for whom the surgical approach and prognosis have been modified. In fact, thanks to specific gravity, PFCLs fill the vitreous cavity proceeding from the posterior pole to the crystalline lens. Consequently, the subretinal fluid is displaced toward the periphery (steamroller effect) so the retina is relocated against the retinal pigment epithelium (RPE) as the PFCL bubble expands, helping the surgeon at the time of the fluid-air exchange. Removing PFCLs from the eye using small-gauge instruments is also very simple. During fluid-air exchange it is possible to aspirate passively through an extrusion cannula the entire PFCL bubble without leaving any drop inside the eye. We usually set the vitrectomy machine with an IOP of 25 mm Hg that is sufficient to aspirate PFCL bubbles.

Intraocular Gases

The intraocular gases in vitreoretinal surgery are important tools used primarily for the ability to provide a postoperative internal tamponade for retinal tears or holes. Many types of gases have been investigated for use in vitreoretinal surgery. Two physical properties of gas, surface tension and buoyant force, are of fundamental importance to understand why gas has become such important surgical tools. The surface tension of a bubble prevents it from passing through the tear; therefore, when the gas bubble is positioned against the tear, the passage of fluid from the vitreous into the subretinal space is blocked and the RPE can reabsorb the subretinal fluid. The surface tension between gas and fluid is around 70 dynes/cm, almost twice that of the surface tension between SO and fluid (40 dynes/cm). Buoyant force is because the specific gravity of gases is lower than that of water and therefore a gas bubble floats into the vitreous cavity. This buoyant force is greatest at the apex of the bubble and weakest at the lower meniscus of the bubble that contacts the retina [3]. The buoyant force is approximately 10 times greater with gas than with an equivalent volume of SO.

Surgical Technique in Microincision Vitreoretinal Surgery

To achieve a gas bubble of adequate size, surgeons should consider that all tractional forces on the retina have to be relieved to flatten the retina. Regarding the exchange, a syringe containing the desired gas mixture is connected to the infusion line and the gas is gently injected inside the eye while a cannula is kept open. In this way the gas, which is heavier than air, falls down and the air is expelled from the open cannula or alternatively from an extrusion cannula. Once the required gas volume is injected, the last cannula is extracted and the patency of sclerotomies is evaluated by irrigating the ocular surface with balanced salt solution. If there is leakage from the sclerotomy, it is usually enough to perform a refilling with a 30-gauge needle through the sclera and massage the sclera with a cotton tip in order to facilitate wound closure. If the IOP is too high (hard eye), a 30-gauge needle (without syringe) can be inserted to let out a small amount of gas from the eye. Wound sealing-related complications are very rare for us. Using 25- or 23-gauge systems, it is sometimes possible to see leakage from one sclerotomy; however, if massage does not work, it is possible to perform a diathermy on the conjunctiva above the sclerotomy to block any leakage [4]. In a series of 16 cases using a 27-gauge system, we did not have any leakage, either with air or balanced salt solution [5].

Postoperative Management of Patients with Intraocular Gas

After surgery for retinal detachment, we usually place patients with their head in a prone position for two reasons. First, it reduces the chances of pupillary block glaucoma or corneal endothelial decompensation. A pupillary block displaces the lens-iris diaphragm forward against the corneal endothelium. In this case an aspiration of a small amount of the gas should be done at the slit-lamp and the intraocular lens must be repositioned behind the iris using a balanced salt solution cannula. Second, gases push the macula against the RPE and displace the subretinal fluid away from the submacular space. In our opinion, this is necessary to avoid macular folds after surgery for a macula-off rhegmatogenous retinal detachment because only pushing the macula against the RPE makes it possible to displace any submacular fluid away from the macula. In fact, the buoyancy of the gas bubble in this posture promotes a smooth attachment of the macula, and after few hours, when the subretinal fluid has been displaced toward the periphery and absorbed through the RPE, the posture is changed according to the position of the tear. In fact, we can accurately direct the buoyant force by simply positioning the patient's head so that the bubble is situated against the retinal break wherever it is located. It is then desirable that gas persists as an effective volume (therapeutic) until the chorioretinal adhesion, resulting from photocoagulation or cryotherapy, becomes complete (approx. 8–14 days).

In phakic patients, the position should keep the gas bubble away from the crystal clear lens to prevent the 'lens feathering' that is the formation of branched opacities at the level of posterior capsular of the lens and develops as a result of hours of continuous contact with the gas, but are reversible if the patient takes a prone position. The presence of such opacity therefore indicates a prone positioning not respected by the patient. In theory the phakic patient should remain in the prone position until the gas bubble decreases to about 20% of the vitreous capacity to avoid the contact of the gas with the posterior face of the lens when the patient stands upright. However, it is also true that in case of a retinal detachment we are forced to place the patient's head in the most appropriate position depending upon the location of the retinal break. Therefore, it is not always possible to leave the patient prone until the gas bubble is reduced to 20%. As a result, it is our practice to perform combined surgery in phakic patients who need a vitrectomy because we know that they will develop a significant cataract within a few months.

Contraindications

There are no absolute contraindications to the use of intraocular gas in MIVS. The use of gas is not recommended in uncooperative patients who will not be able to maintain the required position (SO is better in such cases) and in patients who have to travel by plane or travel to high altitudes.

Complications
One of the main drawbacks regarding the use of MIVS is the high risk of postoperative hypotony and endophthalmitis. Previous publications about 23- and 25-gauge systems reported high rates of hypotony 1 day after surgery when sclerotomies were done with a straight incision [6]. In contrast, by using an oblique incision, other surgeons have had less hypotony [7]; in fact, to date in our clinical practice we rarely see serious hypotony. In a consecutive series where we operated on 16 patients using a new 27-gauge system, we did not have any postoperative hypotony and no patients developed choroidal detachment or required a postoperative supplemental air or gas tamponade [5]. We believe these results are related to the carefully constructed tunnel-based sclerotomies. We usually perform a one step 10° angle sclerotomy (30° with 27-gauge) to achieve a flat and linear scleral wound. In this way, once the microcannulas are removed, it is only necessary to massage the sclera at the entry sites to determine the correct apposition of wound edges to avoid dangerous leakage.

The incidence of elevated IOP ranged from 26 to 59% in patients who underwent vitrectomy and gas fill [8–10]. In most cases, an increase of IOP is transient and can be controlled medically. If still high, it might be necessary to aspirate some gas from the vitreous cavity. Permanent secondary glaucoma is infrequent and most likely results from peripheral angle closure as a result of anterior displacement of the lens-iris diaphragm by a large gas bubble. This change is most frequently seen in patients who are not able to maintain their head in a prone position.

Silicone Oils

Physical and Chemical Properties
SO is made up of a group of hydrophobic polymeric and monomeric compounds constituted of silicon-oxygen bonds (organo-siloxane) that are composed of a linear chain of siloxane repeating units (Si-O) and a variety of radical side groups (hydrocarbon radicals, e.g. methyl, phenyl, vinyl, trifluoroproyl groups) which are attached to the silicon atoms. Thus, each type of SO have specific chemical and physical characteristics because it is possible to have SO with different molecular weights and lengths of the linear chain, as well as different radical side groups. The viscosity of a different type of SO arises from the molecular weight and length of the polymers: increasing an SO's molecular weight results in an increased polymer chain length and consequently an increase in its viscosity [11]. The types of SO currently in use have viscosity ratings from 1,000 to 12,500 cSt.

In order to create a tamponade effect on the superior or inferior retina, SO has the capability to be lighter or heavier than water, a property that arises from the radical side groups. In clinical use, we currently use two classes of SO: SO lighter than water, which are the most commonly used, and SO heavier than water (heavy SO). Like every tamponade, the dynamic of SO in the eye depends on the interaction between buoyancy, interfacial surface tension, and viscosity. Buoyancy arises from the difference in specific gravity between the aqueous (or vitreous) humor and the selected SO. In comparison to water, the gravity of SO is a little lower (0.97) and therefore they float inside vitreous cavity and the upward force is defined as buoyancy. This force is highest at the apex and gradually decreases to zero at the horizontal meniscus. Surface tension is responsible for the shape of the liquid droplets because it describes the forces that tend to keep a bubble as a whole; for 1,000 cSt SO it is 40 mN/m (at 25°C), which is approximately a third of that generated on an air bubble. Viscosity influences the surface tension of an SO bubble: the higher the viscosity, the higher the surface tension. Other factors, however, may decrease the surface tension: viscoelastic solutions, blood, proteins, lipids, ionized solutions (e.g. biological fluids). Therefore, if they are present in the vitreous cavity when a SO is injected, the surface tension decreases and thus leads to emulsification.

Surgical Techniques: Silicone Oil Injection and Removal in MIVS

With modern vitrectomy systems, which are also in even smaller gauges, the injection and the removal of all SO is made using a syringe connected to a pump that is controlled by the surgeon with a foot pedal. Due to Poiseuille's law, which states the flow of a fluid in a tube is proportional to the fourth power of the radius of the tube and inversely proportional to the length of the tube, and due to the high viscosity and the high pressure that is required to infuse SO into the vitreous cavity, special devices have been developed for using them with MIVS. Therefore, the system consists of a large syringe, an infusion line as short as possible, and nondistensible material. A large syringe is required because it needs to be able to handle the high infusion pressure, while a short infusion line is important to reduce the resistance during the injection and removal. The use of nondistensible material is important so that when the injection is stopped no further injections will occur, as the distended tube returns to its normal diameter, forcing more silicone into the eye. Furthermore, there is a perceived need for less viscous SO that can be introduced and removed more easily through smaller instruments and cannulas. However, even if a less viscous oil would be user-friendly, a more viscous oil would be less likely to emulsify. For this reason different types of SO with an increasing extensional viscosity have been studied. Such SO is obtained by the addition of very-long-chain silicone molecules to a common SO. The advantage of an SO with an increasing extensional viscosity would be the increased resistance to emulsification [12] while maintaining its ease of injection into and removal from the vitreous cavity.

There are three surgical techniques to inject SO into the eye: fluid-silicone exchange, air-silicone exchange, and PFCL-silicone exchange (also named direct-exchange). We do not use fluid-silicone exchange because, we believe the risk of undesired subretinal silicone oil drops due to the low surface tension is too high. Air-silicone exchange presupposes that a fluid-air exchange has been done first. In MIVS, there is a diffuse consensus to perform this type of exchange because it is easier to inject SO through a cannula instead of through the infusion line (direct exchange) (fig. 2). However, the choice of air-silicone instead PFCL-silicone exchange depends on two main factors: the eventual presence of a retinectomy or an anterior break. If the break is in the mild periphery or at posterior pole, we usually perform first a fluid-air exchange with internal drainage of subretinal fluid, and then (once the retina is flattened under air) an air-silicone exchange. If a relaxing retinectomy has been done or the retinal break is too anterior (fig. 3), in order to avoid the slippage of the posterior edge of the tear, we prefer to perform a direct exchange between PFCL and SO. In this case we connect the

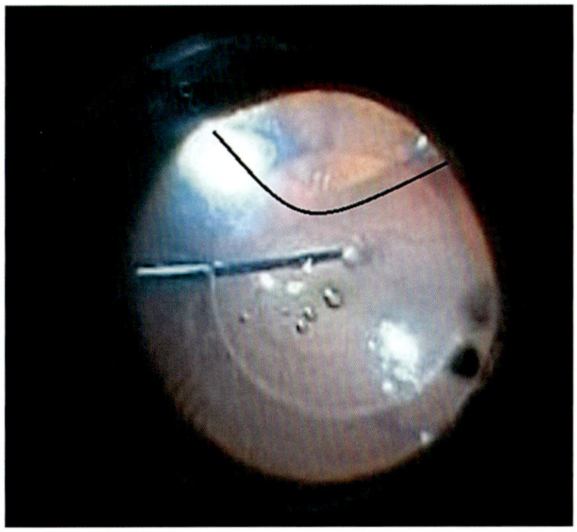

Fig. 2. PFCL-SO exchange. The curved black line indicates the SO entry into the vitreous cavity from the infusion cannula while PFCL is removed using an extrusion cannula.

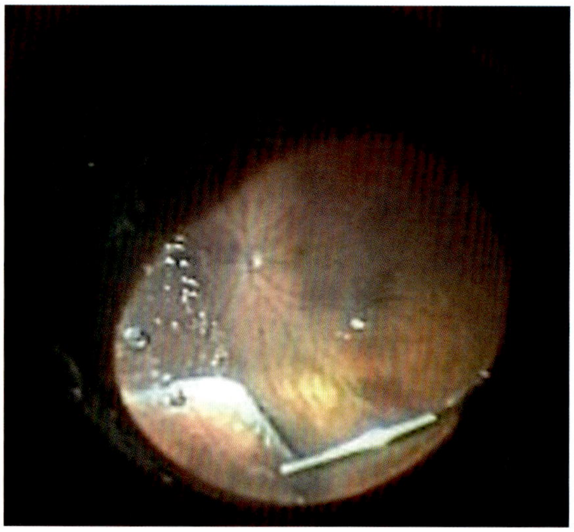

Fig. 3. PFCL-SO exchange for giant retinal tear with retinal detachment. Subretinal fluid removal using extrusion cannula while SO is injected.

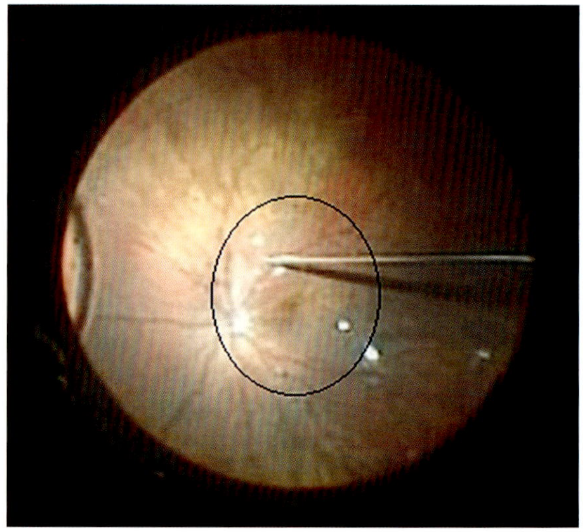

Fig. 4. PFCL-SO exchange. Aspiration of the last amount of PFCL bubble (inside the black ring).

syringe to the infusion line and an extrusion cannula is placed into the vitreous cavity. While a surgeon injects the SO by pushing the foot pedal, either passive or active aspiration may be used to remove the PFCL simultaneously. With 23- and 25-gauge systems, we set the machine with an aspiration rate from 0 to 30 mm Hg and an infusion pressure rate from 0 to 28 Psi (fig. 4). It is important to not exceed 30 Psi of infusion pressure to avoid the disconnection of the infusion line from the eye. This technique is possible with both types of SO (lighter and heavier than water).

Regarding SO removal, we always perform a standard three-port pars plana vitrectomy. We set the machine with an IOP of 20 mm Hg and a vacuum rate from 0 to 650 mm Hg. We currently use the new high-flow extraction sleeve by Alcon (fig. 5), which significantly improves oil extraction times over the old system – up to 5 times faster depending on gauge. The sleeve consists of a silicone tube that is inserted on the head of the trocar cannula (both 23 and 25 gauge) and allows the aspiration of the SO through the trocar cannula (fig. 6). To remove the sleeve from the cannula, it is enough to do a tilt motion, taking care to keep the head of the cannula with a forceps (e.g. Bonn). This technique is possible with both types of SO (lighter and heavier than water). In order to remove the small drops of SO that always remain inside the eye, once the SO bubble has been removed, it is necessary to perform several fluid-air

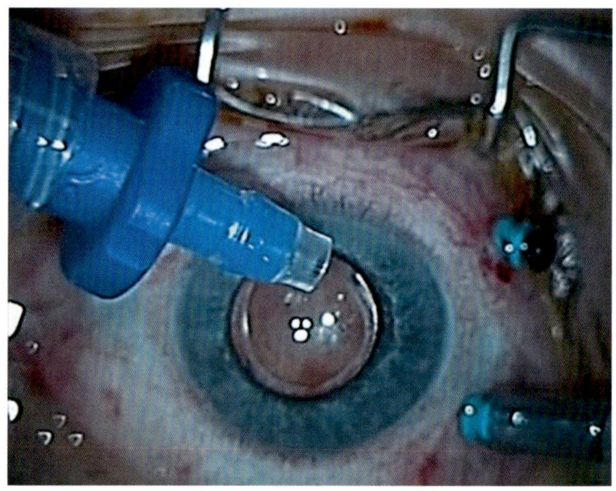

Fig. 5. 25-gauge high-flow extraction sleeve by Alcon.

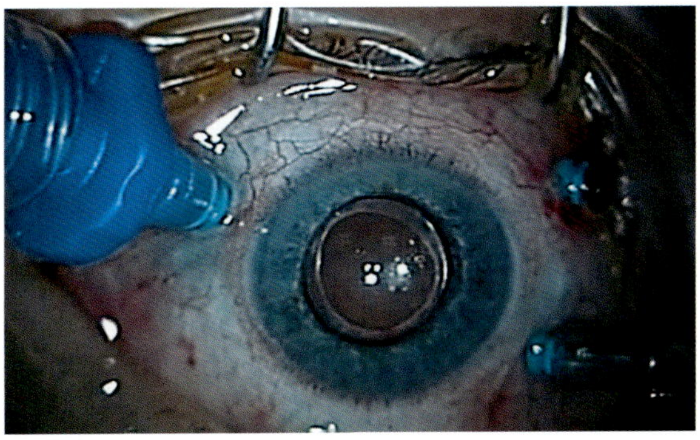

Fig. 6. 25-gauge pars plana vitrectomy for SO removal.

exchanges. In case of emulsified drops in the anterior chamber, it is also very important to remove them through a small corneal incision to minimize the postoperative risk of complications such as silicone keratopathy and secondary glaucoma. In phakic eyes, the decision whether or not to remove the lens depends on the presence of a cataract and the patient's age. If there is a significant cataract, we usually remove the lens during the operation. If the crystalline lens is clear, the decision is based on the age of the patient because in cases of patients older than 50 years we prefer to remove the lens as a significant cataract will develop in few months. We perform a combined phacoemulsification, posterior-chamber intraocular lens implantation and vitrectomy or SO removal.

Indications for Silicone Oil Tamponade

As we have seen with the use of gases, the indications for use of SO at the end of a surgery do not depend on the gauge that is used because the choice to use gases instead of SO depends on the vitreoretinal disease and on the duration of the tamponade that is required. The first indications for SO are therefore complicated retinal detachment due to proliferative vitreoretinopathy (PVR) or viral retinitis, giant retinal tears, trauma, and severe proliferative diabetic retinopathy. New possible indications are now retinal detachment due to macular hole in a highly myopic eye, chronic and persistent macular hole, colobomatous retinal detachment, and chronic uveitis with hypotony; in summary, every time a long-term tamponade is required. In fact, SO has the important advantage to determine long support until the recovery of the retina. In case of retinal detachment, we usually perform SO removal after 3–6 months; we believe this is a sufficient amount of time for the recovery of the eye with minimal risk for the development of PVR. SO is also the first choice for patients that have to fly or for patients that cannot maintain the correct postoperative positioning, such as children or oldest patients.

The Silicone Oil Study [13–15], a prospective, multicenter, randomized controlled clinical trial comparing SO and long-acting gases in the management of eye with severe PVR, concluded that SO was superior to SF_6 and equivalent to C_3F_8. However, when we look at certain subgroups, it appears clear that the use of SO is better in cases of relaxing retinotomy, severe anterior PVR, anticipated difficulty with the postoperative positioning, and the need to fly or travel to higher altitudes. In contrast, the use of C_3F_8 has the relative indications for cases with a poor iris diaphragm due to a high probability of corneal tamponade touch, superior retinal breaks on the posterior edge of a scleral buckle (because gas conforms better than silicone oil to the slope of the buckle), and the presence of a silicone intraocular lens with an open posterior capsule. The rationale for their use in the management of proliferative diabetic retinopathy is the reduction in postoperative hemorrhages and the presence of a severe anterior-segment neovascularization because SO may prevent the flow of vasoproliferative factors into the anterior segment, decreasing the risk of iris rubeosis and neovascular glaucoma. We consider the use of SO for selected cases of macular hole: when there are problems with the postoperative positioning, when air travel is necessary, in one-eyed patients, and in cases of persistent macular hole. SO is used in case of a severely traumatized eye to minimize the risk of postoperative bleeding, maintain retina attachment, and avoid phthisis. Often, several operations are needed to obtain a reasonable anatomical and functional outcome. After SO removal, the high failure rate is generally due to the development of a retinal detachment and/or PVR that require a new operation. In this regard, since it is believed that the proliferative process continues for a longer period of time than in eyes with non-traumatic retinal detachment, it is convenient to leave SO for several months.

In summary, the decision to use SO may be made both before and during the operation. The first and more important parameter of choice is the surgeon's opinion on the time required for the tamponade. Before the operation, it is fundamental to take into consideration the type of vitreoretinal disease (e.g. PVR, high risk of a surgical failure) and the postoperative position. If we know that maintaining the best position after surgery is impossible for the patient (e.g. children), it is better take in consideration to leave SO instead of another tamponade. However, even if we have not planned the use of a permanent tamponade, it is possible to decide during the operation that silicon oil tamponade is needed. For example, the decision of a retinectomy or complication as an intraocular bleeding can indicate the choice of SO.

Complications

Since a variety of complications are possible in case of a vitreoretinal surgery, it is important to understand whether they are associated with the use of SO or related to the underlying pathology or other aspects of surgical intervention. In relation to MIVS, there are not complications related to the use a small-gauge system because the complications that a surgeon can have are the same using both 23/25/27 gauge and 20 gauge. Surgeons have to keep in mind that by using a higher viscosity SO, the time required for SO removal is longer in comparison to a 20-gauge system. However, the duration of the entire operation is not different because, as demonstrated, the start and the close of the operation are faster.

Conclusions

Intraocular tamponades are very useful surgical tools because they are able to simplify the surgical management of many vitreoretinal pathologies. With modern MIVS, the possibility to use such different tamponades has improved the prognosis of several diseases. Whatever the pathology, we have a choice of a variety of tamponades and therefore can array the best intraocular tamponade in relation to the underlying disease. Depending on the situation and the duration of the tamponade, we can decide which of the various characteristics of an endotamponade would be the most important.

References

1 Perfluorocarbon liquids in vitreoretinal surgery; in Ryan JS (ed): Retina, ed 4. Amsterdam, Elsevier Mosby, 2006, vol 3, p 2179.

2 Charles S, Calzada J, Wood B: Vitreous Microsurgery, ed 5. Philadelphia, Wolters Kluwer, Lippincott Williams & Wilkins, 2011, p 62.

3 Intraocular Gases; in Ryan JS (ed): Retina, ed 4. Amsterdam, Elsevier Mosby, 2006, vol 3, p 2167.

4 Reibaldi M, Longo A, Reibaldi A, Avitabile T, Pulvirenti A, Lippolis G, Mininni F, La Tegola MG, Sborgia L, Recchimurzo N, Sborgia C, Boscia F: Diathermy of leaking sclerotomies after 23-gauge transconjunctival pars plana vitrectomy: a prospective study. Retina 2013;33:939–945.

5 Rizzo S, Barca F, Genovesi Ebert F, Di Bartolo E: 27-gauge sutureless microincision vitrectomy surgery for a various retinal pathologies (poster; ID 5794-d0041). ARVO, Seattle, 2013.

6 Acar N, Kapran Z, Unver YB, Altan T, Ozdogan S: Early postoperative hypotony after 25-gauge sutureless vitrectomy with straight incision. Retina 2008;28: 545–552.

7 Hsu J, Chen E, Gupta O, Fineman MS, Garg SJ, Regillo CD: Hypotony after 25-gauge vitrectomy using oblique versus direct cannula insertions in fluid-filled eyes. Retina 2008;28:937–940.
8 Lincoff H, Coleman DJ, Kreissing I: The perfluorocarbon gases in the treatment of retinal detachment. Ophthalmology 1983;90:546–551.
9 Abrams GW, Swanson DE, Sabates WI: The results of sulfur hexafluoride gas in vitreous surgery. Am J Ophthalmol 1982;94:165–171.
10 Sabates WI, Abrams GW, Swanson DE: The use of intraocular gases: the results of sulfur hexafluoride gas in retinal detachment surgery. Ophthalmology 1981; 88:447–454.
11 Silicone oils: physicochemical properties; in Ryan JS (ed): Retina, ed 4. Amsterdam, Elsevier Mosby, 2006, vol 3, p 2199.
12 Williams RL, Day M, Garvey MG, English R, Wong D: Increasing the extensional viscosity of silicone oils reduces the tendency for emulsification. Retina 2010;30:300–304.
13 Silicone Study Group. Silicone Study report 1. Vitrectomy with silicone oil or sulphur hexafluoride gas in eyes with severe proliferative vitreoretinopathy: results of a randomized clinical trial. Arch Ophthalmol 1992;110:779–791.
14 Silicone Study Group. Silicone Study report 2. Vitrectomy with silicone oil or sulphur hexafluoride gas in eyes with severe proliferative vitreoretinopathy: results of a randomized clinical trial. Arch Ophthalmol 1992;110:792–805.
15 Silicone Study Group. Silicone Study report 3. Vitrectomy with silicone oil or perfluoropropane gas in eyes with severe proliferative vitreoretinopathy: results of a randomized clinical trial. Retina 1993;13:278–284.

Francesco Barca
U.O. Chirurgia Oftalmica
Azienda Ospedaliero Universitaria Pisana (AOUP)
via Paradisa 2, IT–56124 Pisa (Italy)
E-Mail barcaf@hotmail.com

Oh H, Oshima Y (eds): Microincision Vitrectomy Surgery. Emerging Techniques and Technology.
Dev Ophthalmol. Basel, Karger, 2014, vol 54, pp 102–107 (DOI: 10.1159/000360455)

Phacovitrectomy

Victor M. Villegas · Aaron S. Gold · Azeema Latiff · Andrea C. Wildner · Fiona J. Ehlies · Timothy G. Murray

Murray Ocular Oncology and Retina, Miami, Fla., USA

Abstract

Recent advances in vitreoretinal surgical technology combined with advances in small-incision cataract surgery have enabled the ophthalmic surgeon to provide combined management of cataract and retinal pathology. Progressive understanding of the inevitability of cataract progression after pars plana vitrectomy along with the negative impact of early cataract progression on visual acuity outcomes have defined the importance of combined cataract surgery and pars plana vitrectomy in improving surgical outcomes. Combining phacoemulsification with intraocular lens placement with vitrectomy has now been shown to decrease visual rehabilitation time in patients with early/visually significant cataracts. These benefits are especially apparent when complex ocular pathology is present and clear visualization during surgery is needed. This report focuses on specific factors pertaining to combined surgery that include patient selection, mechanics of phacovitrectomy, and potential complications. The authors report that utilization of combined phacovitrectomy at their institution has had an outstanding success rate with 95% of the patients achieving 2-line or greater improvements in visual acuity within 6 weeks of surgery. Combined phacovitrectomy is associated with a significant reduction in overall healthcare costs that may become more important in this era of healthcare reform. Finally, rapid adoption of combined phacovitrectomy has occurred internationally, but remains delayed at most institutions in the USA.

Vitreoretinal surgery may be the most technically difficult of all ophthalmologic surgeries as it involves high-tech microsurgical skills to treat intricate pathophysiological mechanisms. The combination of phacoemulsification with intraocular lens (IOL) implantation and microincision pars plana vitrectomy has numerous advantages when complex pathology is present. Multiple authors have described the therapeutic benefits of combined phacovitrectomy, including decreased macular edema, decreased postsurgical vitreous traction, optimized visualization of the posterior segment, and decreased amount of total surgical procedures [1–8].

Phacoemulsification following vitrectomy carries increased risks of posterior capsular tears, zonular dialysis, and loss of lens particles posteriorly [9]. Combining phacoemulsification with vitrectomy speeds visual rehabilitation and decreases the risks and costs associated with a second surgery. This chapter will describe the preferred surgical techniques used by the authors during microincision phacovitrectomy including relevant pathoanatomy.

Patient Selection

Patients with a visually significant cataract that needs maximization of visualization during vitrectomy are considered good candidates for combined phacovitrectomy surgery. Patients with preexisting, but early, lenticular changes who are likely to have visual loss due to cataract progression postoperatively are also excellent candidates. Young patients with clear lenses may not benefit from surgical management of the lens and may be observed after vitrectomy surgery.

Surgical Steps and Mechanics of Phacovitrectomy

A full understanding of the physical principles behind the surgical steps enhances the skills of the vitreoretinal surgeon. A discussion of the steps needed to perform a successful phacovitrectomy follows.

Dilation
Preoperative dilation with both a cycloplegic and sympathomimetic is performed. We routinely use 10% phenylephrine to achieve better visualization of the posterior pole during vitrectomy. Avoidance of long-acting cycloplegic drops may decrease the incidence of posterior synechiae [10].

Trochars
Transconjuctival, sutureless, trochar vitrectomy systems (23/25/27 gauge) have evolved significantly during the last years. Advantages of the 23-/25-/27-gauge systems include improved safety with fewer iatrogenic breaks, reduced operating time, less patient discomfort, less astigmatism, and enhanced visual rehabilitation. However, a single 20-guage sclerostomy may be required to remove intraocular foreign bodies and require the use of a fragmatome.

The advent of valved trochars has improved the fluidics of combined phacovitrectomy by preventing aqueous reflux through an open cannula. Difficulty introducing instruments such as the soft-tipped extrusion cannula through the valved cannula may be experienced. However, this may be managed by the use of the push-pull technique or displacement of the valved leaflets. The stabilization of the fluid dynamics during surgery outweighs any difficulties, especially in complex vitrectomized eyes.

We typically place the trochars at the beginning of surgery prior to phacoemulsification due to better globe stability (fig. 1). Alternatively, in Europe, patients undergo complete phacoemulsification with IOL placement prior to placement of the trochars. The infusion cannula is connected but kept off until the phacoemulsification portion of the procedure is completed to decrease posterior pressure on the posterior capsule. Early trochar placement permits the surgeon to perform a core vitrectomy in cases in which posterior pressure makes the anterior chamber uncomfortably shallow for safe lens manipulation. In cases of posterior capsule tear, it allows for rapid access posterior to the lens for added flexibility during surgery.

Sclerostomies
Conjunctival displacement maximizes that the conjunctiva and scleral wound do not overlap. The displacement of the conjunctiva is critical for the transconjuctival sutureless technique in order

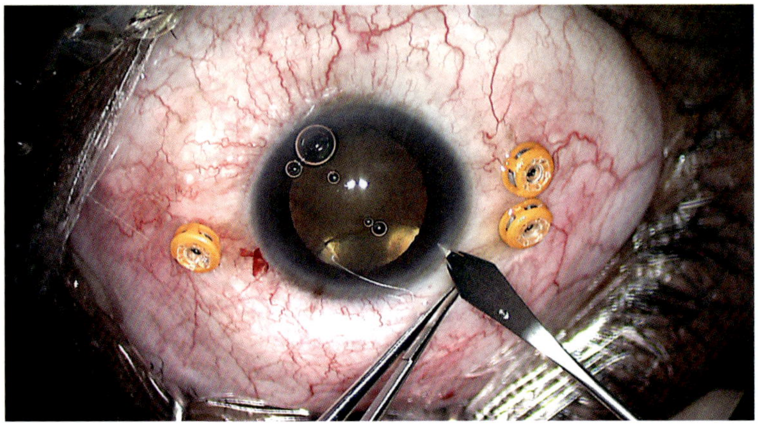

Fig. 1. Trochar placement before the start of phacoemulsification.

to decrease the possibility of having a vitreous wick in the incision site as well as to prevent access of the tear film into the sclerostomy. Furthermore, using an oblique trochar wound incision provides added incision stability and reduces postoperative hypotony.

Sclerostomies should be placed to avoid conjuctival scars, filtering blebs, and regions of abnormal pars plana. The placement should maximize the angle for intraocular access and comfort. The inferotemporal trochar should be placed just below the horizontal meridian to reduce the risk of touching the inferior eyelid when manipulating the globe to visualize the inferior retina.

Corneal Incisions
Corneal incisions (clear cornea phaco wound and paracenetesis) should be placed to maximize the surgical approach to the lens while taking into account existing trochar placement. Choosing the location of the corneal incisions at the steep axis of corneal astigmatism improves astigmatic postoperative correction. A biplanar clear corneal incision is preferred due to corneal wound stability. Closure of the phaco wound with 10-0 Nylon prior to the pars plana vitrectomy minimizes the possibility of iris prolapse and anterior segment instability. Patients without leaks and a biplanar incision can be left sutureless.

Capsulorhexis
The success of the planned phacoemulsification of the cataract is largely dependent on the continuous curvilinear capsulorhexis. We prefer a large capsulorhexis of approximately 6.5 mm to maximize the view postoperatively in patients at risk of developing significant posterior capsule opacification (fig. 2). However, a smaller capsulorhexis may be preferred, especially in cases of toric IOLs or if the posterior capsule is compromised, or a sulcus lens is planned.

Phacoemulsification
Phacoemulsification may be performed before vitrectomy in order to optimize the view of the posterior pole during subsequent vitrectomy. However, in cases where an adequate view is present, cataract extraction may be performed following the vitrectomy. In cases of vitreous hemorrhage, clearing the hemorrhage from the posterior segment in order to elicit an optimal red reflex may be beneficial.

Phacoemulsification should be performed at the iris plane when possible to minimize both corneal edema and posterior capsular breaks. We prefer to use a chop technique in order to minimize ultrasonic energy (fig. 3). However, phacoemulsification techniques vary widely and a sur-

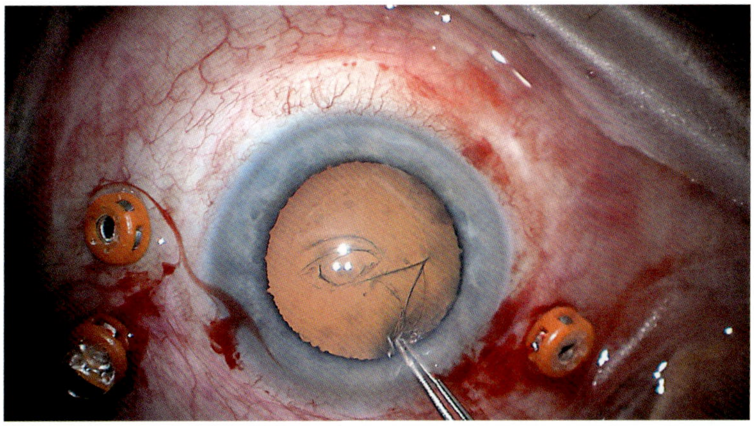

Fig. 2. A large continuous curvilinear capsulorhexis (approx. 6.5 mm) maximizes the view during and after surgery.

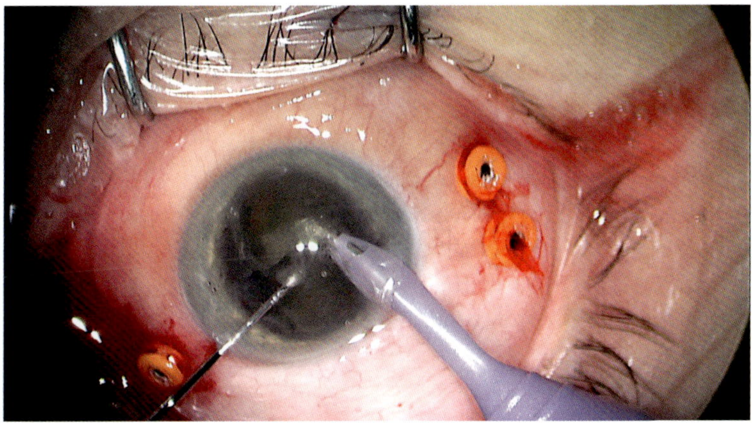

Fig. 3. We perform a chop technique to minimize energy directed towards the endothelium.

geon's choice on technique may vary depending on each patient's unique pathology. Posterior capsule integrity after nuclear and cortical extraction is critical to maximize the refractive outcomes.

Lens

The IOL can be inserted prior to vitrectomy or at the end of the case. The lens should be placed in the capsular bag unless there is any concern about an intact posterior capsule. Sulcus lens placement is recommended if a posterior capsule break is suspected.

Silicone lenses should be avoided. Silicone oil beads and condenses on the surface of the lens when intraocular silicone oil is present. Additionally, during fluid-air exchange, tiny droplets of fluid coat the exposed posterior surface of the silicone lens and impair the surgeon's view. Because of their physical properties, an acrylic IOL is the preferred IOL for most vitreoretinal surgeons.

In cases of severe proliferative vitreoretinopathy, extensive giant breaks, severe uveitis, and trauma, it may be beneficial to perform a lensectomy with capsulectomy to accomplish decompartmentalization of the eye.

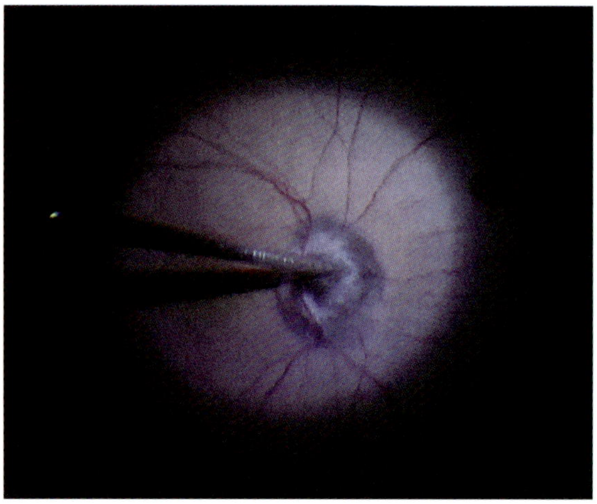

Fig. 4. Fine needle aspiration biopsy of an optic disc melanocytoma that has undergone presumed malignant transformation.

Vitrectomy

Pars plana vitrectomy techniques are tailored to each individual patient. In macular hole surgery, we peel the posterior hyaloid with the vitrector and the internal limiting membrane of the retina is peeled with internal limiting membrane forceps. Longer-acting gases (C_3F_8) can be used to tamponade the hole. During macular pucker surgery, the epiretinal membrane is removed and intravitreal triamcinolone acetonide is injected to treat coexisting macular edema. We perform scleral depression to remove anterior vitreous associated to traction allowing for thorough inspection of the peripheral retina. Any breaks discovered should be treated with a laser. In patients with active neovascularization undergoing vitrectomy, fill-in panretinal photocoagulation should be performed. Patients with posterior segment tumors should undergo release of all vitreoretinal adhesions. We biopsy posterior segment melanomas and atypical nevi after moderate endolaser has been applied for tumor treatment (fig. 4).

Complications

Visually significant opacification of the posterior capsule is the most common postsurgical event after combined phacovitrectomy [10]. In many patients with combined surgery for macular hole or diabetic retinopathy, significant posterior capsular opacification occurs within the first 2 months [11]. Other postoperative findings of combined surgery may include increased intraocular pressure, corneal epithelial defects, corneal edema, vitreous hemorrhage, and retinal detachment.

Conclusion

Utilizing combined phacovitrectomy at our institution has had an outstanding success rate: 95% of our patients have 2-line improvement at 6 weeks after surgery. We have had no cases of hypotony, endophthalmitis, or poor lens placement. The retinal detachment rate is 5% in patients with high-risk characteristics for retinal detachment.

References

1. Parke DW 3rd, Sisk RA, Murray TG: Intraoperative intravitreal triamcinolone decreases macular edema after vitrectomy with phacoemulsification. Clin Ophthalmol 2012;6:1347–1353.
2. Sisk RA, Murray TG: Combined phacoemulsification and sutureless 23-gauge pars plana vitrectomy for complex vitreoretinal diseases. Br J Ophthalmol 2010;94:1028–1032.
3. Jun Z, Pavlovic S, Jacobi KW: Results of combined vitreoretinal surgery and phacoemulsification with intraocular lens implantation. Clin Exp Ophthalmol 2001;29:307–311.

4 Lahey JM, Francis RR, Kearney JJ, et al: Combining phacoemulsification and vitrectomy in patients with proliferative diabetic retinopathy. Curr Opin Ophthalmol 2004;15:192–196.
5 Androudi S, Ahmed M, Fiore T, et al: Combined pars plana vitrectomy and phacoemulsification to restore visual acuity in patients with chronic uveitis. J Cataract Refract Surg 2005;31:472–478.
6 Soheilian M, Mirdehqhan SA, Peyman GA: Sutureless combined 25-gauge vitrectomy, phacoemulsification, and posterior chamber intraocular lens implantation for management of uveitic cataract associated with posterior segment disease. Retina 2008;28:941–946.
7 Lott MN, Manning MH, Singh J, et al: 23-gauge vitrectomy in 100 eyes: short-term visual outcomes and complications. Retina 2008;28:1193–1200.
8 Fine HF, Iranmanesh R, Iturralde D, et al: Outcomes of 77 consecutive cases of 23-gauge transconjunctival vitrectomy surgery for posterior segment disease. Ophthalmology 2007;114:1197–1200.
9 McDermott ML, Puklin JE, Abrams GW: Phacoemulsification for cataract following pars plana vitrectomy. Ophthalmic Surg Lasers 1997;28:558–569.
10 Demetriades AM, Gottsch JD, Thomsen R, et al: Combined phacoemulsification, intraocular lens implantation, and vitrectomy for eyes with coexisting cataract and vitreoretinal pathology. Am J Ophthalmol 2003;135:291–296.
11 Lahey JM, Francis RR, Fong DS, et al: Combining phacoemulsification with vitrectomy for treatment of macular holes. Br J Ophthalmol 2002;86:876–878.

Timothy G. Murray, MD, MBA
Murray Ocular Oncology and Retina
6705 Red Road Suite 412
Miami, FL 33143 (USA)
E-Mail tmurray@murraymd.com

Oh H, Oshima Y (eds): Microincision Vitrectomy Surgery. Emerging Techniques and Technology.
Dev Ophthalmol. Basel, Karger, 2014, vol 54, pp 108–119 (DOI: 10.1159/000360456)

23-Gauge Endoscopic Vitrectomy

S. Chien Wong[a–c] · Thomas C. Lee[d, e] · Jeffrey S. Heier[f]

[a]Moorfields Eye Hospital, [b]Royal Free Hospital, and [c]Great Ormond Street Hospital for Children, London, UK;
[d]Children's Hospital Los Angeles and [e]University of Southern California Eye Institute, Los Angeles, Calif., and
[f]Ophthalmic Consultants of Boston, Boston, Mass., USA

Abstract

Vitreoretinal diseases are exemplified by a wide spectrum of complexities. The purpose of this review is to highlight the potential role of endoscopic vitrectomy in modern microincision vitreoretinal surgery. This is related to the clinically relevant optical properties that are exclusive to endoscopy, namely the ability to bypass anterior segment opacities, visualization of difficult-to-access regions of the retina, the unique surgeon's perspective, and the use of reflected (coaxial) versus transmitted (dissociated) illumination. Indications for endoscopy include posterior pathology with limited-to-no view secondary to anterior segment pathology, difficult-to-assess retroirideal pathologies involving the sclerotomy, pars plana, pars plicata, ciliary sulcus, ciliary body, or peripheral lens, and complex anterior retinal detachments, particularly in pediatric vitreoretinopathies and anterior proliferation. The recent advent of the 23-gauge endoscope significantly increases the utility of endoscopic vitrectomy, making it a potentially important part of the surgical armamentarium alongside conventional viewing systems.

Vitreoretinal diseases requiring surgery present with a wide spectrum of complexities. These range from the relatively uncomplicated, e.g. vitreous opacities and idiopathic epiretinal membrane, to the highly complex, e.g. severe penetrating trauma and rhegmatogenous retinal detachment (RRD), endophthalmitis, and tractional retinal detachment (TRD) secondary to diabetes, familial exudative vitreoretinopathy (FEVR), or retinopathy of prematurity (ROP).

In order for vitreoretinal surgeons to effectively manage the entire spectrum of the diseases, it is arguably necessary to have access to the full surgical armamentarium. Endoscopy is a unique complement to conventional operating microscope-enabled viewing systems (e.g. wide-angle systems), principally due to the unique surgical perspective and access to anterior pathology. The recent development of 23-gauge endoscopy significantly increases the utility of the technique in the current age of microincision vitrectomy surgery.

Instrument Development

The term 'endoscope' is derived from the Greek 'endon', meaning inside, and 'skopin', meaning to view. In 1934, Thorpe [1] developed the first ophthalmic endoscope, which had integrated forceps for intraocular foreign body removal, although this required a separate source of illumination. Shortly thereafter, an endoscope incorporating illumination was developed, although this measured 6.5 mm in width [2]. Visualization was through an eyepiece attached to the external tip of the endoscope. It took over 40 years before Norris and Cleasby [3] developed a 1.7-mm diameter endoscope for intraocular and orbital surgery. In the 1990s, 20-gauge endoscopes were developed for vitreoretinal surgery [4, 5], with the intraocular image projected onto an electronic monitor, as is the case with current technology. In a series of 23 eyes, Volkov et al. [4] demonstrated the feasibility of using the endoscope to circumvent anterior segment opacities and enable vitrectomy.

The general principle of the endoscope is that it acts as an optical conduit, capturing light through an objective lens at its distal end within the human body and transferring the image through an image relay system for viewing by the operator/surgeon. Currently, there are two different ophthalmic designs. The principal difference between the two available ophthalmic endoscope designs lies in the image relay system. GRIN, or gradient index lens systems, uses a short *rigid* housing, with the option of an eyepiece instead of a camera at its proximal end for viewing. The resultant greater light transmission and higher image quality is outweighed by the rather limited intraoperative maneuverability and field of view (FOV), and thus its widespread utility. Fiber optic systems are by far the most widely used, due to the key advantages of smaller diameter instruments and longer *flexible* fibers, culminating in greater maneuverability.

The Endo Optiks (Little Silver, N.J., USA) E2 or E4 fiberoptic systems are most commonly used. In 2011, the 23-gauge endoscope was introduced [6]. Other endoscopes, e.g. by FiberTech Co. Ltd (Tokyo, Japan), are less commonly available, particularly in North America and Europe. At the time of writing, FiberTech does not have a CE mark or FDA approval (pers. commun., Ogawa G and Maekawa Y, Fibertech Co. Ltd, Nov 17, 2013).

Endoscopes are available in 19, 20, and 23 gauge, and incorporate three functions into one probe, namely illumination, viewing, and laser [7, 8]. These functions are driven by a base unit containing a xenon light source, a charge-coupled device camera which captures the image from the fiber optics and projects it on a monitor, and an 810-nm thermal laser. The different gauge sizes determine the number of pixels, thus image resolution, as well as the FOV: 19 gauge = 17,000 pixels, 140° FOV, 20 gauge = 10,000 pixels, 110° FOV, and 23 gauge = 6,000 pixels, 90° FOV. The resolution and FOV of the 23-gauge endoscope suffices for the majority of cases, such as RRD, trauma, and endophthalmitis [9, 10]. In our experience, complex pediatric TRDs (e.g. ROP and FEVR) benefit from the additional resolution of 19-gauge endoscopes, facilitating more aggressive dissection of anterior and retroirideal membranes [7, 8].

Clinically Relevant Optical Properties

Three unique optical properties of endoscopy underpin its irreplaceable and complementary role in vitreoretinal surgery.

Bypassing Anterior Segment Opacities

The endoscope captures the intraoperative view directly from its location in the posterior segment, bypassing the anterior segment of the patient. This obviates the need for clear optical media, enabling potentially time-sensitive vitreoretinal surgery in cases with anterior segment pathology, e.g. RRD in the context of cornea opacity in trauma, endophthalmitis, or anterior segment dysgenesis.

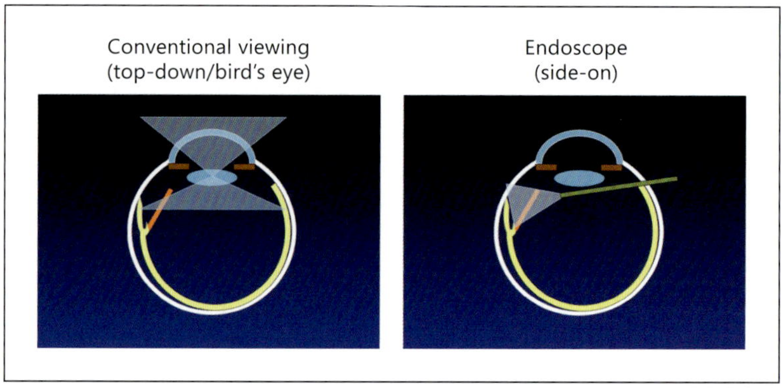

Fig. 1. Surgeon's perspective: illustrative comparison between a conventional top-down (bird's eye) wide-angle viewing system and an endoscopic side-on view, i.e. 90° apart.

Surgeon's Perspective

The unique surgeon's perspective stems from the point at which the intraoperative view is captured, i.e. at the tip of the endoscope close to a sclerotomy versus over the top of the patient's cornea with an operating microscope with conventional systems (fig. 1). This equates to a side-on versus a top-down (or bird's eye) perspective. The side-on perspective conferred by the endoscope is advantageous in visualization of very anterior pathology and optimal visualization of anteroposteriorly orientated pathology.

Visualization of Very Anterior Pathology

Pathology in the space between the vitreous base and posterior iris cannot be visualized with conventional viewing systems. Endoscopy enables unobstructed and undistorted views of that space. The quality of the intraoperative view is identical whether at (1) the center or edge (i.e. no aberration) of the image circle of the endoscope, or (2) the posterior pole or immediately behind the iris, thus setting it apart from conventional viewing systems. Examples of its applicability include managing retained lens matter in the ciliary sulcus causing chronic uveitis [9], proliferative vitreoretinopathy-related ciliary body and cyclitic membrane formation causing ciliary body detachment and chronic hypotony, and anterior scleral penetrating injury causing secondary retinal and/or vitreous incarceration. Another instance is placement of posterior tube shunts. The endoscope allows visualization of the tube in its true position, without scleral depression which often distorts and/or hides potential problems (anterior and postirideal vitreous, residual lens material not visualized with conventional wide-angle systems).

Optimal Visualization of Anteroposteriorly Orientated Pathology

A classic example is TRD in ROP or FEVR, where the retinal detachment (RD) extends anteriorly towards the anterior hyaloid and lens, somewhat parallel to the patient's visual axis. Endoscopy enables visualization of the entire side profile and thus extent of the RD, as opposed to looking at the top edge of the RD with a conventional bird's eye view, thus facilitating safer and more effective tissue dissection [7].

Use of Reflected (Coaxial) versus Transmitted (Dissociated) Light

With endoscopy, illumination and viewing are coaxial, as the point of light emission and capture occur at the same endoscope tip in the vitreous cavity; light *reflects* off ocular tissues into the tip of the endoscope (fig. 2). On the other hand, with conventional viewing systems, illumination and viewing are dissociated, as the points of light emission (endoillumination in the vitreous cavity) and capture (operating microscope) are disparate; light within the vitreous cavity is *transmitted*

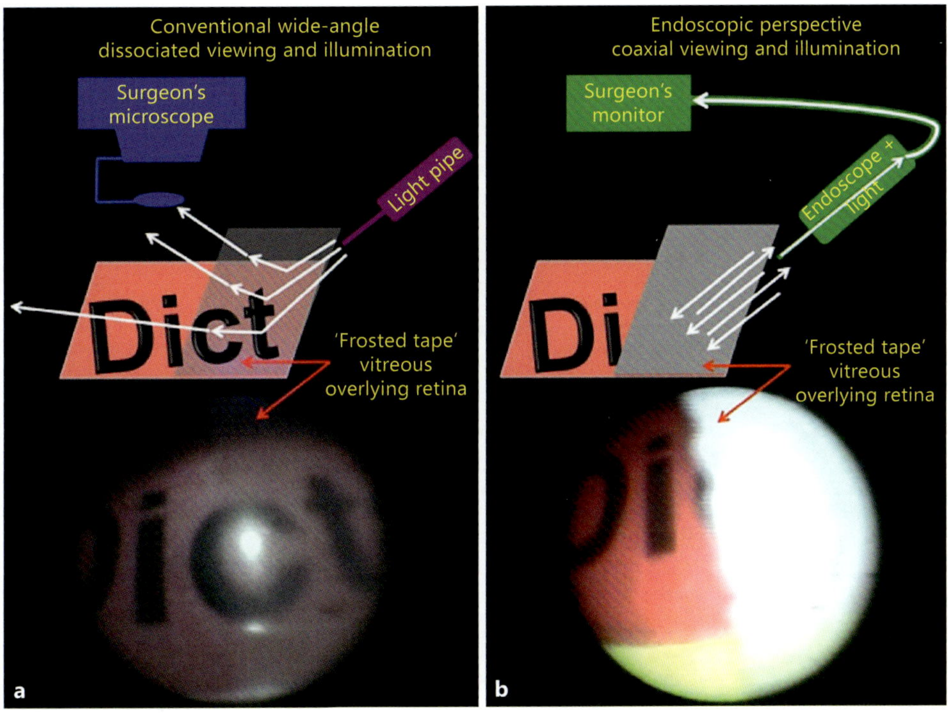

Fig. 2. Cellophane tape experiment simulating the view of the vitreous during pars plana vitrectomy, differentiating transmitted (**a**) from reflected light (**b**). **a** Conventional wide-angle microscope-enabled viewing perspective dissociates the surgeon's visual axis and source of illumination. Light is transmitted through the patient's clear vitreous. The vitreous appears largely transparent, as demonstrated by a good view of the underlying letters. **b** In contrast, with endoscopy, illumination and light capture are coaxial. Light is reflected back into the endoscope, making the vitreous appear more opaque, as demonstrated by the obscuration of the underlying alphabets. Image reproduced with permission from JP Brothers Medical Publishers [30].

through the patient's anterior segment into the operating microscope. This use of reflected light has been shown to make vitreous and membranes appear more opaque although it is otherwise transparent [7].

Clinical Application and Outcomes

Endoscopy has been shown to be efficacious in a wide range of vitreoretinal disorders [9, 11–25]. Table 1 summarizes the outcomes of a number of cases series, with study numbers ranging from 9 to 74. Case reports have been excluded.

Indications for Endoscopic Vitrectomy

In general, any anterior vitreoretinal pathology that is difficult to access and optimally visualize using conventional systems may benefit from endoscopic surgery, whether in isolation or as an adjunct to conventional viewing systems [26]. Classically, endoscopy is used in the presence of significant *anterior segment opacity* such as corneal edema, corneal scarring, or 8-ball hyphema, which is sufficiently dense to preclude adequate visualization of the vitreous cavity using conventional viewing systems. Chun et al. [23] showed that endoscopy has advantages over temporary keratoprosthesis in the context of severe ocular

Table 1. Summary of studies on endoscopic vitrectomy for various indications

Author/s, year	Indication (n of eyes)	Endoscopic procedure
Uram [11], 1992	neovascular glaucoma (10)	ciliary body photocoagulation
Uram [12], 1994	RRD with anterior PVR (10)	PPV
Boscher et al. [13], 1998	retained lens fragments and/or posterior IOL dislocation (30)	PPV
Ciardella et al. [14], 2001	complicated proliferative diabetic retinopathy (9)	PPV
Hammer and Grizzard [15], 2003[a]	chronic hypotony (9)	PPV + ciliary body dissection
Sasahara et al. [16], 2005	IOL dislocation (26)	PPV + transscleral IOL sulcus suture fixation
De Smet and Carlborg [17], 2005	endophthalmitis with coexistent corneal opacities (15)	PPV
Sonoda et al. [18], 2006	subretinal fluid drainage during PPV for RRD (10)	subretinal fluid drainage
De Smet and Mura [32], 2008	RRD with media opacities (9)	PPV
Olsen and Pribila [19], 2011	sutured posterior chamber IOL implantation (74)	transscleral sulcus suture fixation
Tarantola et al. [20], 2011	uncontrolled chronic angle closure glaucoma (19)	PPV + pars plana tube shunt placement
Kita and Yoshimura [21], 2011	RRD with undetected breaks (20)	PPV
Sabti and Raizada [22], 2012	ocular trauma (50)	PPV
Chun et al. [23], 2012	ocular trauma: endoscopy (9) compared to temporary keratoprosthesis (8)	PPV
Heier [9], 2012	RRD (19), vitreous hemorrhage (4), chronic hypotony (5), severe endophthalmitis (2), uncontrolled glaucoma (3)	PPV + pars plana tube shunt (in uncontrolled glaucoma cases)
Ren et al. [24], 2013	Endophthalmitis and RD (21)	PPV
Wong et al. [25], 2013	complex RD in ROP (37): stage 4A (17), 4B (12), 5 (8) [5-CTRRD subgroup (5)]	vitrectomy using pars plicata or scleral limbal approach

PPV = Pars plana vitrectomy; PVR = proliferative vitreoretinopathy; CME = cystoid macular edema; IOL = intraocular lens; IOP = intraocular pressure; LP = light perception; FF = fix and follow; CTRRD = combined TRD-RRD. [a] This series used a GRIN type endoscope; all other series were performed with fiber optic endoscopes.

Result/s	Follow-up, months	Complications (n of eyes)
90% with IOP <21 mm Hg	9	none
60% retinal reattachment	9	none
63% final visual acuity ≥20/40	21	retinal tear (2), CME (2), RD (2)
75% visual improvement	11	retinal tear (1)
67% postoperative IOP >5 mm Hg	not available	none
96% stable or improved visual acuity 0% postoperative IOL dislocation 0% CME	≥3	IOP elevation (1)
100% final retinal reattachment 100% stable or improved vision	≥6	RD (2)
100% retinal reattachment	6	transient retinal heme (2)
89% retinal reattachment 100% stable or improved visual acuity	11	RD (1)
4% IOL decentration 0.7 logMAR (children) and 0.6 logMAR (adult) average postoperative visual acuity improvement	29	IOP elevation (11); corneal decompensation (6); transient vitreous heme (2)
significant reduction in IOP from 31.3 mm Hg to 11.4 mm Hg ($p < 0.001$) at final follow-up visit	62	phthisis (2), shunt retraction (1), shunt blockage (3), suprachoroidal hemorrhage (1)
breaks found in 19/20 (95%) eyes 100% retinal reattachment 100% stable or improved vision	24	none
82% visual acuity improvement 90% retinal reattachment	14	not available
endoscopy vs. keratoprosthesis: shorter time to surgery: median 14 vs. 38 days shorter surgical time: median 2.8 vs. 8.4 h anatomic success: 44% (4/9) vs. 25% (2/8), $p = 0.64$	6	failure: 0% (endoscopy) vs. 38% (3/8) (keratoprosthesis), $p = 0.082$
79% (15/19) retinal reattachment 100% (4/4) vitreous hemorrhage resolution 40% (2/5) hypotony resolution 50% (1/2) endophthalmitis resolution and recovery of hand motions vision 100% (3/3) successful tube shunt placement	not available	none
62% visual acuity better than LP	≥18	recurrent infection (2)
Anatomic: 68% (25/37) primary success (partial or complete reattachment) 80% (4/5) in stage 5-CTRRD 78% (29/37) qualified success (stabilization or reattachment) 100% (5/5) in stage 5-CTRRD Vision: 70% (23/33) FF or better 85% (28/23) LP or better 100% (5/5) LP for better in stage 5-CTRRD: 40% (2/5) LP, 60% (3/5) FF	37	phthisis (6)

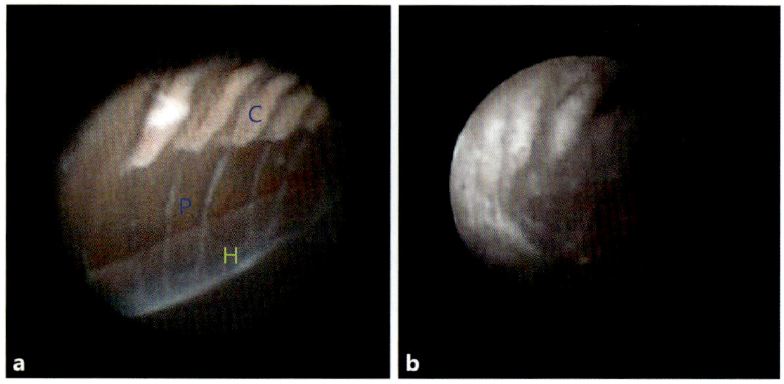

Fig. 3. a Intraoperative view with a 19-gauge endoscope. Child with aphakic glaucoma and RRD. Normal anterior anatomical structures are clearly visualized. C = Ciliary processes; P = pars plana; H = hyaloid (anterior hyaloid face). Note that the anterior hyaloid face is seen very clearly, due to the use of reflected rather than transmitted light. Image reproduced with permission from Lippincott Williams & Wilkins [31]. **b** Intraoperative view with a 23-gauge endoscope of an adult patient with a view of the pars plicata.

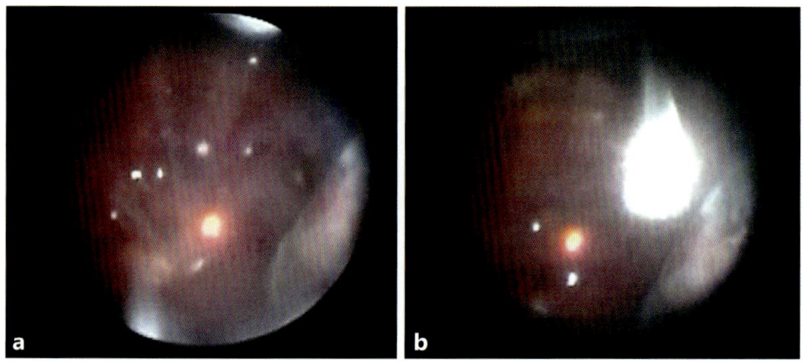

Fig. 4. Intraoperative view with a 19-gauge endoscope. In this case of RRD repair, vitreous became incarcerated into the sclerotomy port during perfluorocarbon liquid injection. **a** Vitreous can be seen as 'folds' from the inside of the sclerotomy, extending towards the edge of the image circle in this figure. **b** Following release of vitreous incarceration, there was immediate relief of traction and the 'folds' are no longer seen. Image reproduced with permission from JP Brothers Medical Publishers [30].

trauma (table 1). As patients were able to have surgery earlier (median reduction: 24 days), eyes that had endoscopy were less likely to have progressed to RD by the time of primary surgery. In addition, surgical times were shorter with endoscopy (median reduction: 5.6 h). Ben-nun [27] suggested that endoscopy can obviate the need for temporary keratoprosthesis, and thus a penetrating keratoplasty altogether, by enabling timely vitreoretinal surgery yet allowing sufficient time for the cornea to potentially recover.

Endoscopy's value is highlighted by enabling direct visualization of difficult-to-access areas of the posterior segment (fig. 3). In the ciliary sulcus, endoscopy can facilitate complete capsulectomy in uveitics (particularly children) during vitreolensectomy, and complete removal of retained lens matter causing chronic uveitis in pseudophakes [10], potentially ruling out chronic endophthalmitis and thus a more complex surgical procedure. At the internal lip of a sclerotomy, vitreous incarceration can, for the first time, be directly seen as folds emanating from the sclerotomy or trocar, enabling targeted and complete release by a vitrector (fig. 4). Endoscopy is also indicated in ciliary body and retroirideal pathologies, e.g. cyclitic membranes causing ciliary body detachment, chronic hypotony, and potentially phthisis bulbi. Additionally, it can be helpful for directly visualizing sutured haptics of malpositioned intraocular lenses at the pars plana or pars plicata, as these can be entrapped within significant fibrosis adjacent to the vitreous base (fig. 5); resultant traumatic haptic removal increases the risk of iatrogenic retinal break and detachment. Pars plana-based

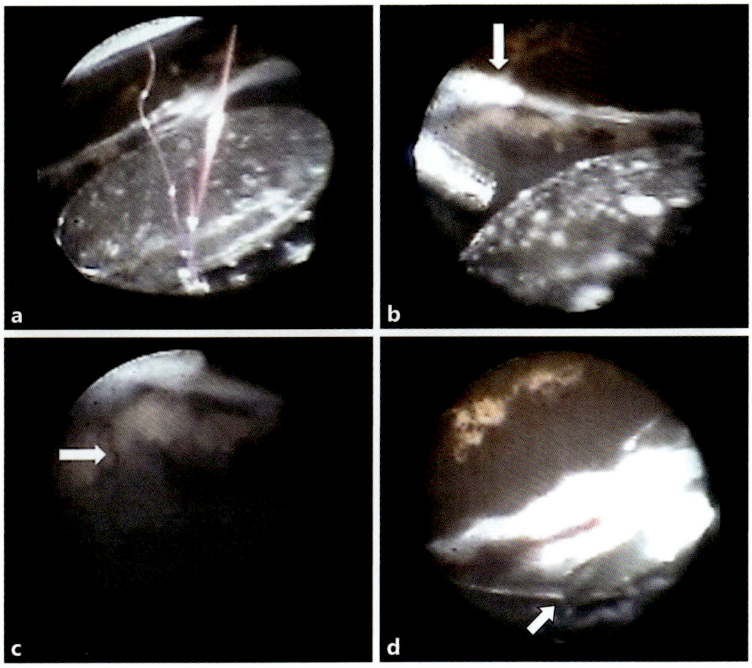

Fig. 5. Intraoperative view with a 19-gauge endoscope. **a** Case of a subluxed, opacified sutured sulcus intraocular lens. **b** During intraocular lens removal, the inferior haptic was encased in a tunnel of fibrosis (white arrow). **c** Close up view of fibrosis with attachment to retina posteriorly as evidenced by retinal vessels (white arrow). This increases the risk of creating a retinal break. The proximity of retina to the intraocular lens haptic could well have been missed by a conventional viewing system due to its very anterior position. **d** 23-gauge scissors were used to segment the optic-haptic junction rather than pulling it in one piece. Image reproduced with permission from JP Brothers Medical Publishers [30].

glaucoma shunts may be needed in advanced glaucoma. These frequently become occluded by vitreous or residual lens material despite careful vitrectomy around the site of shunt placement aided by scleral indentation. As has been mentioned elsewhere [10], indentation distorts the normal anatomy during vitrectomy, thus potentially masking any residual vitreous. Endoscopy enables direct visualization (without scleral indentation) of the undistorted vitreous anatomy with the shunt in place, enabling more precise and complete vitreous clearance.

Subretinal surgery is occasionally indicated to remove clinically relevant proliferative vitreoretinopathy bands (fig. 6), and less commonly choroidal neovascular membranes. The endoscope can be used to access these by tracking along the subretinal surface from a relatively small retinotomy at a remote site, facilitating more thorough removal of pathology (fig. 6).

Endoscopy is advantageous to conventional viewing systems when clear corneal trocar placement is necessary. Specifically, with conventional viewing systems, the viewing lens (contact or non-contact, e.g. BIOM) can obstruct the maneuverability of vertically positioned instruments when manipulation of posterior pathology is required. Endoscopy circumvents this problem as the lens and image relay system are within the endoscope itself. Clinical indications for clear corneal vitrectomy include significant scleromalacia, history of necrotizing scleritis, total TRD in ROP or FEVR, and RD in retinoblastoma-treated eyes [28], precluding safe posterior segment trocar placement.

Endoscopic cyclophotocoagulation (ECP) is typically used from an anterior segment approach, with or without cataract surgery, to laser ablate ciliary processes to achieve long-term reduction in intraocular pressure [29]. In cases of highly refractory glaucoma, more extensive ECP, also known as 'ECP plus', can be performed from the vitreous cavity, extending laser ablation of ciliary processes from its posterior edge to the pars plicata.

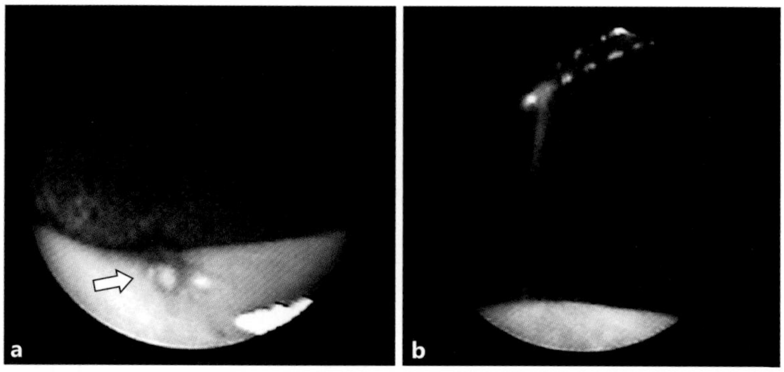

Fig. 6. Intraoperative view with a 19-gauge endoscope. A case of combined TRD-RRD with subretinal bands. **a** An underlying subretinal band was engaged posterior to the main arcades, a reasonable distance away from the edge of the limited 3-o'clock retinectomy. The endoscope enabled the surgeon to track posteriorly along the undersurface of the retina while avoiding the need to extend the retinectomy. Exposed retinal pigment epithelium is seen superiorly. **b** Subretinal band removed with the 23-gauge serrated forceps. Image reproduced with permission from JP Brothers Medical Publishers [30].

Pediatric Vitreoretinal Surgery

Endoscopy has been shown to have unique applicability in complex pediatric vitreoretinal surgery [7, 8, 25]. Highly elevated pediatric vitreoretinal pathologies can occur, e.g. TRD in ROP or FEVR and posterior persistent fetal vascular syndrome, where the retina can be drawn up along the primary hyaloidal stalk. In the former, extensive retrolental plaque can preclude adequate visualization of the underlying retina, complicated by multiple undulating retinal folds. In the latter, it can be difficult to identify where a dragged retina ends along the hyaloidal stalk, which is essential for safe transection of the stalk. Endoscopy can circumvent both of these problems by enabling direct visualization of the peaks and troughs of retinal folds under retrolental plaques, and revealing the entire side profile of a hyaloidal stalk and its relationship to the retina, respectively (fig. 7). Pediatric TRDs can extend anteriorly, very close to the lens and pars plicata, with a high risk of iatrogenic retinal break or lens trauma during sclerotomy formation with a blade. Endoscopy can directly guide the safe passage of a sclerotomy blade (fig. 8).

Surgical Technique and Pearls and Pitfalls

Setup

A standard 3-port technique is used. The Endo Optiks 23-gauge endoscope can be inserted through a standard trocar system. If higher resolution is necessary (e.g. in pediatric TRDs), 19- or 20-gauge endoscopes can be used. Assuming the surgeon is positioned at the head of the patient, the endoscope base unit and adjoining LCD monitor are placed immediately adjacent to the side of the bed anywhere along its length at a point that is most conveniently within the line of sight of the surgeon. This gives the surgeon access to both viewing systems only requiring a slight turn of the head to switch between the operating microscope and LCD monitor.

Pearls and Pitfalls

Leveling the Image

Before inserting the endoscope into the eye, ensure that the image on the LCD screen is level by rotating the proximal (base unit) end of the endoscope. Focus the on-screen image by rotating the adjacent black collar.

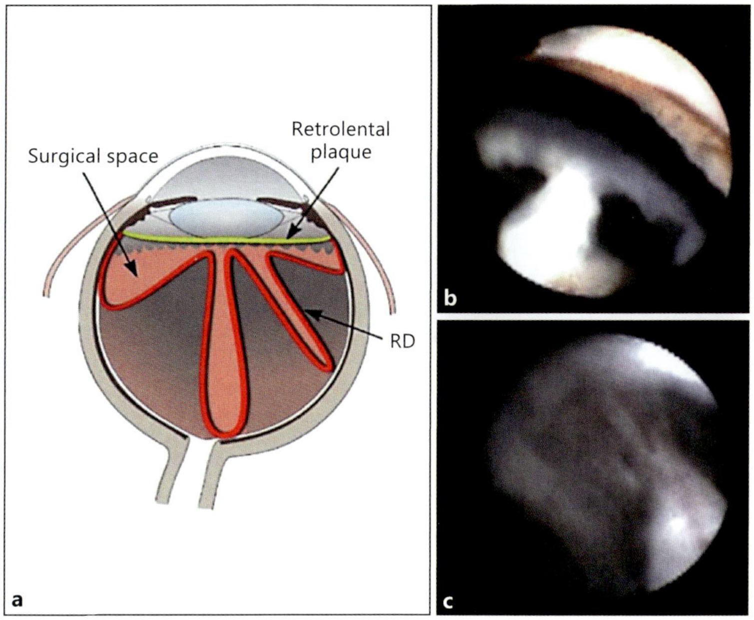

Fig. 7. Intraoperative view with a 19-gauge endoscope. **a** Illustration of total TRD in the setting of FEVR or ROP showing anteroposterior orientation of the TRD. **b** A case of total TRD from FEVR showing a top-down view of the retrolental plaque; it is difficult to visualize and address the TRD with conventional wide-angle viewing systems. **c** In the same case, a side-on view enabled by the endoscope, bypassing the retrolental plaque. The underlying fibrovascular membranes and extensive TRD can be appreciated. Image reproduced with permission from JP Brothers Medical Publishers [30].

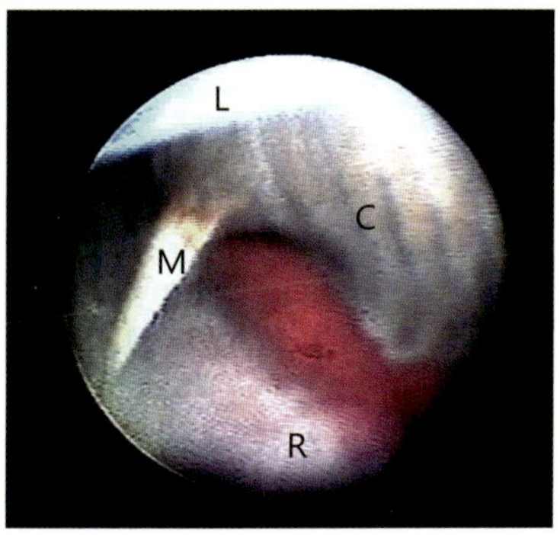

Fig. 8. Intraoperative view with a 19-gauge endoscope. This is a neonate with stage 4B ROP (macular involving TRD). Anterior TRD is present. There is a much smaller space than normal for safe sclerotomy placement without lacerating the lens or retina due to an immature pars plana and anterior TRD. L = Lens; M = MVR blade (20 gauge); C = ciliary processes; R = retina. Image reproduced with permission from Lippincott Williams & Wilkins [31].

Optimizing the Intraocular Image

Orientation. One of the main challenges in the initial learning curve is staying orientated within the surgical field. The key to success is a critical awareness of rotation of the endoscope, which is in contradistinction to conventional viewing systems where rotation of the illumination probe is largely irrelevant. Maintaining orientation inside the eye at all times reduces the risk of inadvertent iatrogenic ocular trauma and optimizes surgical manipulation. The straight rather than curved endoscope probe is preferred, as the latter adds a further axis of rotation which can be quite disorientating. Begin with an extraocular view of the globe in a vertical position prior to entry (such that you are looking at the eye from the side with the corneal apex being the highest point on the screen). Immediately upon entering the vitreous cavity, orientate the on-screen view such that the patient's lens is at the top (12-o'clock position), with the iris-lens diaphragm on a horizontal plane. This is useful for maintaining orientation when manipulating the anterior retina and adjacent structures. On approaching the posterior pole, keep the inferior or superior retina at the top of the screen, depending on surgeon preference; the former is the view we are accustomed to with conventional viewing systems. Do not hesitate to intermittently reorientate by seeking out the iris-lens diaphragm.

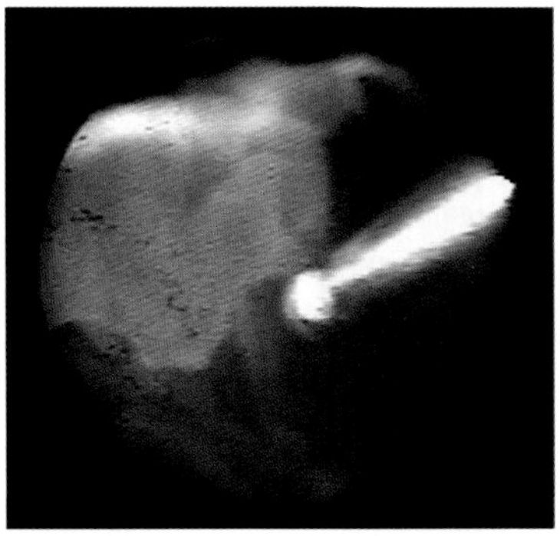

Fig. 9. Vitrectomy being performed in the safe zone of the center of the image circle with a 19-gauge endoscope.

Magnification. Magnification is a direct function of the distance of the endoscope from the point of interest. Due to the high magnification that is achievable, it is possible to fill the entire LCD screen with the image of the tip of a 23-gauge vitrector, i.e. a diameter no larger than 0.6 mm. In addition, one could be within 100 μm of the retina, or ciliary body, and be lulled into a false sense of security due to the image size. It is important to bear these in mind when manipulating vitreous and preretinal membranes (e.g. with vitreous cutter or forceps) close to the retina or uvea, as it is all too easy to get a false sense of security and distance from sensitive anatomical structures, potentially leading to iatrogenic ocular trauma such as a choroidal hemorrhage or retinal break.
Illumination. In contrast to conventional viewing systems, regular adjustment of illumination levels is necessary. The optimal amount of light required is heavily dependent on the distance between the point of interest and the endoscope. In particular, an image whiteout can occur with high illumination when close to a point of interest. Illumination intensity is adjustable via a dedicated foot pedal or at the base unit (assistant required).
Safe Surgical Zone. The on-screen image has a round border relating to the shape at the endoscope tip. The center of the image is the safest area for surgical manipulation, as one can fully visualize the surrounding structures along the circumference of the image circle. It is important to maintain the area of interest in the center by making small adjustments to the endoscope position (fig. 9). Surgical maneuvers at the edge of the image circle significantly increases the risk of inadvertent iatrogenic trauma at the edge or outside the FOV, thus potentially going unnoticed.
Overcoming the Learning Curve. The learning curve relates to three principal factors: (1) a lack of stereopsis, (2) dissociation between the surgeon's hand movement and the intraoperative view, as the surgeon is looking at an LCD screen rather than down at an operating microscope and directly at the surgical instruments, and (3) maintaining intraocular orientation (see above). In the first 10–20 cases, it is highly recommended to have both the endoscope and a conventional wide-angle viewing system set up, so as to enable one to quickly switch to the more familiar microscope to regain orientation and to learn other nonstereoscopic visual clues. It is thus preferable that the first cases have clear optical media. Additionally (particularly if starting with cases with media opacity), gradually increase surgical movements and actions to facilitate technique adoption. It is also useful to practice in a wet-lab type setup with an artificial eye (to avoid cross-species issues with animal eyes).

Conclusion

Endoscopy has a distinct role in vitreoretinal surgery that is complementary to conventional viewing systems. This relates to the unique properties of the endoscope, particularly the ability to bypass media opacities, the vastly different surgeon's perspective, and the ability to visualize areas of the eye that may not be possible with conventional viewing systems. With the recent advent of 23-gauge endoscopy, this technique is undoubtedly a valuable addition to the modern microincision vitreoretinal armamentarium.

References

1 Thorpe HE: Ocular endoscope. An instrument for the removal of intravitreous nonmagnetic foreign bodies. Trans Am Acad Ophthalmol Otolaryngol 1934; 39:422–424.
2 Thorpe HE: Nonmagnetic intraocular foreign bodies. JAMA 1945;127:197–204.
3 Norris JL, Cleasby GW: An endoscope for ophthalmology. Am J Ophthalmol 1978;85:420–422.
4 Volkov VV, Danilov AV, Vassin LN, et al: Flexible endoscopes. Ophthalmoendoscopic techniques and case reports. Arch Ophthalmol 1990;108:956–957.
5 Eguchi S, Araie M: A new ophthalmic electronic videoendoscope system for intraocular surgery. Arch Ophthalmol 1990;108:1778–1781.
6 Endo Optiks I: Press release: Endo Optiks, Inc. develops triple-function 23 gauge laser endoscope. 2011.
7 Wong SC, Lee TC: Chapt 13; in Hartnett, ME (ed): Pediatric Retina. Philadelphia, Lippincott Williams & Wilkins, 2013, pp 125–130.
8 Wong SC, Lee TC: Endoscopic vitrectomy in children. Retina Times 2012;30: 18–20.
9 Heier J: 23-gauge endoscopic vitrectomy for complicated retinal diseases. Am Soc Retinal Specialists Annu Meet, Las Vegas, 2012.
10 Heier J, Chen C: Small-gauge endoscope facilitates difficult cases. Retina Today 2012, pp 56–58.
11 Uram M: Ophthalmic laser microendoscope endophotocoagulation. Ophthalmology 1992;99:1829–1832.
12 Uram M: Laser endoscope in the management of proliferative vitreoretinopathy. Ophthalmology 1994;101:1404–1408.
13 Boscher C, Lebuisson DA, Lean JS, et al: Vitrectomy with endoscopy for management of retained lens fragments and/or posteriorly dislocated intraocular lens. Graefes Arch Clin Exp Ophthalmol 1998;236:115–121.
14 Ciardella AP, Fisher YL, Carvalho C, et al: Endoscopic vitreoretinal surgery for complicated proliferative diabetic retinopathy. Retina 2001;21:20–27.
15 Hammer ME, Grizzard WS: Endoscopy for evaluation and treatment of the ciliary body in hypotony. Retina 2003;23: 30–36.
16 Sasahara M, Kiryu J, Yoshimura N: Endoscope-assisted transscleral suture fixation to reduce the incidence of intraocular lens dislocation. J Cataract Refract Surg 2005;31:1777–1780.
17 De Smet MD, Carlborg EA: Managing severe endophthalmitis with the use of an endoscope. Retina 2005;25:976–980.
18 Sonoda Y, Yamakiri K, Sonoda S, et al: Endoscopy-guided subretinal fluid drainage in vitrectomy for retinal detachment. Ophthalmologica 2006;220: 83–86.
19 Olsen TW, Pribila JT: Pars plana vitrectomy with endoscope-guided sutured posterior chamber intraocular lens implantation in children and adults. Am J Ophthalmol 2011;151:287–296.e2.
20 Tarantola RM, Agarwal A, Lu P, et al: Long-term results of combined endoscope-assisted pars plana vitrectomy and glaucoma tube shunt surgery. Retina 2011;31:275–283.
21 Kita M, Yoshimura N: Endoscope-assisted vitrectomy in the management of pseudophakic and aphakic retinal detachments with undetected retinal breaks. Retina 2011;31:1347–1351.
22 Sabti KA, Raizada S: Endoscope-assisted pars plana vitrectomy in severe ocular trauma. Br J Ophthalmol 2012;96:1399–1403.
23 Chun DW, Colyer MH, Wroblewski KJ: Visual and anatomic outcomes of vitrectomy with temporary keratoprosthesis or endoscopy in ocular trauma with opaque cornea. Ophthalmic Surg Lasers Imaging 2012;43:302–310.
24 Ren H, Jiang R, Xu G, et al: Endoscopy-assisted vitrectomy for treatment of severe endophthalmitis with retinal detachment. Graefes Arch Clin Exp Ophthalmol 2013;251:1797–1800.
25 Wong SC, Say E, Lee TC: Outcomes of endoscopic vitrectomy for retinal detachment in retinopathy of prematurity. Am Acad Ophthalmol Annu Meet, New Orleans, 2013.
26 Yonekawa Y, Papakostas TD, Marra KV, et al: Endoscopic pars plana vitrectomy for the management of severe ocular trauma. Int Ophthalmol Clin 2013;53: 139–148.
27 Ben-nun J: Cornea sparing by endoscopically guided vitreoretinal surgery. Ophthalmology 2001;108:1465–1470.
28 Lee TC, Wong SC, Say E: Outcomes of clear corneal endoscopic vitrectomy for vitreoretinal complications following retinoblastoma treatment. Retina Soc 46th Annu Sci Meet, Beverly Hills, 2013.
29 Francis BA, Kwon J, Fellman R, et al: Endoscopic ophthalmic surgery of the anterior segment. Surv Ophthalmol 2014;59:217–231.
30 Wong SC, Say E, Lee TC: Endoscopic vitrectomy; in Ho AC, Garg S (eds): Expert Techniques in Ophthalmic Surgery, ed 1. Philadelphia, JP Brothers Medical Publishers, 2014.
31 Wong SC, Lee TC: Endoscopic vitrectomy. Endoscopy and endoscope-assisted vitreous surgery in infants and children; in Harnett ME (ed): Pediatric Retina, ed 2. Philadelphia, Lippincott Williams & Wilkins, 2013, pp 125–130.
32 De Smet MD, Mura M: Minimally invasive surgery-endoscopic retinal detachment repair in patients with media opacities. Eye (Lond) 2008;22:662–665.

S. Chien Wong
Moorfields Eye Hospital
162 City Road
London EC1V 2PD (UK)
E-Mail chien22@yahoo.com

Oh H, Oshima Y (eds): Microincision Vitrectomy Surgery. Emerging Techniques and Technology.
Dev Ophthalmol. Basel, Karger, 2014, vol 54, pp 120–125 (DOI: 10.1159/000360457)

Chromovitrectomy and Vital Dyes

Hiroshi Enaida[a, b] · Toshio Hisatomi[b] · Shintaro Nakao[b] · Yasuhiro Ikeda[b] · Shigeo Yoshida[b] · Tatsuro Ishibashi[b]

[a]Department of Ophthalmology, Saga University Faculty of Medicine, Saga, [b]Department of Ophthalmology, Graduate School of Medical Sciences, Kyushu University, Fukuoka, Japan

Abstract

It is important to secure visibility during microsurgery. In vitreous surgery, staining and peeling of the internal limiting membrane with vital dyes, such as indocyanine green, have been widely performed since 2000, and surgical outcomes have improved in some vitreoretinal disorders such as macular holes and epiretinal membranes. It has been subsequently shown that triamcinolone acetonide is an adjuvant that is extremely effective for intraoperative vitreous visualization. In recent years, the term 'chromovitrectomy' has been used for performance of a vitrectomy using these surgical adjuvants for improved visibility. While there have been reports that an auxiliary chromovitrectomy with vital dyes is very effective, the question of retinal toxicity with use of these dyes remains. Therefore, a new safer vital dye, i.e. brilliant blue G, was developed and applied in clinical use. Chromovitrectomy using these adjuvants is an important technique that has low invasiveness and is very safe and very helpful in microincision vitrectomy surgery.

Intraoperative visibility is particularly important during detailed operations, such as peeling of the internal limiting membrane (ILM), and for sufficient vitrectomy. The ILM is (on average) 2.5 μm thick. It is a very thin and transparent basement membrane of Müller cells. In a vitrectomy, peeling of the ILM without any adjuvant requires a very high level of skill. The usefulness of ILM staining and peeling with indocyanine green (ICG) in macular hole surgery was reported in 2000 and the use of this method immediately spread throughout the world [1, 2]. It not only significantly improved the closure rate in macular hole cases, but was subsequently used in other cases of vitreoretinal disorders such as epiretinal membranes (ERMs) and diabetic retinopathy.

Fluorescein sodium was reported as being used in experimental staining of the vitreous in 1978 [3]. Although clinical application of this technique was eventually carried out [4], it did not become widespread. A new method of visualization of the vitreous using triamcinolone ace-

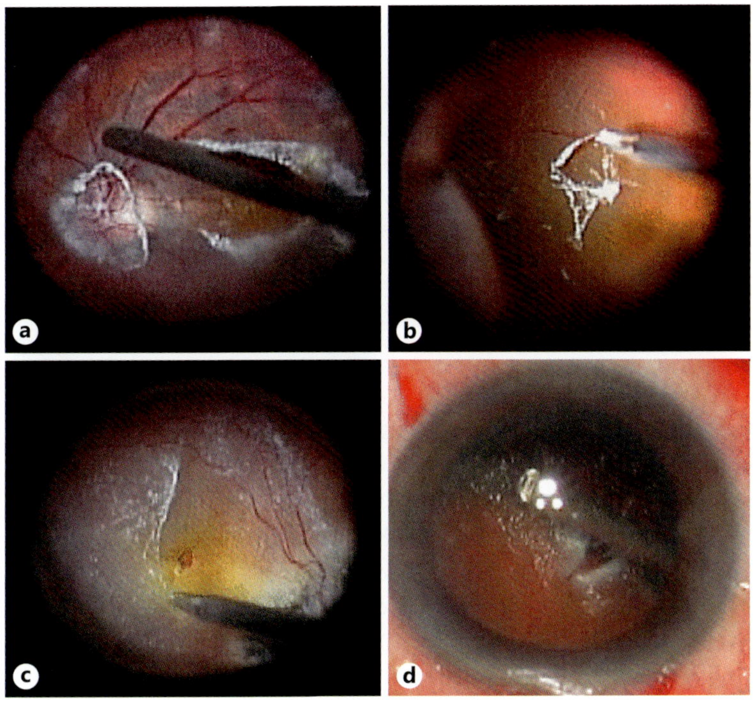

Fig. 1. Visualization of the vitreous with TA granules in MIVS. **a** Posterior vitreous detachment created by suction with a vitrectomy cutter using a TA injection in a diabetic macular edema case. The vitreous was satisfactorily visualized by TA granules and the surgical procedure was easily performed. **b**, **c** Moreover, the TA injection-assisted removal of the ERM or the residual posterior hyaloids was easily performed in cases with retinal detachment. In a peripheral vitrectomy, a TA suspension was injected towards the peripheral vitreous. **d** Visible TA granules on the peripheral vitreous were removed as thoroughly as possible by shaving with the cutter.

tonide (TA) was introduced in 2000 [5]. This technique was extended worldwide by Sakamoto and colleagues [6–10] after 2002.

In recent years, a surgical technique that involves visualization of the ILM and vitreous using various surgical adjuvants has been termed 'chromovitrectomy' [11]. Furthermore, chromovitrectomy has been recognized as an important surgical technique in microincision vitrectomy surgery (MIVS).

Visualization of the Vitreous Using Triamcinolone Acetonide

If a vitrectomy is insufficient, critical complications may result, such as proliferative vitreoretinopathy. When an operation with a low invasion system like MIVS is performed, it is important to perform an efficient positive vitrectomy. Improvement in the visibility of the vitreous is important for a short operation time. TA has been used to assist the visualization of the vitreous during vitrectomy [5, 6]. TA-assisted vitrectomy has been accepted as the primary course of treatment for various vitreoretinal diseases [5–10].

The general surgical procedure of TA-assisted vitrectomy is as follows. After a standard core vitrectomy is performed, a small amount of adjusted TA solution (MaQaid; Wakamoto Pharmaceutical Co., Ltd., Tokyo, Japan) is gently injected with a 27-gauge needle into the vitreous cavity. The vitreous is visualized by trapping the TA granules. Thereby, a posterior vitreous detachment can be performed easily (fig. 1a). The residual posterior hyaloid membrane and ERM-attached TA granules are removed using surgical microforceps (fig. 1b, c). Visible TA granules on the vitreous base are removed as thoroughly as possible by shaving with a high-speed cutter in retinal detachment cases (fig. 1d). When the vitreous base is shaved, more sufficient excision can be attained by repeated pouring of TA onto the vitreous base and peripheral vitreous.

Moreover, there is also the merit of a pharmacological effect with TA. TA is a water-insoluble steroid that inhibits various postoperative inflammatory reactions. Previous studies have reported good results following vitrectomy using TA for various vitreoretinal diseases such as refractory uveitis and proliferative vitreoretinopathy [8, 10].

Staining the Internal Limiting Membrane Using Vital Dyes

Alterations in the structure of the retina due to cellular proliferation may cause distortion of the ILM, leading to the formation of an ERM and macular hole. Removal of the ILM can successfully alleviate these vitreoretinal disorders; however, difficulties in visualization of the virtually translucent ILM can present technical challenges in this procedure. Staining of the ILM is therefore one of the most important developments in surgery for the treatment of vitreoretinal disorders. The development of ICG [1, 2] and trypan blue (TB) [12] staining has greatly facilitated the peeling of the ILM and ERM in the treatment of various vitreoretinal diseases.

The general surgical procedure of ILM staining with ICG is as follows. The prepared ICG solution is gently injected into the vitreous cavity and immediately washed out with a balanced salt solution. In cases with macular holes following the creation of a posterior vitreous detachment, the ILM is instantly stained a clear green. Following removal of the ILM using ILM forceps, the difference in the retinal surface color between the area from which the ILM has been removed and the surrounding area is clearly visible (fig. 2a). The stainability of the ILM with ICG can be very good, and it can also allow easy removal of the ILM. With this technique, the surgical outcomes have improved in some diseases [13, 14]. Moreover, this ICG staining technique has created a basis for the development of chromovitrectomy [11]. Drug approval has not been obtained for ICG, and, generally, it is used off-label.

TB differs in dyeing characteristics compared with ICG. Although the stainability of the ILM is inferior with TB compared with ICG, the stainability of the ERM is good [12]. TB can be used as a clinical application (Membrane Blue®; DORC, Zuidland, the Netherlands). However, numerous recent clinical and experimental reports have suggested that intravitreal injections of ICG and TB can cause retinal damage [15–20].

Other new dyeing agents are Patent blue (PB) [21] and bromophenol blue [22]. PB and bromophenol blue have the same dyeing characteristics as TB, and affinity over the ERM is high without any adverse effects. However, these adjuvants require additional techniques during the staining process, such as fluid-air exchange. PB can be used as a clinical application (Blueron®; Fluoron GmbH, Ulm, Germany).

Brilliant blue G (BBG) was introduced as a new surgical dye for ILM staining during vitrectomy in 2006 [23]. The stainability of BBG is very good for the ILM (fig. 2b), but not for the ERM or residual posterior hyaloids. The staining method with prepared BBG is the same as that for ICG and is very simple. Moreover, enhancement of the staining color tone of BBG becomes possible by sharp-cut filter insertion (fig. 2c, d) [24, 25]. Therefore, an improvement in visibility is obtained.

Many clinical studies using BBG have recently been performed in many countries. In these reports, BBG improved visualization of the ILM, enabled peeling, and allowed surgery to be performed successfully [26–30]. Furthermore, adverse effects induced by the toxicity of BBG have not been reported in previous clinical studies [26–30].

Since 2010, BBG could be used as a clinical application (ILM-Blue®; DORC; fig. 2e). ILM-Blue contains 4% polyethylene glycol. The dose of BBG

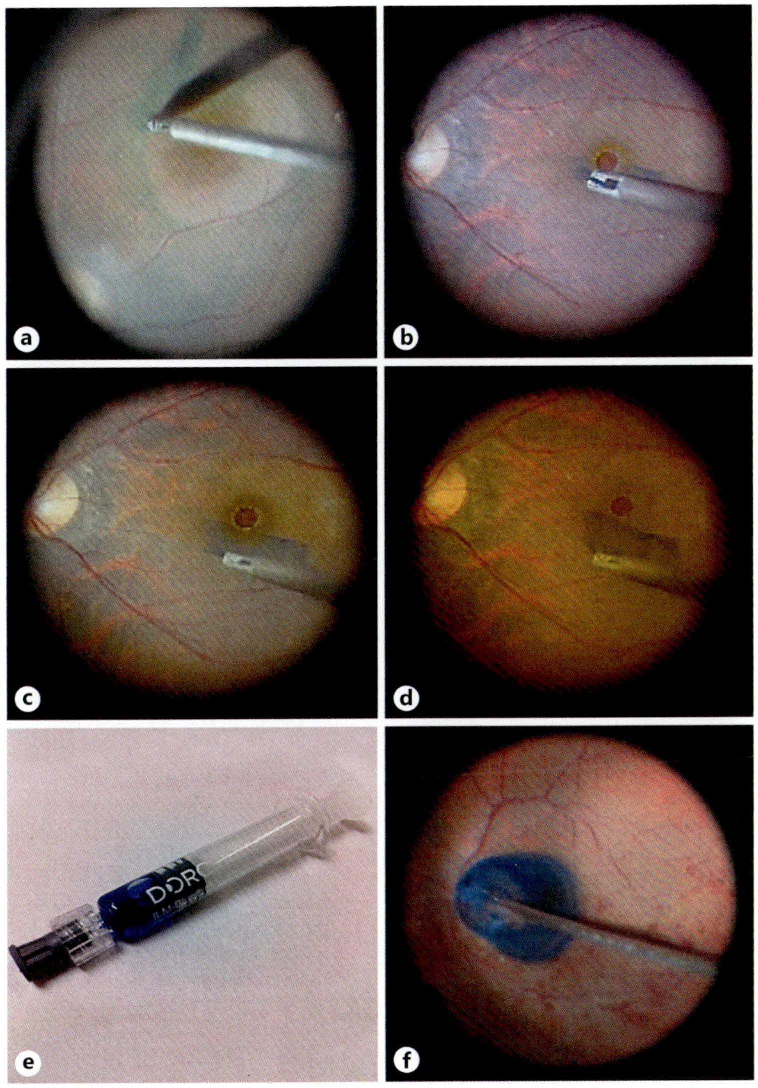

Fig. 2. Staining and peeling of the ILM with vital dyes. In cases with macular holes, the flap of the ILM was clearly visible during ILM peeling with ICG (**a**; Courtesy of Kazuaki Kadonosono, MD) and BBG staining (**b**). Moreover, there was an apparent color difference obtained with sharp cut filters in this case between the BBG-stained and non-stained areas (**c**, **d**) in the BBG staining case. Visibility was thereby further improved. The BBG-stained ILM was easily removed (**b–d**). **e** The formulation of BBG was performed by DORC as ILM-Blue. ILM-Blue was injected into the vitreous cavity. **f** Unnecessary BBG was prevented from diffusing to the interior of the eye because of the presence of 4% polyethylene glycol, which was easy to wash out after injection. This point also holds for ILM peeling in MIVS.

is 0.25 mg/ml. As a result, BBG is prevented from diffusing to the interior of the vitreous cavity (fig. 2f) and is easy to wash out after injection [31]. The amount of residual BBG in the vitreous cavity at the end of surgery is very small [32]. ILM-Blue is easy and fast to wash out, and is a very useful adjuvant in MIVS. Furthermore, the mixture of BBG and TB can also be used as a clinical application (MembraneBlue-Dual®; D.O.R.C.) and is widely used in the European Union.

Advantages of Chromovitrectomy in Microincision Vitrectomy Surgery

MIVS has become a standard type of vitrectomy globally. It is a safe procedure and the vitreous and ILM, including the vitreoretinal surface, can be observed satisfactorily during vitrectomy. Efficient surgery is attained with chromovitrectomy and the operation time is also shortened. The advantage of MIVS is therefore clear.

Some believe an even more effective surgical adjuvant can be developed and chromovitrectomy will continue to develop with MIVS.

Disclosure Statement

BBG/Hiroshi Enaida, Toshio Hisatomi, and Tatsuro Ishibashi are the inventors of patent application 'Staining composition for staining an ophthalmic membrane' (US7731941/EP1819366/4200222JP). Kyushu University holds the patent. Kyushu University licensed the patent of BBG to the bio-venture company, Aqumen Biopharmaceuticals NA Inc. (Fukuoka, Japan). Eventually, the license was granted to the Dutch Ophthalmic Research Center International BV (DORC) from Aqumen.

The remaining authors declare no conflicts of interest.

References

1 Kadonosono K, Itoh N, Uchio E, et al: Staining of internal limiting membrane in macular hole surgery. Arch Ophthalmol 2000;118:1116–1118.
2 Burk SE, Da Mata AP, Snyder ME, et al: Indocyanine green-assisted peeling of the retinal internal limiting membrane. Ophthalmology 2000;107:2010–2014.
3 Abrams GW, Topping T, Machemer R: An improved method for practice vitrectomy. Arch Ophthalmol 1978;96:521–525.
4 Yao Y, Wang ZJ, Wei SH, et al: Oral sodium fluorescein to improve visualization of clear vitreous during vitrectomy for proliferative diabetic retinopathy. Clin Experiment Ophthalmol 2007;35: 824–827.
5 Peyman GA, Cheema R, Conway MD, et al: Triamcinolone acetonide as an aid to visualization of the vitreous and the posterior hyaloid during pars plana vitrectomy. Retina 2000;20:554–555.
6 Sakamoto T, Miyazaki M, Hisatomi T, et al: Triamcinolone-assisted pars plana vitrectomy improves the surgical procedures and decreases the postoperative blood-ocular barrier breakdown. Graefes Arch Clin Exp Ophthalmol 2002;240: 423–429.
7 Enaida H, Hata Y, Ueno A, et al: Possible benefits of triamcinolone-assisted pars plana vitrectomy for retinal diseases. Retina 2003;23:764–770.
8 Sonoda KH, Enaida H, Ueno A, et al: Pars plana vitrectomy assisted by triamcinolone acetonide for refractory uveitis: a case series study. Br J Ophthalmol 2003;87:1010–1014.
9 Yamakiri K, Sakamoto T, Noda Y, et al: Reduced incidence of intraoperative complications in a multicenter controlled clinical trial of triamcinolone in vitrectomy. Ophthalmology 2007;114: 289–296.
10 Ueno A, Enaida H, Hata Y, et al: Long-term clinical outcomes and therapeutic benefits of triamcinolone-assisted pars plana vitrectomy for proliferative vitreoretinopathy: a case study. Eur J Ophthalmol 2007;17:392–398.
11 Rodrigues EB, Meyer CH, Kroll P: Chromovitrectomy: a new field in vitreoretinal surgery. Graefes Arch Clin Exp Ophthalmol 2005;243:291–293.
12 Feron EJ, Veckeneer M, Parys-Van Ginderdeuren R, et al: Trypan blue staining of epiretinal membranes in proliferative vitreoretinopathy. Arch Ophthalmol 2002;120:141–144.
13 Gandorfer A, Messmer EM, Ulbig MW, et al: Indocyanine green selectively stains the internal limiting membrane. Am J Ophthalmol 2001;131:387–388.
14 Haritoglou C, Eibl K, Schaumberger M, et al: Functional outcome after trypan blue-assisted vitrectomy for macular pucker: a prospective, randomized, comparative trial. Am J Ophthalmol 2004;138:1–5.
15 Enaida H, Sakamoto T, Hisatomi T, et al: Morphological and functional damage of the retina caused by intravitreous indocyanine green in rat eyes. Graefes Arch Clin Exp Ophthalmol 2002;240: 209–213.
16 Sippy BD, Engelbrecht NE, Hubbard GB, et al: Indocyanine green effect on cultured human retinal pigment epithelial cells: implication for macular hole surgery. Am J Ophthalmol 2001;132:433–435.
17 Uemura A, Kanda S, Sakamoto Y, et al: Visual field defects after uneventful vitrectomy for epiretinal membrane with indocyanine green-assisted internal limiting membrane peeling. Am J Ophthalmol 2003;136:252–257.
18 Gandorfer A, Haritoglou C, Gass CA, et al: Indocyanine green-assisted peeling of the internal limiting membrane may cause retinal damage. Am J Ophthalmol 2001;132:431–433.
19 Veckeneer M, van Overdam K, Monzer J, et al: Ocular toxicity study of trypan blue injected into the vitreous cavity of rabbit eyes. Graefes Arch Clin Exp Ophthalmol 2001;239:698–704.
20 Haritoglou C, Gandorfer A, Schaumberger M, et al: Trypan blue in macular pucker surgery: an evaluation of histology and functional outcome. Retina 2004;24:582–590.
21 Mennel S, Meyer CH, Tietjen A, et al: Patent blue: a novel vital dye in vitreoretinal surgery. Ophthalmologica 2006; 220:190–193.
22 Haritoglou C, Schumann RG, Strauss R, et al: Vitreoretinal surgery using bromphenol blue as a vital stain: evaluation of staining characteristics in humans. Br J Ophthalmol 2007;91:1125–1128.
23 Enaida H, Hisatomi T, Hata Y, et al: Brilliant blue G selectively stains the internal limiting membrane/brilliant blue G-assisted membrane peeling. Retina 2006;26:631–636.
24 Enaida H, Ikeda Y, Yoshida S, et al: Clinical evaluation and feasibility of changing intraoperative visibility with a novel viewing filter system for human eye. Retina 2013;33:1923–1930.

25 Enaida H, Yoshida S, Nakao S, et al: Improved brilliant blue G staining of the internal limiting membrane with sharp cut filters of a novel viewing filter system. Ophthalmologica 2013; 230(suppl 2):27–32.
26 Shimada H, Nakashizuka H, Hattori T, et al: Double staining with brilliant blue G and double peeling for epiretinal membranes. Ophthalmology 2009;116: 1370–1376.
27 Henrich PB, Haritoglou C, Meyer P, et al: Anatomical and functional outcome in brilliant blue G assisted chromovitrectomy. Acta Ophthalmol 2010;88: 588–593.
28 Schumann RG, Gandorfer A, Eibl KH, et al: Sequential epiretinal membrane removal with internal limiting membrane peeling in brilliant blue G-assisted macular surgery. Br J Ophthalmol 2010;10: 1369–1372.
29 Kenawy N, Wong D, Stappler T, et al: Does the presence of an epiretinal membrane alter the cleavage plane during internal limiting membrane peeling? Ophthalmology 2010;117:320–323.
30 Baba T, Hagiwara A, Sato E, et al: Comparison of vitrectomy with brilliant blue G or indocyanine green on retinal microstructure and function of eyes with macular hole. Ophthalmology 2012;119: 2609–2615.
31 Veckeneer M, Mohr A, Alharthi E, et al: Novel 'heavy' dyes for retinal membrane staining during macular surgery: multicenter clinical assessment. Acta Ophthalmol 2013, Doi: 10.1111/aos.12208, Epub ahead of print.
32 Enaida H, Kumano Y, Ueno A, et al: Quantitative analysis of vitreous and plasma concentrations of brilliant blue G after use as a surgical adjuvant in chromovitrectomy. Retina 2013;33: 2170–2174.

Hiroshi Enaida, MD
Department of Ophthalmology
Saga University Faculty of Medicine
5-1-1 Nabeshima, Saga 849-8501 (Japan)
E-Mail enaida2002@yahoo.co.jp

Oh H, Oshima Y (eds): Microincision Vitrectomy Surgery. Emerging Techniques and Technology.
Dev Ophthalmol. Basel, Karger, 2014, vol 54, pp 126–134 (DOI: 10.1159/000360458)

Pharmacovitrectomy

Rosa Dolz-Marco[a] • Roberto Gallego-Pinazo[a] •
Manuel Díaz-Llopis[b] • J. Fernando Arévalo[c, d]

[a]Department of Ophthalmology, University and Polytechnic Hospital La Fe, and [b]Faculty of Medicine, University of Valencia, Valencia, Spain; [c]Retina Division, Wilmer Eye Institute, Johns Hopkins University School of Medicine, Baltimore, Md., USA; [d]Vitreoretina Division, King Khaled Eye Specialist Hospital, Riyadh, Saudi Arabia

Abstract

Pharmacovitrectomy refers to a particular approach consisting of the intravitreal injection of drugs that can modify the anatomical and/or biochemical composition of the vitreous and retina. It constitutes a field in permanent expansion, particularly with pharmacologic vitreolysis and vascular endothelial growth factor inhibition.

The anatomy of the eye enables the retinal physician to access the vitreous cavity with minimally invasive techniques without significant damage to the ocular tissues. The development of intravitreal injections of a variety of therapeutic agents constitutes a field in permanent expansion. The term 'pharmacovitrectomy' refers to the possibility of inducing anatomical or biochemical changes in the vitreous or retina by using intravitreal injection of drugs that might complement or prevent a surgical vitrectomy. Among the different possibilities, the use of vitreolytic and antiangiogenic agents has been extensively studied and has become a very important topic in the field of pharmacovitrectomy.

The authors have no proprietary or financial interest in any products or techniques described in this article.

Pharmacologic Vitreolysis

The understanding of vitreoretinal interface anatomy and pathology has been dramatically transformed with the advent of optical coherence tomography [1, 2]. A clear example of this development is the new classification of vitreomacular adhesion, traction, and macular hole based on optical coherence tomography images [3].

Throughout our lifetime, several changes in the vitreous structure take place, leading to progressive vitreous liquefaction. These changes are associated with a concurrent weakening of vitreoretinal adhesion and may progress to partial or complete posterior vitreous detachment (PVD) characterized by the collapse of the vitreous body and separation from the retina [4]. Anomalous PVD results from vitreous liquefaction without concurrent complete separation of vitreoretinal adhesion. The abnormal development of PVD is involved in the pathogenesis of different vitreoretinopathies such as retinal detachment, macular hole, and macular pucker, and it may play an important role in proliferative diabetic retinopathy and age-related macular degeneration [5].

The treatment of vitreomacular tractional abnormalities has been widely reported, mainly with surgical procedures [5]. Sebag [6] coined the term 'pharmacologic vitreolysis' in 1998. Since then, several intravitreally administered agents activated against the molecular substrate responsible for vitreomacular adhesion have been used in animal models, but only a few have been tested in humans and those have been with variable outcomes. We may differentiate two mechanisms of action: liquefactant drugs (vitreous liquefaction) and interfactant drugs (dehiscence at the vitreoretinal interface) [7]. The main characteristics of the currently tested molecules are summarized in table 1.

The main benefits of enzymatic vitreolysis compared with pars plana vitrectomy (PPV) include the possibility to avoid conventional invasive surgery and thus the complications related to this procedure, and preservation of the vitreous gel inside the vitreous activity. On the other hand, the potential problems of enzymatic vitreolysis compared with PPV include variabilty of anatomical outcomes and efficacy limited to selected cases.

The two vitreolytic molecules with the best level of evidence are plasmin and ocriplasmin (formerly known as microplasmin). Autologous plasmin enzyme is a serine protease that hydrolyses a variety of glycoproteins including laminin and fibronectin, two major components of the vitreoretinal interface [8]. Collagen type IV, present in the internal limiting membrane, is not degraded by plasmin, thus allowing a separation of the posterior hyaloid without damaging the retina. It requires plasminogen to be activated.

Several pilot studies have reported the safety and efficacy of autologous plasmin enzyme in vitreoretinal adhesion pathologies (traumatic and nontraumatic macular hole [9, 10], retinopathy of prematurity [11], tractional diabetic macular edema [12], diabetic retinopathy [13], branch retinal vein occlusion [14], and X-linked retinoschisis [15]) (fig. 1–3). No enzyme-related complications have been reported.

The main limitation of autologous plasmin enzyme is that it is extremely unstable due to its inactivation via autolysis or by binding α_2-antiplasmin. In addition, as no commercial plasminogen is available, different publications have reported varied mechanisms for serine plasminogen obtention and activation of serine plasmin [7].

Ocriplasmin (Jetrea; ThromboGenics Inc., Iselin, N.J., USA) is the only drug approved to treat symptomatic vitreomacular adhesion syndrome. Ocriplasmin is a truncated form of the human plasmin obtained from microplasminogen produced in a *Pichia pasoris* expression system by recombinant DNA technology. Ocriplasmin has proteolytic activity against fibronectin and laminin, both present at the vitreoretinal interface.

The Microplasmin Intravitreal Administration in Patients with Vitreomacular Traction (MIVI-TRUST Study Group) phase III clinical trial showed positive results compared with placebo regarding PVD induction rate with resolution of vitreomacular adhesion and macular hole closure [16, 17]. In addition, best-corrected visual acuity (BCVA) was better in the group injected with ocriplasmin. Minimal adverse events (photopsias, floaters, and conjunctival hemorrhage) were reported. The results are summarized in table 2.

The future development of nonenzymatic agents may enhance the efficacy of pharmacologic vitreolysis without retinal damage. Furthermore, the usefulness of vitreolysis in patients with age-related macular degeneration and diabetic macular edema should be explored in order to improve the prognosis of these patients [18].

Table 1. Summary of the main characteristics of the current vitreolytic tested molecules

Molecule		Target	Mechanism	Trials	Results and Indications
Tissue plasminogen activator	serine protease	converts plasminogen into plasmin	liquefactant and interfactant	human models	postvitrectomy fibrin formation and subretinal hemorrhage; negative results regarding vitreolysis
Nattokinase	serine protease (produced by *Bacillus subtilis*)	fibrinolytic	liquefactant and interfactant	animal models	inconclusive results
Chondroitinase	protease	degrade chondroitin sulfate (glycosaminoglycan)	liquefactant and interfactant	animal models	negative results
Dispase	protease	cleaves fibronective, collagen IV and I	interfactant	animal and human models	positive PVD results, but important adverse events (lens subluxation, proliferative vitreoretinopathy, cataract, and retinal toxicity)
Hyaluronidase	protease	dissolves hyaluronan network of the vitreous gel	liquefactant	phase III clinical trial	efficacy of purified bovine hyaluronidase (Vitrase) in vitreous hemorrhage resolution; negative results regarding vitreolysis
Collagenase	protease (derived from *Clostridium histoliticum*)	cleaves collagen II vitreous network	liquefactant	animal and human models	reports of serious adverse events
Nonenzymatic agents (Vitreosolve)	urea-derived molecule	unknown	unknown	phase II/III clinical trial	45% of PVD induction with 1st injection (day 0); 75% of PVD induction with 2nd injection (day 30)
Autologous plasmin enzyme	serine protease	laminin and fibronectin	liquefactant and interfactant	animal and human models (pilot studies)	traumatic and nontraumatic macular hole, retinopathy of prematurity, tractional diabetic macular edema, diabetic retinopathy, branch retinal vein occlusion
Ocriplasmin (microplasmin)	recombinant form of a serine protease	laminin and fibronectin	liquefactant and interfactant	phase III clinical trial	symptomatic vitreomacular adhesion syndrome and macular hole

In this sense, both diabetic maculopathy and retinopathy may be influenced by the vitreous status. Although PPV has been used, certain cases may benefit from medical approaches that preserve the vitreous gel. The spectrum of vitreomacular interface disease in diabetic patients include a myriad of changes that should be differentiated as some are potentially treatable with vitreolytic agents, while others might not respond to this approach. Typical vitreomacular traction syndromes and thickened and taut posterior hyaloid membrane [19] constitute two examples that might benefit from a medical approach as the posterior hyaloid is

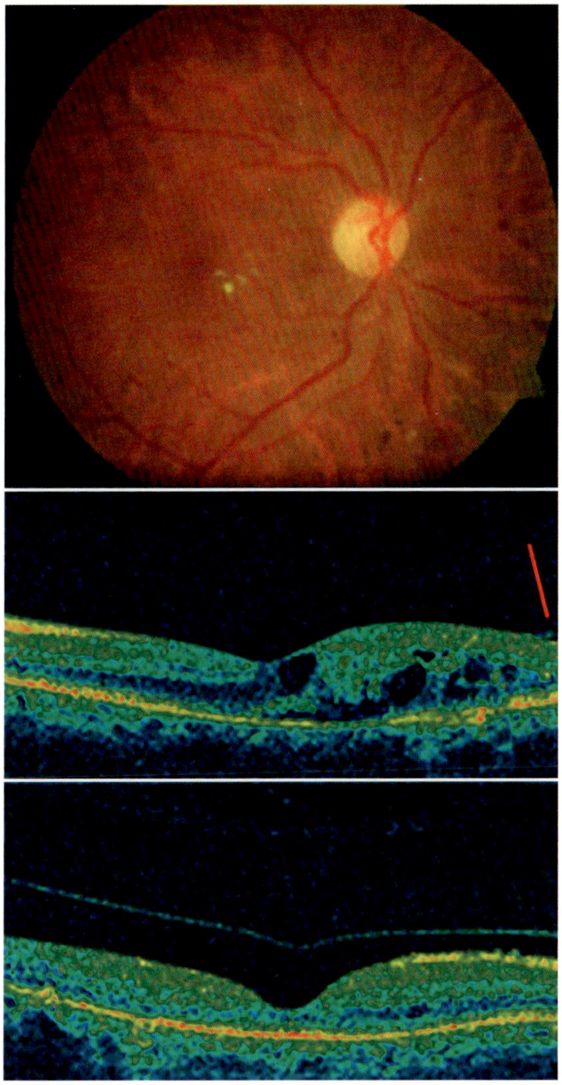

Fig. 1. Complete PVD and complete resolution of macular edema in a diabetic patient treated with autologous plasmin.

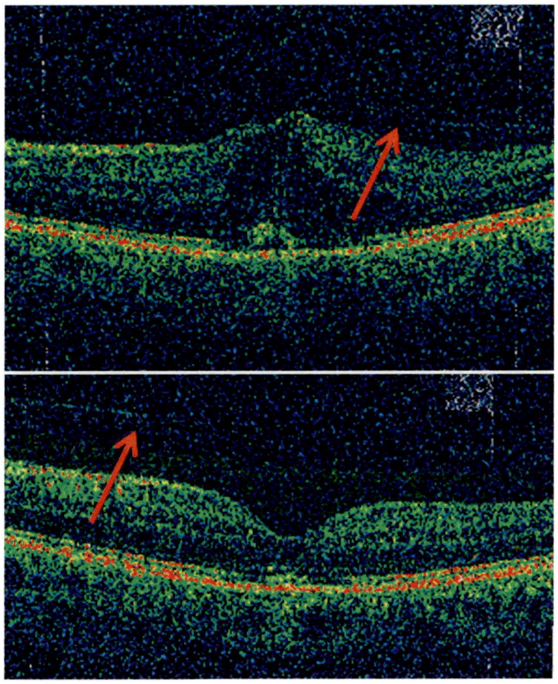

Fig. 2. Ocular coherence tomography showing a diffuse and refractory diabetic macular edema treated with autologous plasmin. The red arrows mark the posterior hyaloid before and after treatment.

the main cause of the anatomical disturbance of the macula. However, the indication of such treatment in the presence of epimacular membranes or postoperative taut internal limiting membrane [20] may result in complete failure as they are not directly related to hyaloidal traction.

Intravitreal Antiangiogenic Agents as an Adjuvant to Vitrectomy

Numerous publications have reported the clinical outcomes of intravitreal injections of vascular endothelial growth factor (VEGF) inhibitors, mainly bevacizumab (Avastin; Genentech Inc., South San Francisco, Calif., USA) as an adjuvant treatment to PPV in the management of proliferative diabetic retinopathy. These drugs can induce regression of the vascular component of fibrovascular proliferations [21–23]. On the other hand, this same effect can also induce development or progression of tractional retinal detachment (TRD) due to changes in the fibrovascular proliferation composition. El-Sabagh et al. [24] evaluated histopathologically the effects of intervals between preoperative in-

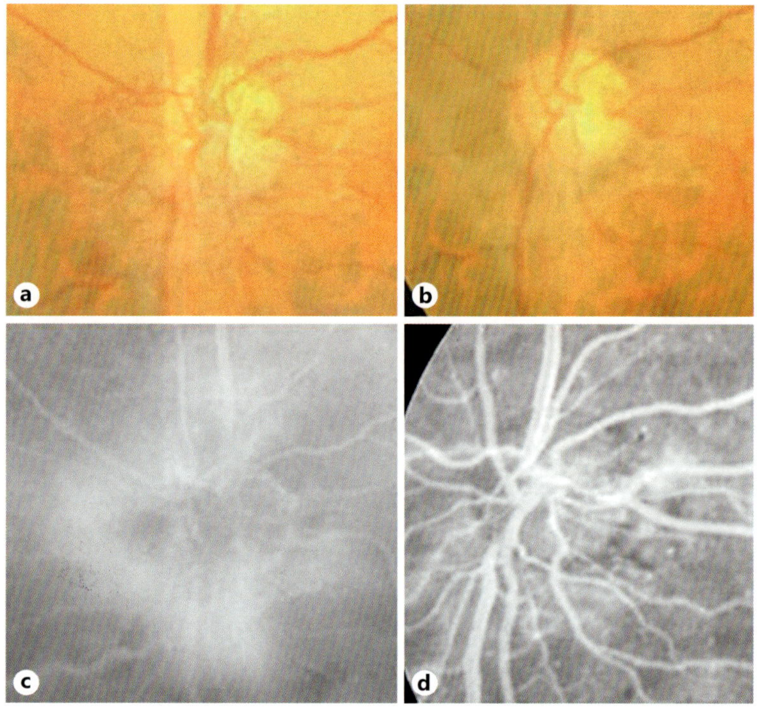

Fig. 3. Regression of the new vessels of the optic disc in a treated eye with plasmin. **a**, **b** Color images before and after treatment. Fluorescein angiogram shows the active vessels (**c**) and the important but not complete resolution of leakage (**d**).

Table 2. Summary of the main anatomical outcomes of the intravitreal injection of ocriplasmin reported in the MIVI-TRUST Study Group phase III clinical trial [17]

	Ocriplasmin, %	Placebo, %	p
Vitreomacular adhesion resolution	26.50	10.10	<0.001
Total posterior vitreous detachment	13.40	3.70	<0.001
Nonsurgical closure of macular holes	40.60	10.60	<0.001

travitreal injection of bevacizumab (IVB) and surgery on the components of removed diabetic fibrovascular proliferative membranes. They found evidence that a fibrotic switch in these tissues was induced following IVB, and that at approximately 10 days post-IVB the vascular component in the proliferation was markedly reduced, whereas the contractile components including smooth muscle actin and collagen were not yet abundant but nevertheless predominant.

A retrospective review by Arévalo et al. [25] provided evidence that 5.2% of eyes with proliferative diabetic retinopathy developed or had progression of TRD after IVB (fig. 4). The mean time from the injection to TRD was 13 days, showing a significant agreement with the results by El-Sabagh et al. [24]. Oshima et al. [26] found a significant progression in 18% of TRD as soon as 7 days after bevacizumab, whereas Pokroy et al. [27] also identified worsening of the TRD following bevacizumab in 8.8% of cases.

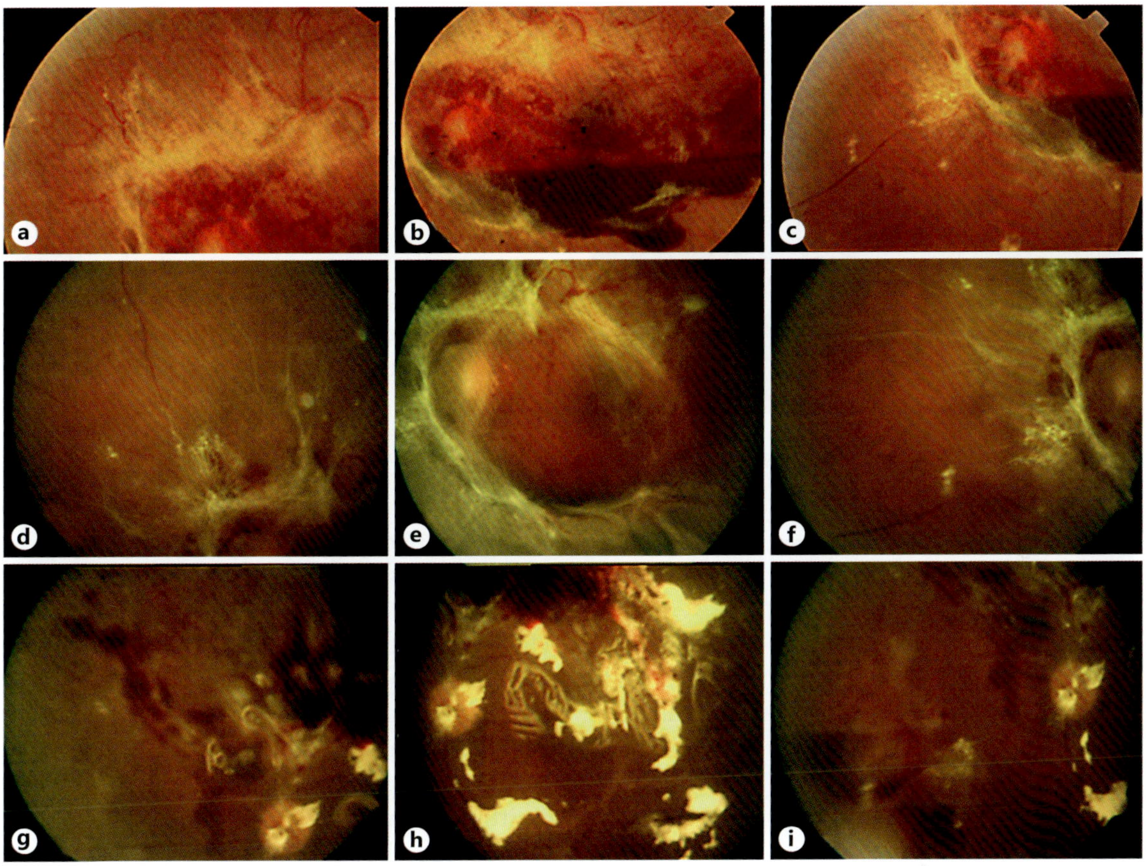

Fig. 4. a–c Color photographs before IVB. Severe proliferative diabetic retinopathy with abundant fibrovascular tissue and subhyaloid hemorrhage. The retina is attached and BCVA is 20/80. **d–f** Color photographs 10 days after 2.5 mg of IVB demonstrating dense fibrous tissue contraction, and TRD with macular involvement. BCVA is hand motions at 2 m. **g–i** Same eye, 8 days after vitrectomy. The retina is reattached and the BCVA is 20/120 with silicone oil tamponade.

Caution should be exercised in eyes with advanced PDR since a rapid involution of the fibrovascular proliferation may lead to the development or the progression of a TRD. Out of 698 eyes, Arévalo et al. [28] recently identified 25 (3.5%) that developed or had progression of TRD following IVB in eyes with PDR. Of the 25 eyes that developed or had progression of TRD, 19 (73%) received a dose of 1.25 mg (out of 626 injections: 3%), and 6 (27%) had received a dose of 2.5 mg (out of 72 injections: 8.3%). The mean time from injection to TRD was of 11 ± 7.5 days (range: 5–32). The short time between the injection and TRD suggests a cause-and-effect relationship. The earliest development or progression of TRD occurred 5 days after the injection. Timely surgery should be anticipated following IVB. Therefore, to be on the safe side, if bevacizumab is to be used as an adjunct to vitrectomy, surgery should be performed no later than 4 days after injection.

The mean baseline BCVA was a logMAR of 1.4 ± 0.7 (range: 0.2–2.9). At TRD development or progression, the mean BCVA dropped to a logMAR of 1.9 ± 0.6 (range: 0.3–2.9). This difference was statistically significant compared to

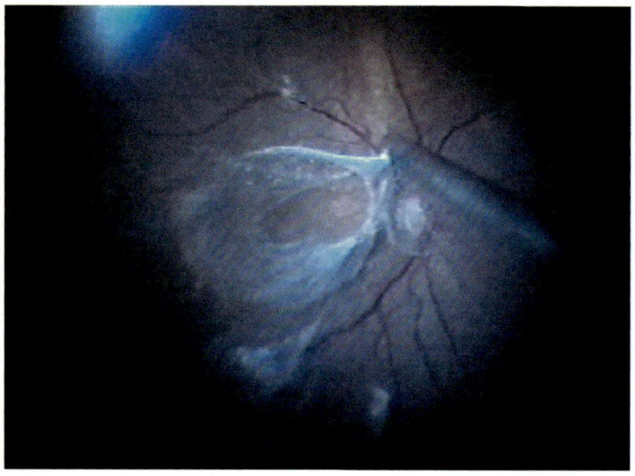

Fig. 5. The main indication for the use of intravitreal triamcinolone acetonide in vitreoretinal surgery is to better visualize the vitreous and facilitate PVD as seen in the intraoperative image during vitrectomy.

baseline BCVA (p = <0.0001). One patient developed a retinal break as a result of the increased traction, and a combined total tractional-rhegmatogenous retinal detachment was apparent 3 weeks after IVB.

Twenty-two eyes underwent vitrectomy. Vitrectomy was performed a mean of 18.8 ± 11.5 days after IVB. TRD was managed with vitrectomy, membranectomy, photocoagulation, and extended intraocular tamponade with gas in all patients that underwent surgery. The final mean BCVA after surgery was a logMAR of 1.4 (range: 0.2–2.9; mean ETDRS equivalent: 20/400, range: 20/32 to NLP), which was statistically significant compared to TRD BCVA (p = 0.012). Subgroup analysis of final BCVA after vitrectomy demonstrated that 12 (54.5%) out of 22 eyes improved two or more ETDRS lines of BCVA when compared to TRD BCVA.

In our study, risk factors for TRD after IVB included more than 15 years from the diagnosis of diabetes mellitus (p = 0.009; OR = 0.30; 95 CI: 0.10–0.83; RR = 0.35), more than 13 days from injection to vitrectomy (p = 0.0001; OR = 9.9; 95 CI: 3.4–29; RR = 6.9), and the use of a higher dose (2.5 mg) of bevacizumab (p = 0.022; OR = 2.7; 95 CI: 1.05–7.18; RR = 2.38) [28]. Despite this complication, intravitreal injections of VEGF inhibitors previous to PPV in patients with proliferative diabetic retinopathy have positively been shown to improve the following intraoperative and postoperative outcomes [21–31]: decrease in the incidence of intraoperative bleeding, decrease in the frequency of endodiathermy, decrease in the time of surgery required, decrease in the postoperative time of reabsorption of blood decrease in the incidence of recurrent vitreous hemorrhage, and improvement of final visual outcomes.

Intravitreal Triamcinolone Acetonide as a Coadjuvant to Vitrectomy

The main indication for the use of intravitreal triamcinolone acetonide in vitreoretinal surgery is to better visualize transparent membranes in the vitreous cavity and the retinal surface, such as vitreous collagen bundles and the internal limiting membrane or epiretinal membranes (fig. 5) [32]. The goal of achieving a complete removal of the vitreous and the posterior hyaloid membrane is essential in cases of proliferative vitreoretinopathies complicating a rhegmatogenous or TRD, and in epimacular membrane surgeries. On the other hand, following posterior capsule violation during phacoemulsification, the injection of triamcinolone acetonide in the anterior chamber may aid in visualization of vitreous and thus its accurate removal, resulting in decreased postoperative complications [33, 34].

Conclusion

Enzymatic vitrectomy performed by the intravitreal injection of autologous plasmin or ocriplasmin has been shown to be effective and can be considered a good alternative as the initial therapeutic option in diabetic patients before performing other treatments such as intravitreal injections of anti-VEGF or steroids, surgical vitrectomy, or laser. Further studies are necessary to assess efficacy and safety for a longer term and the most convenient therapeutic strategy, including association of treatments, in diabetic patients to get better and more permanent results. In addition, intravitreal injections of VEGF inhibitors before PPV in proliferative diabetic retinopathy constitute a beneficial approach, but the progression and development of TRD should be taken into account and the PPV scheduled 4 days after IVB to avoid further complications. Finally, triamcinolone acetonide may enhance the visualization of the vitreous and the posterior hyaloid facilitating their complete removal during PPV.

References

1 Bishop PN: Structural macromolecules and supramolecular organisation of the vitreous gel. Prog Retin Eye Res 2000;19: 323–344.
2 Stalmans P, Duker JS, Kaiser PK, Heier JS, Dugel PU, Gandorfer A, Sebag J, Haller JA: Oct-based interpretation of the vitreomacular interface and indications for pharmacologic vitreolysis. Retina 2013;33:2003–2011.
3 Duker JS, Kaiser PK, Binder S, de Smet MD, Gaudric A, Reichel E, Sadda SR, Sebag J, Spaide RF, Stalmans P: The International Vitreomacular Traction Study Group Classification of Vitreomacular Adhesion, Traction, and Macular Hole. Ophthalmology 2013;120: 2611–2619.
4 Le Goff MM, Bishop PN: Adult vitreous structure and postnatal changes. Eye (Lond) 2008;22:1214–1222.
5 Sebag J: Molecular biology of pharmacologic vitreolysis. Trans Am Ophthalmol Soc 2005;103:473–494.
6 Sebag J: Pharmacologic vitreolysis. Retina 1998;18:1–3.
7 Bandello F, La Spina C, Iuliano L, Fogliato G, Parodi MB: Review and perspectives on pharmacological vitreolysis. Ophthalmologica 2013;230:179–185.
8 Uemura A, Nakamura M, Kachi S, Nishizawa Y, Asami T, Miyake Y, Terasaki H: Effect of plasmin on laminin and fibronectin during plasmin-assisted vitrectomy. Arch Ophthalmol 2005;123: 209–213.
9 Margherio AR, Margherio RR, Hartzer M, Trese MT, Williams GA, Ferrone PJ: Plasmin enzyme-assisted vitrectomy in traumatic pediatric macular holes. Ophthalmology 1998;105:1617–1620.
10 Sakuma T, Tanaka M, Inoue M, Mizota A, Souri M, Ichinose A: Efficacy of autologous plasmin for idiopathic macular hole surgery. Eur J Ophthalmol 2005;15: 787–794.
11 Tsukahara Y, Honda S, Imai H, Kondo N, Fujii S, Yokoyama N, Hirata A, Kawaji T, Fukushima M, Tanihara H, Negi A: Autologous plasmin-assisted vitrectomy for stage 5 retinopathy of prematurity: a preliminary trial. Am J Ophthalmol 2007;144:139–141.
12 Sakuma T, Tanaka M, Inoue J, Mizota A, Souri M, Ichinose A: Use of autologous plasmin during vitrectomy for diabetic maculopathy. Eur J Ophthalmol 2006; 16:138–140.
13 Hirata A, Takano A, Inomata Y, Yonemura N, Sagara N, Tanihara H: Plasmin-assisted vitrectomy for management of proliferative membrane in proliferative diabetic retinopathy: a pilot study. Retina 2007;27:1074–1078.
14 Udaondo P, Díaz-Llopis M, García-Delpech S, Salom D, Romero FJ: Intravitreal plasmin without vitrectomy for macular edema secondary to branch retinal vein occlusion. Arch Ophthalmol 2011;129:283–287.
15 Wu WC, Drenser KA, Capone A, Williams GA, Trese MT: Plasmin enzyme-assisted vitreoretinal surgery in congenital X-linked retinoschisis: surgical techniques based on a new classification system. Retina 2007;27:1079–1085.
16 de Smet MD, Gandorfer A, Stalmans P, Veckeneer M, Feron E, Pakola S, Kampik A: Microplasmin intravitreal administration in patients with vitreomacular traction scheduled for vitrectomy: the MIVI I trial. Ophthalmology 2009;116:1349–1355.
17 Stalmans P, Benz MS, Gandorfer A, Kampik A, Girach A, Pakola S, Haller JA, MIVI-TRUST Study Group: Enzymatic vitreolysis with ocriplasmin for vitreomacular traction and macular holes. N Engl J Med 2012;367:606–615.
18 Jackson TL, Nicod E, Angelis A, Grimaccia F, Prevost AT, Simpson AR, Kanavos P: Vitreous attachment in age-related macular degeneration, diabetic macular edema, and retinal vein occlusion: a systematic review and metaanalysis. Retina 2013;33:1099–1108.
19 Thomas D, Bunce C, Moorman C, Laidlaw AH: Frequency and associations of a taut thickened posterior hyaloid, partial vitreomacular separation, and subretinal fluid in patients with diabetic macular edema. Retina 2005;25:883–888.
20 Gentile RC, Milman T, Eliott D, Romero JM, McCormick SA: Taut internal limiting membrane causing diffuse diabetic macular edema after vitrectomy: clinicopathological correlation. Ophthalmologica 2011;226:64–70.
21 Rizzo S, Genovesi-Ebert F, Di Bartolo E, Vento A, Miniaci S, Williams G: Injection of intravitreal bevacizumab (Avastin) as a preoperative adjunct before vitrectomy surgery in the treatment of severe proliferative diabetic retinopathy (PDR). Graefes Arch Clin Exp Ophthalmol 2008;246:837–842.
22 Modarres M, Nazari H, Falavarjani KG, Naseripour M, Hashemi M, Parvaresh MM: Intravitreal injection of bevacizumab before vitrectomy for proliferative diabetic retinopathy. Eur J Ophthalmol 2009;19:848–852.

23 Ahmadieh H, Shoeibi N, Entezari M, Monshizadeh R: Intravitreal bevacizumab for prevention of early postvitrectomy hemorrhage in diabetic patients: a randomized clinical trial. Ophthalmology 2009;116:1943–1948.
24 El-Sabagh HA, Abdelghaffar W, Labib AM, Mateo C, Hashem TM, Al-Tamimi DM, Selim AA: Preoperative intravitreal bevacizumab use as an adjuvant to diabetic vitrectomy: histopathologic findings and clinical implications. Ophthalmology 2011;118:636–641.
25 Arévalo JF, Maia M, Flynn HW Jr, Saravia M, Avery RL, Wu L, Eid Farah M, Pieramici DJ, Berrocal MH, Sanchez JG: Tractional retinal detachment following intravitreal bevacizumab (Avastin) in patients with severe proliferative diabetic retinopathy. Br J Ophthalmol 2008;92: 213–216.
26 Oshima Y, Shima C, Wakabayashi T, Kusaka S, Shiraga F, Ohji M, Tano Y: Microincision vitrectomy surgery and intravitreal bevacizumab as a surgical adjunct to treat diabetic traction retinal detachment. Ophthalmology 2009;116: 927–938.
27 Pokroy R, Desai UR, Du E, Li Y, Edwards P: Bevacizumab prior to vitrectomy for diabetic traction retinal detachment. Eye (Lond) 2011;25:989–997.
28 Arevalo JF, Sanchez JG, Saldarriaga L, Berrocal MH, Fromow-Guerra J, Morales-Canton V, Wu L, Maia M, Saravia MJ, Bareno J: Retinal detachment after bevacizumab. Ophthalmology 2011;118: 2304.e3–e7.
29 Yeh PT, Yang CM, Lin YC, Chen MS, Yang CH: Bevacizumab pretreatment in vitrectomy with silicone oil for severe diabetic retinopathy. Retina 2009;29: 768–774.
30 da R Lucena D, Ribeiro JA, Costa RA, Barbosa JC, Scott IU, de Figueiredo-Pontes LL, Jorge R: Intraoperative bleeding during vitrectomy for diabetic tractional retinal detachment with versus without preoperative intravitreal bevacizumab (IBeTra study). Br J Ophthalmol 2009;93:688–691.
31 Yang CM, Yeh PT, Yang CH, Chen MS: Bevacizumab pretreatment and long-acting gas infusion on vitreous clear-up after diabetic vitrectomy. Am J Ophthalmol 2008;146:211–217.
32 Couch SM, Bakri SJ: Use of triamcinolone during vitrectomy surgery to visualize membranes and vitreous. Clin Ophthalmol 2008;2:891–896.
33 Arbisser LB, Charles S, Howcroft M, Werner L: Management of vitreous loss and dropped nucleus during cataract surgery. Ophthalmol Clin North Am 2006;19:495–506.
34 Chang CJ, Chiang SY, Chen CL, Wang TY: Clinical outcomes of combined sutureless vitrectomy with triamcinolone stain to manage vitreous loss resulting from posterior capsule rupture during phacoemulsification. J Cataract Refract Surg 2006;32:2054–2059.

J. Fernando Arévalo, MD, FACS
Chief of Vitreoretinal Division
King Khaled Eye Specialist Hospital
Al-Oruba Street, PO Box 7191, Riyadh 11462 (Saudi Arabia)
E-Mail arevalojf@jhmi.edu

Oh H, Oshima Y (eds): Microincision Vitrectomy Surgery. Emerging Techniques and Technology.
Dev Ophthalmol. Basel, Karger, 2014, vol 54, pp 135–146 (DOI: 10.1159/000360459)

Suprachoroidal Buckling

Ehab N. El Rayes

Retina Department, Institute of Ophthalmology, Cairo, Egypt

Abstract

Purpose: To evaluate the feasibility of suprachoroidal buckling procedure using a suprachoroidal catheter, or cannula, as a new approach to treating different forms of retinal detachment, including myopic traction maculopathy, myopic macular holes, and peripheral retinal breaks by creating a suprachoroidal indentation (buckling effect) using a suprachoroidal filler. ***Methods:*** We used specially designed devices, guided in the suprachoroidal space to reach the target space (retinal tear). Then we injected a suprachoroidal filler (long-lasting hyaluronic acid) to indent the choroid creating a suprachoroidal buckle to close retinal tears and support the retina. This was done to both central (myopic macular) holes in areas of the staphyloma as well as for treating peripheral retinal breaks. This technique can be used alone or during vitrectomy. ***Results:*** In myopic patients, retinal layer restoration was achieved in all eyes with myopic foveoschisis. Of the 12 eyes, 10 with macular hole detachment (83%) showed closure of the holes in association with the resolution of the detachment; 2 eyes showed resolution of the detachment and flattening of the edge of the holes, but with incomplete closure on optical coherence tomography. Eight eyes (66.6%) showed improvement in visual acuity by one or more lines with no recurrence of retinal detachment over the 24-month follow-up period. The indentation effect was sufficient over the 24-month follow-up period. For peripheral retinal breaks, tears treated with this technique were all adequately buckled and closed from one procedure. A well-controlled location and support distribution of the buckle was possible through the suprachoroidal space. The buckling effect was enough to seal the tears and support the chorioretinal scarring time needed for tear healing. This also could be controlled by the filler duration time (filler type). The procedure was safe and relatively simple in reaching the treatment area and injecting it. ***Conclusion:*** The indentation effect achieved by the suprachoroidal approach can be used as a method for managing myopic foveoschisis and myopic macular hole with detachment even in eyes with failed primary vitrectomy, counteracting the role of posterior staphyloma in the role of the disease. This technique is also feasible for treating retinal tears, supporting the retina, and treating selected forms of retinal detachment including subsilicone inferior recurrent retinal detachment. It can be done separately or in association with vitrectomy procedures. It adds to our surgical options in treating selected cases of rhegmatogenous retinal detachment and avoids some potential problems of episcleral buckles as well as vitrectomy in selected cases of rhegmatogenous retinal detachment.

The use of scleral buckles in conjunction with chorioretinal adhesions around the break forms the basis of therapy for many cases of uncomplicated rhegmatogenous retinal detachment (RRD). Other techniques for repair include vitrectomy and a gas tamponade or repair by pneumatic retinopexy. RRD is repaired by preventing intravitreal fluid access to the subretinal space via retinal breaks [1]. Fulfilling this base, scleral buckling brings the retina into contact with the treated choroid around retinal tears [2]. This is done by indenting both the sclera and the choroid to the retina; in doing so, a mechanical ocular motility disturbance can happen depending on the size and location of the buckle placement. Although scleral buckling can be indicated for most primary RRDs, it may result in some vision-threatening complications due to the direct depression of the sclera with the buckle and/or the size and location of buckle placement, such as mechanical ocular motility disturbance secondary to an extraocular muscle imbalance, corneal contour changes, and chorioretinal circulatory disturbances [3–5]. Because the therapeutic concept of scleral buckling is to bring the retina into contact with the treated choroid around retinal tears, the sclera itself may not necessarily be involved in the indentation. Based on this idea, we have developed a novel technique called suprachoroidal buckling, which uses a specially designed catheter and cannula to inject and place a suprachoroidal filler [long-lasting hyaluronic acid (HA) solution] in the suprachoroidal space, indenting the choroid alone to close the retinal tear through the suprachoroidal space [6]. This filler, which indents the choroid and creates a suprachoroidal buckling effect to close tears or support the retina, can be used instead of suturing a scleral buckle. The indentation effect achieved with the suprachoroidal approach can also be used as an alternative to episcleral macular buckling for managing challenging myopic traction maculopathy (MTM). In this chapter, we introduce the procedure and discuss preliminary outcomes of suprachoroidal buckling for treating different forms of RRDs with peripheral breaks and challenging MTMs complicated with large staphylomas.

Suprachoroidal Space

The suprachoroidal space represents a potential transition zone in the choroid (inner boundary and scleral outer boundary). The space consists of collagen fiber, elastic fibers, fibrocytes, melonocytes, ganglion cells, and nerve plexuses. Bipolar and multipolar cells with some nerve filaments are also present, especially in the peripheral suprachoroidal space [7–12]. A total of two long posterior ciliary arteries and short posterior ciliary arteries enter the sclera approximately 3–4 mm from the optic nerve [13–18]. The long posterior ciliary arteries run anterior to the suprachoroidal space along the nerve in the horizontal meridian to branch near the ora serrata. The short posterior ciliary arteries pierce the sclera and continue a very short distance in the suprachoroidal space before entering the peripapillary choroid. The vortex veins draining the choroid are located 2.5–3.5 mm behind the equator (14–15 mm from the limbus) between the recti muscles in four quadrants, and are closer to the vertical meridian than the horizontal [1]. Choroidal thickness averages 250 μm posteriorly to 100 μm anteriorly, being thickest at the macula (average 250 μm), and can be as thin as 80 μm in severe high myopia in the macula area.

Principles of Suprachoroidal Devices and Materials

We currently use one of two devices to create a suprachoroidal buckle. The first is the EL Rayes Flextip Catheter (MedOne Surgical; fig. 1a, b), which is roughly 550 μm with illumination capability. It can be connected to a regular bright illumination light source that illuminates a 38-gauge light fiber when placed in the suprachoroidal space for identifying the tip of the inserting cannula and guidance in the suprachoroidal space. The other end of the Y-connector on the catheter is connected to high-pressure tubing to deliver the filler (forms of HA) to the target area creating the choroidal dome (buckling

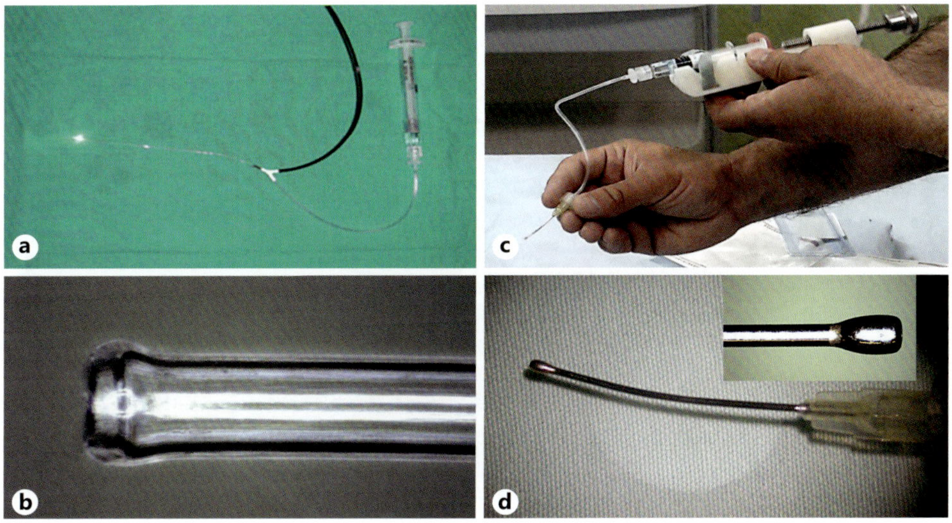

Fig. 1. Suprachoroidal catheter and cannula for suprachoroidal filler injection. **a** EL Rayes Flextip Catheter (MedOne Surgical) showing the two arms of the Y connector, one arm to the light source and the other to the filler injector ampule. It can be connected to a regular bright illumination light source that illuminates a 31-gauge optic fiber in the catheter for identifying the tip of the inserting cannula when placed in the suprachoroidal space. **b** The tip of the catheter with dome safety design for choroidal protection. **c** Nonilluminated 20-gauge curved metal cannula (EL Rayes) with an olive-shaped tip for injecting the filler and creating a suprachoroidal buckling effect for peripheral breaks, the picture shows the complete assembley with connector and scew injector carrying the filler syring. **d** Olive tip design for indentation and safety.

effect). The tip of the catheter has an atraumatic expansion tip for safety manipulations in the suprachoroidal space (fig. 1b). The catheter can be used to treat posteriorly located pathology such as myopic vitreomacular interface disorders or posterior located breaks. It can also be used to treat peripheral retinal breaks at the 1- or 2-o'clock positions.

The second device we use for creating peripheral or anterior retinal buckles is the El Rayes Curved Suprachoroidal Cannula (MedOne Surgical; fig. 1c, d), which is a nonilluminated 20-gauge curved solid cannula with an olive tip for injecting the filler for creating a suprachoroidal buckle. The olive tip is also used as a choroidal depressor to gently indent the choroid and localize the breaks prior to injection. We have used different materials to create the suprachoroidal buckle. When we started using this technique, we were concerned about the duration of the filler causing the separation. We first used dermal filler cross-linked HA 20 mg/ml (Restylane Perlane), which is special because of its high degree of natural entanglements that create a long-lasting biocompatible gel network resistant to degradation compared with regular cross-linked HA (off-label use). We have found that it can be injected with ease into the suprachoroidal space, is well-tolerated by the patients, and can last for 14 months. It is interesting to point out that we are now using Healon5 (HA; 23 mg/ml; stabilized gel; Abbott Medical Optics Inc., Santa Ana, Calif., USA), which has less bonding and shows stability for 2–3 weeks in the suprachoroidal space for peripheral retinal breaks. We believe that the issue of 'how long' (duration) is no longer a problem because the stabilization, bonding technology, and higher cross-linking solve the duration issues and create a gel of superior strength. Therefore, depending on the nature of the pathology, we can

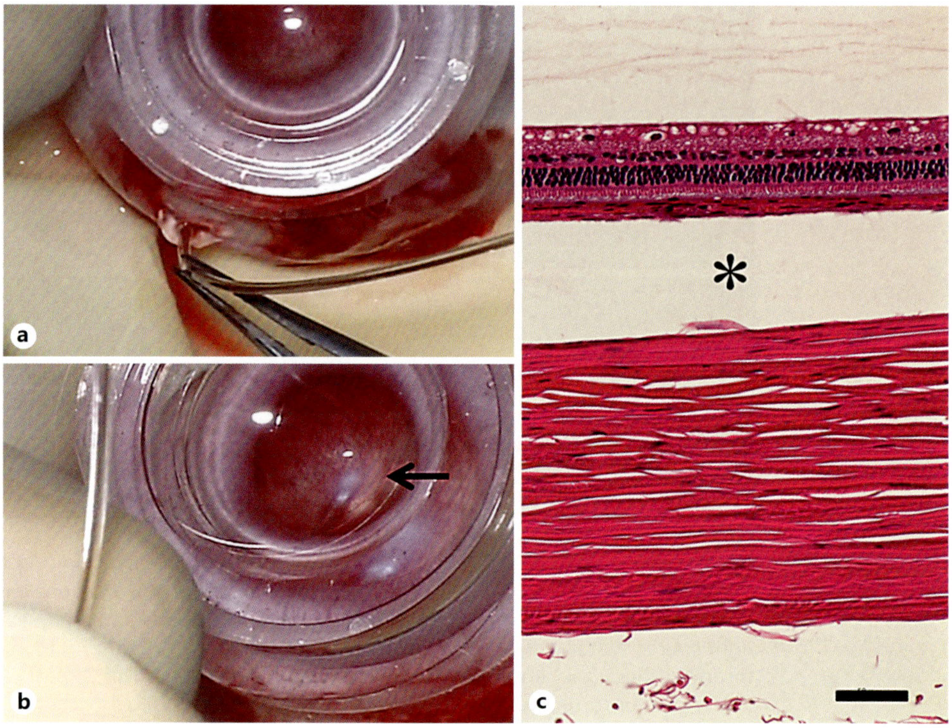

Fig. 2. Suprachoroidal buckling in rabbit eyes. **a** Suprachoroidal catheter inserted into the suprachoroidal space through a 2-mm scleral incision. **b** The illuminated tip (black arrow) of the catheter can be seen underneath the retina through a magnifying contact lens. **c** Histologic examination 3 months after surgery demonstrates clear separation of the choroid from the sclera (asterisk) with intact morphology in the chorioretinal layer. Bar = 50 µm.

choose the type that we will inject. Experimental work has been done in creating suprachoroidal buckles on rabbits and has been successful in safely and gradually separating the choroid [19] (fig. 2).

Suprachoroidal Buckling for Myopic Vitreomacular Interface Disorders

Management of MTM has focused on eliminating epiretinal traction forces by means of vitrectomy with or without ILM peeling [13–18, 20]. One report modified the ILM peeling to a foveal non-peeling technique [21] in an attempt to avoid the complication of ILM peeling in highly myopic eyes, including macular hole (MH) formation or even extrafoveal hole formation [22]. Macular buckling is a well-established technique that supports the posterior scleral wall, releasing the traction forces on the vitreomacular interface in the area of the staphyloma. Several reports have shown favorable results using different forms of episcleral macular buckles in managing MTM [23–25]. Also, Mateo et al. [26] showed a favorable outcome in managing myopic foveoschisis, comparing two different types of episcleral macular buckles in association with vitrectomy. Yet there is a learning curve, with proper localization of the buckles in proper localization of the buckles and fixation in some cases of extremely thin scleral and long axial length of the globe being a challenge.

In this section we show the technique of creating a choroidal buckle through the suprachoroidal space in managing vitreoretinal interface problems in myopic patients. This technique bypasses the difficulties of scleral buckling in the macular area by direct controlled delivery of the buckle-like effect (indentation) in the target area. In a prospective noncomparative study of 23 eyes of 23 patients with MTM-related problems, 11 eyes had myopic foveoschisis, 4 of which were associated with lamellar MH and foveal detachment, and 12 eyes had myopic MH with posterior pole retinal detachment, 5 of which the holes had failed primary repair by vitrectomy before inclusion in this trial. All patients had myopia more than 10 diopters in the phakic or last known refraction before cataract extraction before enrollment if they were pseudophakic.

The surgical procedure for all patients was a standard 3-port, 25-gauge pars plana vitrectomy and dissection of the posterior hyaloid. No ILM peeling was performed. This was followed by a conjunctival incision 4 mm behind the limbus at the 12-o'clock position. A 3-mm circumferential sclerotomy was performed to expose the choroid. Choroidal displacement at the site, using viscoelastic, was done to gain space to introduce the suprachoroidal catheter. We used a flextip suprachoroidal catheter, which was connected to a bright light source at one socket and cross-linked to 20 mg/ml of HA (Perlane Restylane filler) at the other connection port. The catheter was primed with the filler up to the tip before the introduction to the eye. The catheter tip was then fed through the sclerotomy, pushing posteriorly against the sclera to slide on the scleral wall in the suprachoroidal space. The microscope wide-field indirect viewing system was used to view and guide the catheter to the target tissues (posterior staphyloma). Care was taken while attempting to cross the edges of the staphyloma because the choroid is extremely thin, especially at the superior edge of the staphyloma, and tends to curve posteriorly. Before crossing this site, we injected a small amount of filler to dissect and lift the choroid at the edge before pushing the catheter into the posterior staphyloma. Once we placed the catheter in the suprachoroidal space underneath the target tissue (foveoschisis or MH), we injected the filler to dissect the thin choroid toward the retina, creating an indentation effect and bypassing the staphyloma space. This effect restores the normal contour of the choroid or even indents it to a convex configuration supporting the retina. The tip of the catheter is seen underneath the choroid as a light spot, denoting the site of the beginning of the indentation. This step is done under a direct contact lens viewer with the microscope to control the site and desired contour of the buckling effect. In cases of myopic hole with posterior pole detachment, the choroidal elevation has a piston effect, gradually pushing some of the fluid out of the hole. This step has to go slowly and be controlled to avoid sudden expansion so as to avoid excessive expansion and stretching of the short posterior ciliary vessels. The aim of the choroidal elevation is to achieve the normal contour of the globe and support the retina with even a slight indentation effect. Any residual epiretinal surface traction is detected and removed because it is easier to grasp and remove on a support retina than in a detached schitic form. After closure of the sclerotomy site and trocar removal, a 15% sulfur hexafluoride (SF_6) gas bubble was injected after fluid-air exchange.

Retinal layer restoration was achieved in all 11 eyes with myopic foveoschisis (improvement in the thickness). This occurred gradually over a period of 2–6 weeks postoperatively, with no recurrence over the 24 months of follow-up. Visual acuity improved by 1 line or more in 9 eyes (81.8%), and 2 eyes (18%) showed no change in baseline visual acuity. In the 9 eyes showing improvement in visual acuity, 6 eyes (66%) showed gain in reading ability. In the patients with MH detachment, 10 eyes (83%) showed closure of the holes in association with the resolution of the detachment (fig. 3). Two eyes (16.6%) showed resolution of the detachment and flattening of the edge of the holes but with incomplete closure on optical coherence tomography; 8 eyes (66.6%)

showed improvement in visual acuity by 1 or more lines with no recurrence of retinal detachment over the 24-month follow-up period [27].

Regarding complications, we had 2 cases of choroidal hemorrhage. One was at the edge of the staphyloma in a myopic foveoschisis patient; the patch of hemorrhage was small outside the arcades and did not need any intervention. It was controlled by increasing intraocular pressure intraoperatively, and the procedure was continued and completed. The other was in a case of myopic hole and also occurred while attempting to cross the edge of the staphyloma. The blood was displaced away from the foveal area by the effect of the filler injection (dome displacement) and needed a tissue plasminogen activator injection in reintervention to displace the blood, with no effect on the buckling effect. We learned to inject a small bubble of the filler at the staphyloma edge in very high myopic cases before attempting to cross the edge of the deep staphyloma. This step lifts and protects the choroid and decreases the incidence of hemorrhage. The overall indentation effect was sufficient in creating a choroidal buckling effect as of month 36 (fig. 3 and 4). Hyperpigmentation [heaping of retinal pigment epithelium (RPE)] surrounding the edge of the indentation was noted in 2 eyes and was noted to fade over the 12-month follow-up period (fig. 4).

Suprachoroidal Buckling for Peripheral Breaks

Suprachoroidal buckling can be performed with or without vitrectomy. In most cases, a chandelier light (25 gauge or smaller) is placed at the 12-o'clock position or in any other quadrant if the tears are at 12 o'clock; then an operating microscope is combined with a wide-angle viewing system for fundus examination. The tear site can easily be identified and marked under wide-angle fundus viewing with direct illumination from the chandelier. The conjunctiva in the quadrant of the tear is incised, and a 2- to 3-mm circumferential sclerotomy is created 4 mm from the limbus to expose the choroid. After this, the choroid is displaced by injecting some viscoelastic fluid to form a 1-mm pocket to create a space for the introduction of the suprachoroidal catheter or cannula. The catheter is threaded through the sclerotomy into the suprachoroidal space in the direction of the tear location, pushing against the scleral wall in the suprachoroidal space. The wide-angle system is then flipped again to see the fundus with the chandelier light and the location of the tip of the catheter in relation to the tear (fig. 5). Once the light from the catheter is under the middle of the tear, the injection of the HA solution is initiated, causing a controlled choroidal indentation that expands in height and direction depending on the desired location and height, typically 0.05–0.1 ml of suprachoroidal gel, depending on the size of the break and height of buckle needed. This causes the indentation effect for 2–3 weeks as studied by ultrabiomicroscopy images of the treatment area (fig. 5e). This is accompanied by anterior chamber paracentesis or subretinal fluid drainage, and is necessary to adjust the intraocular pressure. The use of the catheter helps in targeting posteriorly located breaks irrelevant to the anterior location of the sclerotomy. If one or more tears are close to each other (1- to 2-o'clock positions), these can be buckled using the same entry site. Once the tear is closed by the suprachoroidal buckle, the catheter is withdrawn from the sclera and the sclerotomy is closed with sutures. The tear can then be treated by indirect laser ophthalmoscopy (fig. 5).

Another treatment option to create chorioretinal adhesion is cryoretinopexy, which should be performed in advance of the suprachoroidal buckling. An air or SF_6 gas bubble may be used depending on the site, size, and location of the break. As an alternative to the illuminated flextip catheter, we successfully used a nonilluminated 20-gauge curved cannula with an olive tip for injecting the filler and creating a suprachoroidal buckling effect. The advantage of the olive tip is that it acts as a choroidal depressor (fig. 1d). However, this cannula is for peripheral pathology

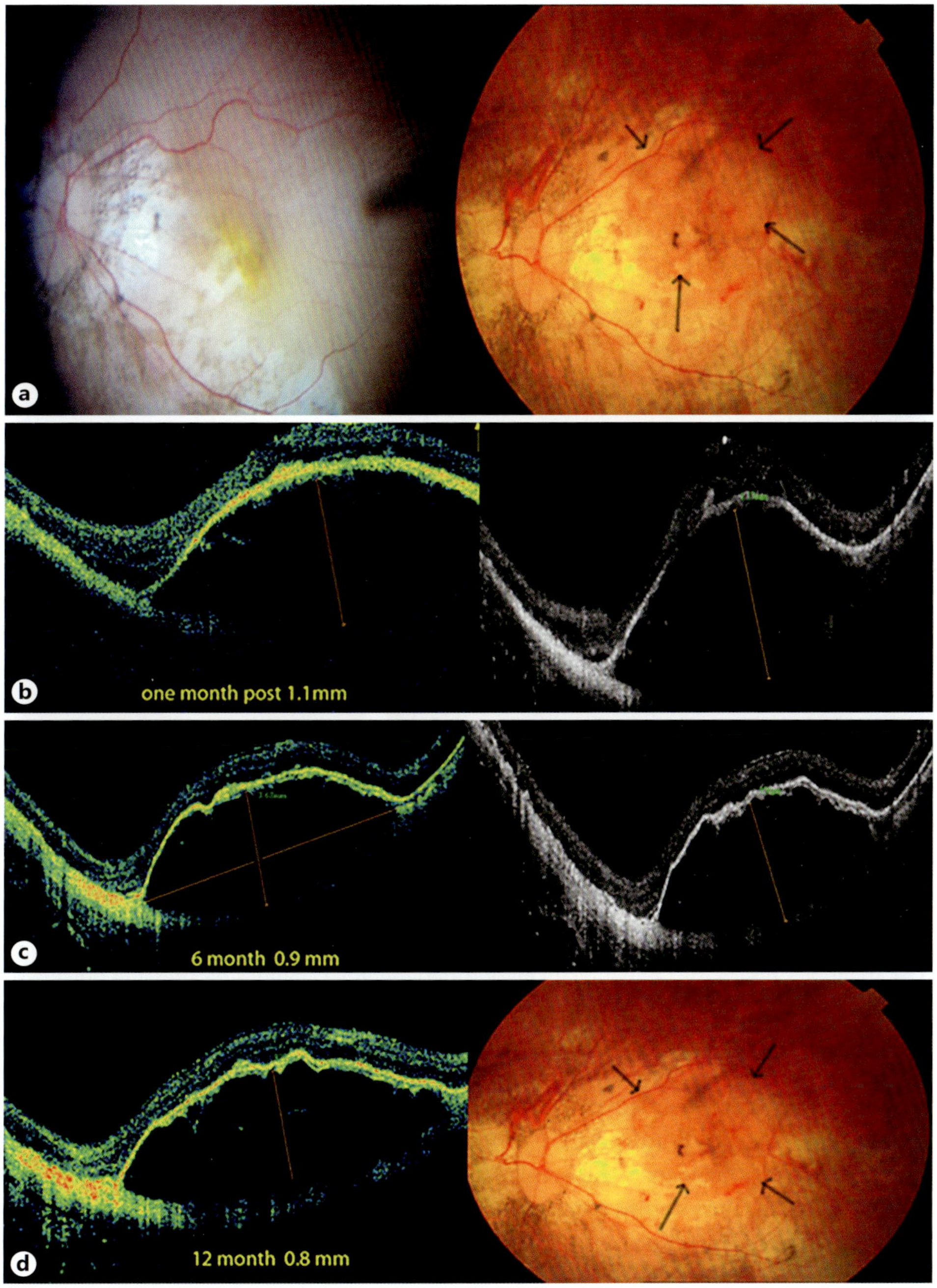

Fig. 3. A patient with failed vitrectomy surgery for myopic MH. **a** Preoperative fundus photograph on the left and postoperative photograph on the right showing the scleral buckling effect marked by arrows with the hole closed. **b** One-month choroidal indentation height is 1.1 mm. **c** At 6 months, choroidal indentation is 0.9 mm. **d** At 12 months, it is 0.8 mm and the equivalent indentation on the right is to be noted.

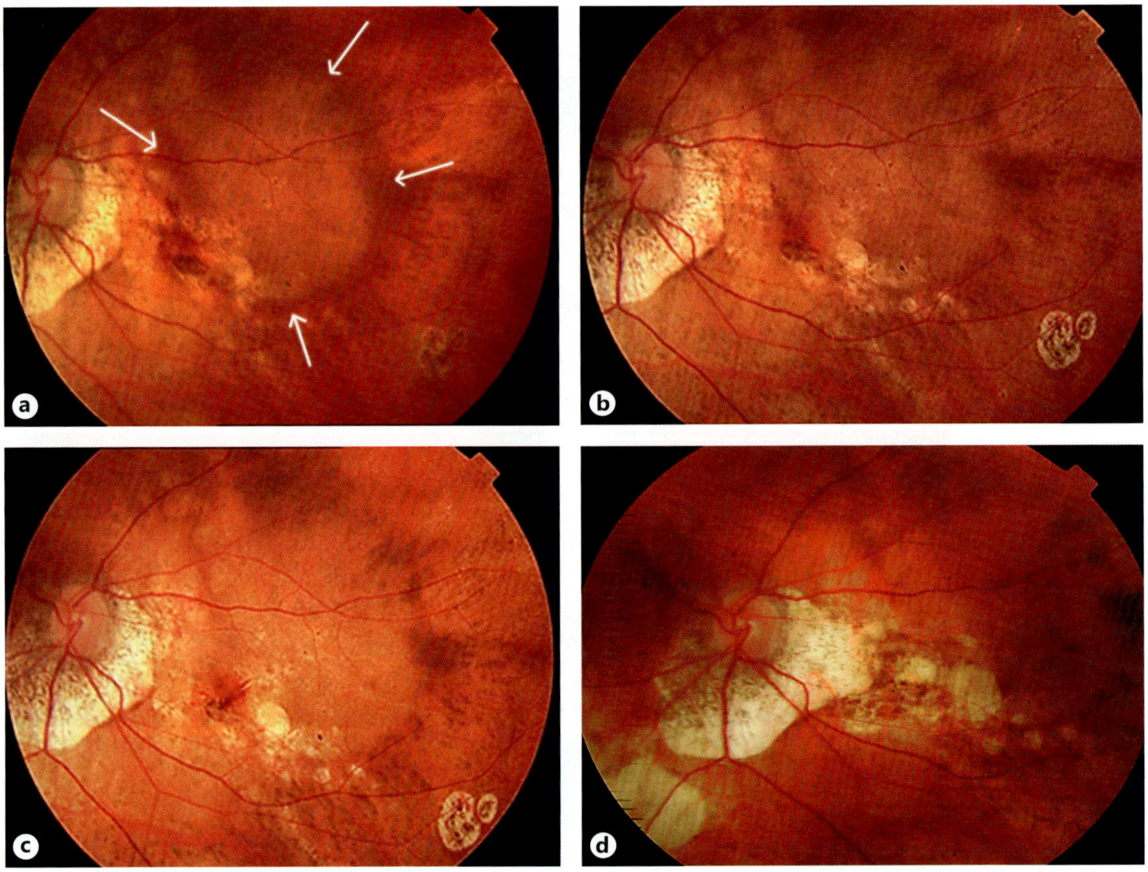

Fig. 4. Serial color fundus photography of a patient with macular suprachoroidal buckling. **a** One-month postoperatively, the area of demarcation is shown by the arrows in the photograph. **b** At 6 months postoperatively, the area of demarcation is fading. **c** At 12 months, interruption of the demarcation (less heaping-like effect) is noted. **d** At 36 month, notice the peripapillary myopic degenerative changes progressing outside the area buckled and involutional changes happened to the CNV at the margin of the buckled area.

only; it is not recommended past the equatorial region. The cannula is introduced in a similar manner as the catheter over the breaks and used to gently depress the choroid localizing the overlying breaks. The injection is then started from the syringe attached to the cannula, creating the buckling effect. The main advantage of the cannula is that it can access tears up to the 3-o'clock position on either side of the sclerotomy. This can create a circumferential buckling effect up to 180° from one single sclerotomy incision. This is particularly helpful when doing inferior buckles or subsilicon retinal detachment when you need inferior circumferential retinal support or in supporting a giant retinal break (GRB; fig. 6).

Discussion

Retinal detachment treatment is based on the closure of the retinal tears as a key issue as well as eliminating the traction forces on the retina or indenting the chorioscleral wall to close the retina. Certainly, scleral buckles help to reduce vitreous

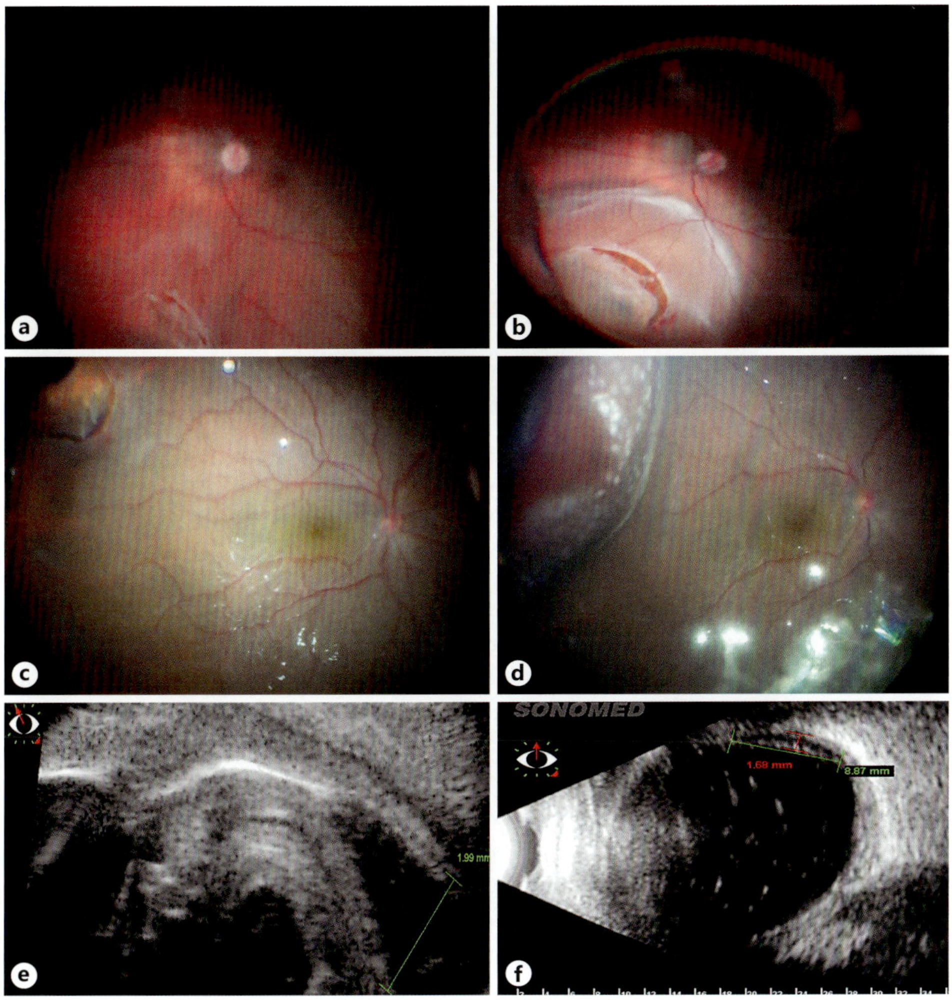

Fig. 5. a Composite picture. **b** Pretreatment fundus photograph of a patient with a lower nasal tear in the 2-o'clock position and retinal detachment. **c** Intraoperative picture after the injection with creation of a suprachoroidal buckle. **d** Pretreatment photograph of a case with upper temporal break. **e** Postsuprachoroidal buckling ultrasound biomicroscopy of the same patient 10 days after the operation showing a 1.9-mm choroidal indentation measured by the green calipers. **f** Ultrasound (B-scan) of the same area showing the clear filler, detaching the choroid marked by the measurement calipers.

traction and diminish the flux of vitreous fluid through retinal tears, thus promoting reposition of the retina to the RPE [28]. Achieving this goal through the suprachoroidal space avoids some of the difficulties associated with episcleral buckles.

We developed the peripheral break suprachoroidal buckling technique after our initial experience in suprachoroidal buckles for myopic vitreomacular interface problem management [27]. In this chapter on the technique, we show that it is possible to create a choroid-only (without sclera) buckle, efficiently closing the retinal tear and supporting the retina [6]. The use of a catheter to achieve this gives us the option of a small incision

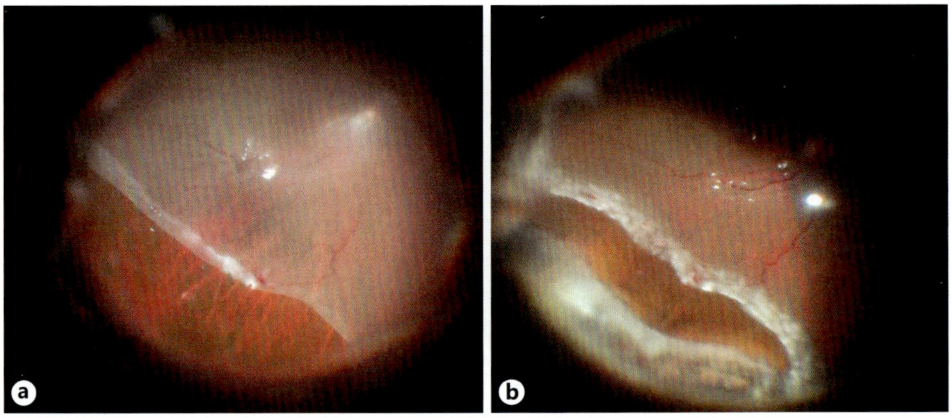

Fig. 6. Color photograph of a patient with GRB. **a** Note GRB after flattening it under PFO. **b** Intraoperative view after creating a suprachoroidal buckle to the edges; note the dome creation supporting the edges of the break.

with navigation in the suprachoroidal space to reach target tissue independent of its location.

The limitation of 1 incision is that we can only treat single tears or a group of tears in the 1- to 2-o'clock position, depending on their location (superior or inferior). With the use of a cannula we can close the opened retinal breaks with silicone oil in cases of inferior silicon oil recurrent retinal detachment, and we use it to create a choroidal buckling support effect in some cases of recurrent inferior retinal detachment and even support GRBs (fig. 6). Certainly, posteriorly located breaks are an indication to use the catheter to reach these breaks to avoid long radial episcleral buckles. Also in a phakic eye, retinal detachment in young myopes is an option to avoid vitreous base shaving over a single break by the cutter vitrectomy behind the lens and also to avoid refraction change by an episcleral buckle for those who did have refractive surgical correction. We have also learned that it is possible to augment the height of existing episcleral buckles by injecting over the overlying choroid (over the buckle) or creating a radial choroidal extension to an existing episcleral buckle. The cannula showed superior results to the flextip catheter in treating groups of breaks at the 3-o'clock position, side-to-side manipulation to buckle breaks within 180°, and to custom draw segmental or circumferential buckles. It was also superior to the flextip catheter in guiding it in inferior detachment and subsilicon recurrent retinal detachment.

It was interesting to find in the literature thoughts on choroidal indentation reported by Poole and Sudarsky in 1986 [30]. Today, we have a broad range of substances to use as a suprachoroidal buckle, depending on how long we need chorioretinal indentation to achieve chorioretinal adhesion or if we need long-term retinal support; therefore, the choice of filler can be selected according to the pathology. We have also shown that this technique can be done with (in part) vitrectomy or as a separate approach, illuminating the fundus by just a chandelier, with the ability to indent and direct the chandelier light to the peripheral tear and complete the procedure without the need of any intravitreal instruments.

We believe that suprachoroidal buckling using catheter-guided fillers can be a surgical option for the repair of selected cases of retinal detachment with good chorioretinal closure of tears. The buckling height and location is controllable by the amount and site of filler (HA) injection, as well as avoiding potential problems of scleral buckles in the posteriorly located break and thin sclera. Treatment options in the literature for myopic foveoschisis and myopic MH have focused on considering that surface vitreoretinal traction is perhaps the primary mechanism for the development of MTM, and thus pars plana vitrectomy with or without ILM peeling to remove the source of traction is a logical intervention [13–16, 20]. Yet this approach fails in some cases, and recurrence of foveoschisis or even MH development after pars plana vitrectomy and ILM peeling can occur [30, 31].

Looking to the mechanism of traction in a more inclusive way of management, supporting the retina and halting or bypassing the global elongation is another logical method of solving this problem. Several authors [24–26] have shown the use of episcleral macular buckling in patients with high myopia complicated by foveoschisis-associated MH and retinal detachment, with even more favorable results with macular buckling compared with vitrectomy in the report from Ando et al. [23]. The aim of the macular buckling approach is to release both the traction caused by posterior staphyloma and the anterior posterior traction caused by the vitreous cortex on the inner retina. It also brings the RPE closer to the retina, reinforcing the weak adherence between RPE and the neurosensory retina [26, 32].

Certainly, episcleral macular buckling has a learning curve for avoiding difficulties in buckle placement, alignment, extrusion, thin scleral problem and choroidal hemorrhages, and postoperative esotropia. The hypothesis behind it is that we need to restore the normal contour of the choroid supporting the retinal contour by separating the choroid from the elongating sclera and thus releasing traction on the retinal layers, especially in cases over 30 mm of axial length where the retina is less likely to yield to the bulb-like elongated sclera and choroid or in cases of failed primary vitrectomy despite inner surface traction relief. In such cases, both episcleral and suprachoroidal macular buckling are better logical solutions. Although it bypasses the difficulties in buckle placement and fixation in thin sclera, we still have to deal with the problem of a thin choroid to avoid hemorrhage. This has been done in part by developing the atraumatic tip design catheter, as well as proper atraumatic guidance with close attention to choroidal dissection at the edge of the staphyloma.

As we know from the literature, Yamagishi et al. [33] reported that the choroid was markedly thin at the upper border of the inferior staphyloma, and we might consider doing an inferior crossing technique to see if it is safer. We also believe that we do not have much choroidal circulatory changes at the choroidal indentation because the cushion-like effect creating the indentation has less mechanical pressure or deformation to the circulation compared with the silicone explants as well as this area of the choroid has very high blood supply from the 15–20 short ciliary vessels. We also learned to target restoring the normal global contour rather than create a dome hight effect that might cause choroidal circulatory disturbance. We have noted 2 cases of hyperpigmentation at the edge the indentation that we believe to be more related to heaping of the RPE at the edge of the dome, but it decreased in effect over the follow-up period (fig. 4). The procedure was relatively safe with proper attention and respect of ocular tissues in this disease as well as with the appropriate training and experience. Absence of recurrence of the problem over the initial 1-year follow-up period encouraged us to consider and add this procedure to our surgical options in managing vitreomacular interface disorders in sever myopia.

In summary, the results of our studies of both myopic vitreomacular interface problems as well as selected forms of retinal detachment, in conjunction with data from animal experiments, encourage us to conclude that suprachoroidal buckling with or without PPV may be a promising less-invasive treatment option for uncomplicated RRDs and refractory MTMs. It is feasible to add it to the options available for treating retinal detachment with buckling in a simplified procedure using the microscope.

References

1 The repair of rhegmatogenous retinal detachment. American Academy of Ophthalmology. Ophthalmology 1990; 97:1562–1572.

2 Schepens CL, Okamura ID, Brockhurst RJ: The scleral buckling procedures 1. Surgical techniques and management. AMA Arch Ophthalmol 1957;58:797–811.

3 Sewell JJ, Knobloch WH, Eifrig DE: Extraocular muscle imbalance after surgical treatment for retinal detachment. Am J Ophthalmol 1974;78:321–323.

4 Smiddy WE, Loupe DN, Michels RG, Enger C, Glaser BM, de Bustros S: Refractive changes after scleral buckling surgery. Arch Ophthalmol 1989;107: 1469–1471.

5 Yoshida A, Feke GT, Green GJ, et al: Retinal circulatory changes after scleral buckling procedures. Am J Ophthalmol 1983;95:182–188.

6 El Rayes EN, Oshima Y: Suprachoroidal buckling for retinal detachment. Retina 2013;33:1073–1075.

7 Hogan MJ, Alvarado JA, Weddell JE: Histology of the human eye: an atlas and textbook. Philadelphia, WB Saunders, 1971.

8 Le Douarin N: A biological cell labeling technique and its use in experimental embryology. Dev Biol 1973;30:217–222.

9 Mund ML, Rodrigues MM, Fine BS: Light and electron microscopic observations on the pigmented layers of the developing human eye. Am J Ophthalmol 1972;73:167–182.

10 McMahon RT: Anatomy, congenital anomalies, and tumors; in Peyman GA, Sanders DR, Goldberg MF (eds): Principles and Practice of Ophthalmology. Philadelphia, WB Saunders, 1980.

11 Duke Elder S, Wybar KC: System of Ophthalmology: The Anatomy of the Visual System. St Louis, Mosby, vol 2, 1961.

12 Yanoff M, Fine BS: Ocular Pathology, ed 2. Philadelphia, JB Lippincott, 1982.

13 Ikuno Y, Tano Y: Vitrectomy for macular holes associated with myopic foveoschisis. Am J Ophthalmol 2006;141:774–776.

14 Kwok AK, Lai TY, Yip WW: Vitrectomy and gas tamponade without internal limiting membrane peeling for myopic foveoschisis. Br J Ophthalmol 2005;89: 1180–1183.

15 Spaide RF, Fisher Y: Removal of adherent cortical vitreous plaques without removing the internal limiting membrane in the repair of macular detachment in highly myopic eyes. Retina 2005;25:290–295.

16 Kuhn F: Internal limiting membrane removal for macular detachment in highly myopic eyes. Am J Ophthalmol 2003;136:477–481.

17 Shimada N, Sugamoto Y, Ogawa M, et al: Foveal sparing internal limiting membrane peeling for myopic traction maculopathy. Am J Ophthalmol 2012; 154:693–701.

18 Kanda S, Uemura A, Sakamoto Y, Kita H: Vitrectomy with internal limiting membrane peeling for macular retinoschisis and retinal detachment without macular hole in highly myopic eyes. Am J Ophthalmol 2003;136:177–180.

19 Oshima Y, El Rayes E, Matsumura N, Sakaguchi H: Suprachoroidal buckling technique. Retina Today 2013;71–76.

20 Yeh SI, Chang WC, Chen LJ: Vitrectomy without internal limiting membrane peeling for macular retinoschisis and foveal detachment in highly myopic eyes. Acta Ophthalmol 2008;86:219–224.

21 Ho TC, Chen MS, Huang JS, et al: Foveal non peeling technique in internal limiting membrane peeling of myopic foveoschisis surgery. Retina 2012;32:631–634.

22 Steven P, Laqua H, Wong D, Hoerauf H: Secondary paracentral retinal hole following internal limiting membrane removal. Br J Ophthalmol 2006;90:293–295.

23 Ando F, Ohba N, Touura K, Hirose H: Anatomical and visual outcomes after episcleral macular buckling compared with those after pars plana vitrectomy for retinal detachment caused by macular hole in highly myopic eyes. Retina 2007;27:37–44.

24 Ripandelli G, Coppe AM, Fedeli R, et al: Evaluation of primary surgical procedures for retinal detachment with macular hole in highly myopic eyes: a comparison of vitrectomy versus posterior episcleral buckling surgery. Ophthalmology 2001;108:2258–2264, discussion 2265.

25 Theodossiadis GP, Theodossiades PG: The macular buckling procedure in the treatment of retinal detachment in highly myopic eyes with macular hole and posterior staphyloma: mean follow-up of 15 years. Retina 2005;25:285–289.

26 Mateo C, Jelstrup AB, Navarro R, Corcostegui B: Macular buckling for eyes with myopic foveoschisis secondary to posterior staphyloma. Retina 2012;32:1121–1128.

27 El Rayes EN: Suprachoroidal buckling in managing myopic vitreoretinal interface disorders: one-year data. Retina 2014; 34:129–135.

28 Wilkinson CP, Rice TA: Michel's Retinal Detachment, ed 2. St Louis, Mosby, 1997.

29 Poole TA, Sudarsky D: Suprachoroidal implantation for treatment of retinal detachment. Ophthalmology 1986;93: 1408–1412.

30 Shukla D, Dhawan A: Foveoschisis after vitrectomy for myopic macular hole with secondary retinal detachment. Eye 2009;23:2124–2125.

31 Kobayashi H, Kishi S: Vitreous surgery for highly myopic eyes with foveal detachment and retinoschisis. Ophthalmology 2003;110:1702–1707.

32 Ichibe M, Yoshizawa T, Murakami K, et al: Surgical management of retinal detachment associated with myopic macular hole: anatomic and functional status of the macula. Am J Ophthalmol 2003; 136:277–284.

33 Yamagishi T, Koizumi H, Yamazaki T, Kinoshita S: Choroidal thickness in inferior staphyloma associated with posterior serous retinal detachment. Retina 2012;32:1237–1242.

Prof. Ehab El Rayes, MD, PhD
Retina Department, Institute of Ophthalmology
35 Salah Salem Street, Suite 702, El Obour Bldg.
11371 Cairo (Egypt)
E-Mail erayes1@hotmail.com

Oh H, Oshima Y (eds): Microincision Vitrectomy Surgery. Emerging Techniques and Technology.
Dev Ophthalmol. Basel, Karger, 2014, vol 54, pp 147–149 (DOI: 10.1159/000360460)

Intraocular Optical Coherence Tomography

Marco Mura[a] • Francesco Barca[b]

[a]Academic Medical Center, University of Amsterdam, Amsterdam, The Netherlands;
[b]U.O. Chirurgia Oftalmica, Azienda Ospedaliero Universitaria Pisana (AOUP), Pisa, Italy

Abstract

Since its introduction as a diagnostic instrument, optical coherence tomography (OCT) has become an essential instrument for ophthalmologists as it offers accurate details on both the vitreoretinal interface and the retinal layers. Initially designed as a pre- and post-operative instrument, today we are attending to its introduction as an intraoperative tool. Inspired by the intravascular use of the OCT, we developed a prototype spectral domain OCT probe for intraocular use. It is therefore possible to make dynamic real-time scans from the vitreous and retina at the posterior pole and in the peripheral retina. This type of endo-OCT may therefore help surgeons during surgical procedures, making them safer and more accurate.

In the last decade, optical coherence tomography (OCT) has changed the way ophthalmologists diagnose and treat vitreoretinal diseases. Pre- and postoperative OCT examinations have led to a better understanding of the pathophysiology and prognosis in vitreoretinal diseases [1, 2]. Image resolution and scanning speed have substantially improved with the recent introduction of spectral domain OCT, providing structural details of the retina and vitreoretinal interface at an almost histological level [3]. The use of OCT during vitreoretinal surgery has been described before in the form of hand-held probes or microscope-mounted OCT systems [4, 5]. This intraoperative use of the OCT has proven to be useful in the decision-making process during surgery, resulting in improved technical performance and ultimately a better outcome for the patients [6].

In recent years, OCT has become an irreplaceable tool for the diagnosis, management, and prognosis of many vitreoretinal diseases [1–3]. However, the idea of having OCT as an adjuvant during surgery is relatively new [4, 5]. The first report describing the use of a hand-held OCT device was published in 2009 [7–9]. Recently, Binder et al. [5] reported the application of a standard OCT system mounted in the operating microscope. Due to its inherent technical limitations, microscope-mounted OCT has mainly been used to obtain scans of the central macular area, to assess the completeness of the macula peeling of epiretinal membrane and internal limiting membrane and to identify local iatrogenic damage after membrane peeling. This device can also be used to assess the presence of subretinal fluid in the macula area in cases of retinal detachment.

Of course, static microscope-mounted standard OCT devices offer only limited possibilities in a dynamic surgical environment. The devices described by Binder et al. [5] and Ray et al. [4] do not have the possibility to examine more peripheral areas of the eye, which can be imaged very well with an intraocular probe.

An intraocular probe can offer dynamic examination and real-time imaging during surgery without the need for a tracking system and an image stabilization system. We have used a prototype intraocular probe to assess several patients during retina surgery [10]. The device is a 23-gauge side-scanning spectral domain OCT probe in a 20-gauge catheter. The device works at wavelength of 1,300 nm, it has a 15-micron axial resolution, 6-mm field of view, and 4 mm of working distance (fig. 1).

With the OCT prototype, the following was possible:

(1) Detection of the presence of otherwise invisible membranes, e.g. epiretinal membrane proliferation
(2) Identification of subretinal membranes otherwise not visible due to the presence of substantial retinal edema and thickened retina
(3) Confirming the completeness of membrane removal in patients with epiretinal and subretinal membrane proliferation
(4) Identification of small retinal breaks, especially in patients with very light colored fundi impossible to detect with a standard internal search
(5) Identification and localization of a cleavage plane in patients with tractional retinal detachment and combined tractional retinal detachment-rhegmatogenous retinal detachment
(6) Detection of residual subretinal fluid, perfluorocarbon, or silicone oil in the macula area and peripherally in an air-filled eye or an eye with hazy optical media

An intraocular OCT probe offering dynamic scan capabilities could also be useful in various steps of the surgical procedure. The identification of epiretinal proliferation makes it possible to perform epiretinal membrane peeling in these patients without the use of any staining that could potentially be toxic, especially in a detached retina. Furthermore, identification of early proliferative vitreoretinopathy or the presence of remnants of a posterior hyaloid can be very difficult even with the use of staining adjuvants.

The possibility of identifying and removing proliferative tissue from the subretinal space with the help of real-time OCT images reduces the need for larger retinotomies (fig. 2). This decreases unnecessary iatrogenic damage and leads to

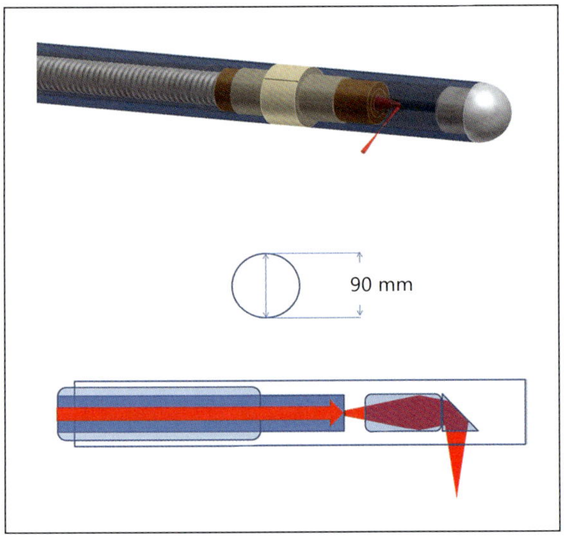

Fig. 1. Schematic representation of a side-scanning OCT probe.

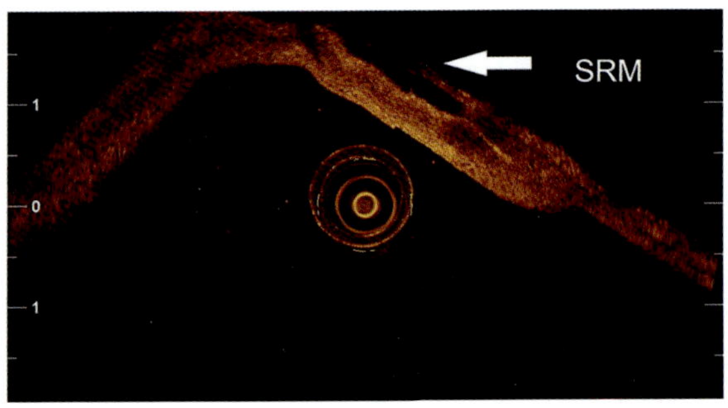

Fig. 2. Intraocular OCT image of the subretinal membrane (SRM).

less exposed retinal pigment epithelium and diminished induction of inflammation through the use of a laser – all positive effects that may lead to a better outcome for the patient.

The possibility of an intraocular OCT probe for scanning is also advantageous in cases of opacified media or in air-filled eyes where the visibility is poor. In those cases, visualization of the retina becomes challenging, and it becomes impossible to identify, for example, residual perfluorocarbon liquid or the presence of subretinal perfluorocarbon liquid/oil/fluid, which if not properly removed can lead to retinal folds and poor visual prognosis.

The possibility to perform OCT-guided vitreous body removal provides certainty over the complete removal of all possible vitreous tractions. As a common procedure, vitreous shaving is performed in patients with the aid of triamcinolone, but following this procedure a significant amount of vitreous is seen to be left in place when checked with the intraocular OCT probe.

Small retinal breaks can sometimes be missed, especially in patients with very light pigmented fundi. In these patients a scan of the periphery with the intraocular OCT probe can highlight the presence of the breaks.

In cases of fibrovascular proliferation, such as proliferative diabetic retinopathy, it can sometimes be challenging to find the correct cleavage plane, but intraoperative OCT can show a clear identification of such planes to guide the dissection. That means safer removal of fibrovascular tissue from the retinal surface, reducing the chance of iatrogenic damage.

In conclusion, an intraocular endoprobe can provide the surgeon with extremely important information, helps him in the decision-making progress (especially in more complex retinal pathology), and allows him to perform OCT-guided surgical maneuvers with potential improvement of the precision and safety of the procedure that could lead to better surgical outcomes.

References

1. Adhi M, Duker JS: Optical coherence tomography – current and future applications. Curr Opin Ophthalmol 2013;24: 213–221.
2. Sakata LM, Deleon-Ortega J, Sakata V, Girkin CA: Optical coherence tomography of the retina and optic nerve – a review. Clin Experiment Ophthalmol 2009;37:90–99.
3. Kiernan DF, Mieler WF, Hariprasad SM: Spectral-domain optical coherence tomography: a comparison of modern high-resolution retinal imaging systems. Am J Ophthalmol 2010;149:18–31.
4. Ray R, Barañano DE, Fortun JA, Schwent BJ, Cribbs BE, Bergstrom CS, Hubbard GB 3rd, Srivastava SK: Intraoperative microscope-mounted spectral domain optical coherence tomography for evaluation of retinal anatomy during macular surgery. Ophthalmology 2011; 118:2212–2217.
5. Binder S, Falkner-Radler CI, Hauger C, Matz H, Glittenberg CG: Clinical applications of intrasurgical SD-optical coherence tomography. ARVO Meeting Abstracts 2010;51:268.
6. Huang LL, Hirose T: Portable optical coherence tomography in management of vitreoretinal diseases: current developments, indications, and implications. Semin Ophthalmol 2012;27:213–220.
7. Scott AW, Farsiu S, Enyedi LB, Wallace DK, Toth CA: Imaging the infant retina with a hand-held spectral-domain optical coherence tomography device. Am J Ophthalmol 2009;147:364–373.
8. Muni RH, Kohly RP, Sohn EH, Lee TC: Hand-held spectral domain optical coherence tomography finding in shaken-baby syndrome. Retina 2010; 30(4 suppl):S45–S50.
9. Chong GT, Farsiu S, Freedman SF, et al: Abnormal foveal morphology in ocular albinism imaged with spectral-domain optical coherence tomography. Arch Ophthalmol 2009;127:37–44.
10. Mura M, Barca F, Chung R, Tan HS, Engelbrecht LA, de Bruin M, Verbraak F: Use of a new intra-ocular spectral domain OCT in vitreo-retinal surgery. Am J Ophthalmol 2013, submitted.

Marco Mura
Academic Medical Center, University of Amsterdam
Meibergdreef 9
NL–1105AZ Amsterdam (The Netherlands)
E-Mail m.mura@amc.uva.nl

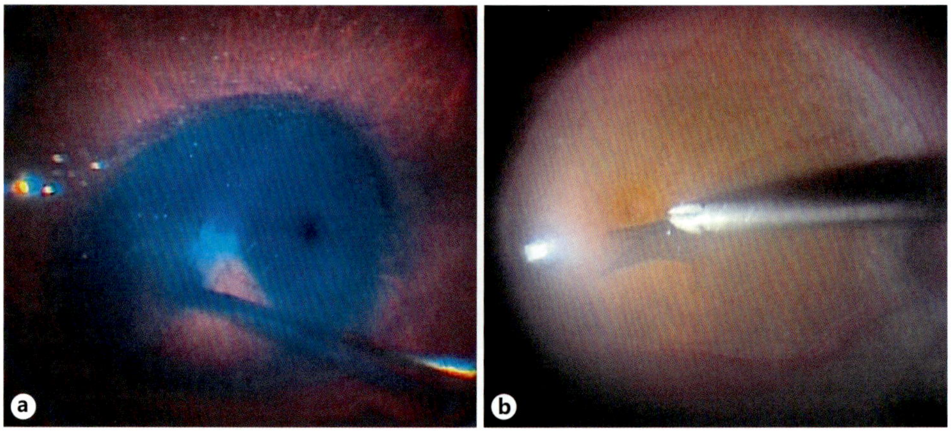

Fig. 3. a Staining of the ILM with BBG (ILM Blue®). Note that the injected BBG solution spontaneously sinks and accumulates within the posterior pole by its gravity since it contains 4% polyethylene glycol as a component. **b** ILM peeling started by direct grasping using a 27-gauge asymmetrical forceps.

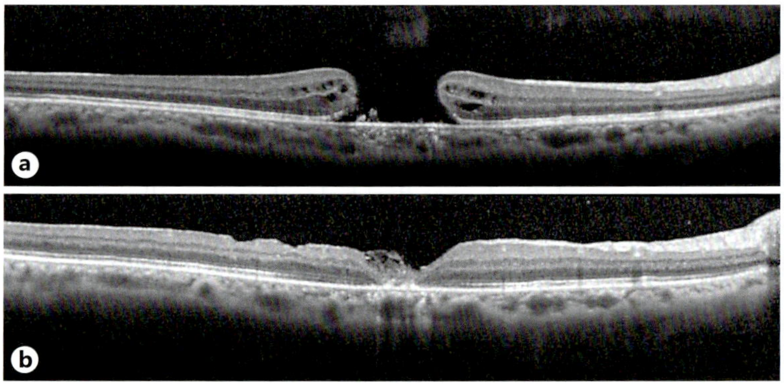

Fig. 4. Inverted ILM peeling. **a** Preoperative OCT image of a large macular hole with a base diameter of 1,364 μm. **b** Postoperative OCT image at 3 months showing the ILM remnants completely filled the original hole.

hole closure was confirmed with sufficient image quality, but later on reopens during the same admission.

Recent Advancements

Inverted ILM Peeling Technique

Preoperative macular hole size is a critical determinant of anatomic success [10, 31]. To overcome surgical failures in larger-sized macular holes, Michalewska et al. [32] reported a surgical technique called inverted ILM peeling (fig. 4). In their report, the remnant of an incompletely peeled ILM was left and then inverted upside-down to cover the macular hole. With this technique, they have shown that even in cases with a macular hole size larger than 400 μm the success rate in terms of hole closure reached as high as 98%, whereas the rate obtained with conventional complete ILM peeling was 81%. More recently, Kuriyama et al. [33] reported that this technique also exhibited an excellent success rate in cases of macular holes associated with pathologic myopia.

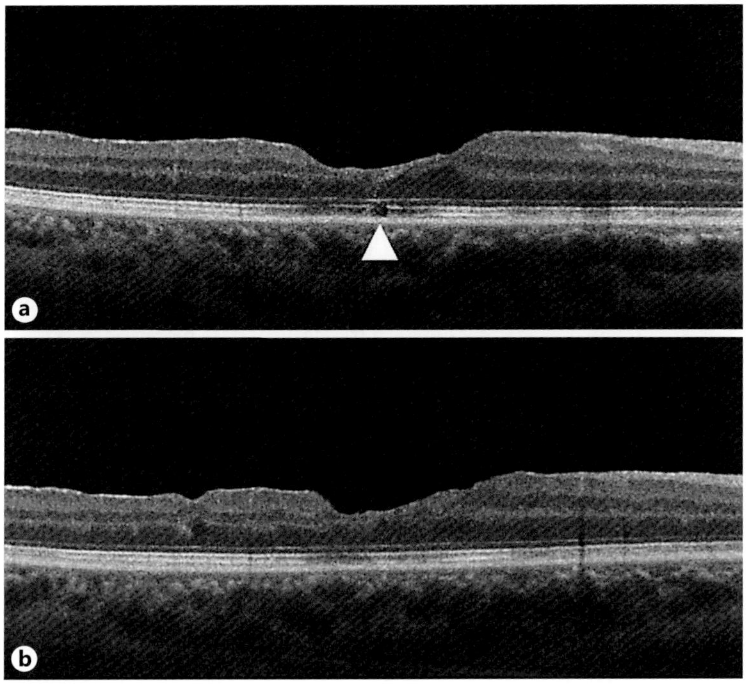

Fig. 5. Postoperative changes of outer retinal structure. **a** Restored external limiting membrane line and discontinuous IS/OS junction line (arrowhead) on OCT 3 months postoperatively. **b** Continuous lines of both the external limiting membrane and IS/OS on OCT 4 months postoperatively.

Postoperative Restoration of Retinal Structures Documented on Optical Coherence Tomography

Visual improvement and recovery from distortion are known to be gradual after macular hole surgery; however, the potential mechanisms have not been explored. Wakabayashi et al. [34] reported that based on postoperative OCT findings the recovery of the external limiting membrane line first occur and is then followed by that of the inner segment/outer segment (IS/OS) junction line (fig. 5). They also showed that patients in whom these structures are in good condition tended to have better visual prognosis. Christensen reported that the discontinuity of the IS/OS line with a diameter of more than 1,500 μm 3 months after surgery was associated with poorer visual acuity after 12 months than less extensive discontinuity [35]. In contrast, subfoveal fluid after 3 months had no effect on the final visual outcome in that study. Accordingly, surgeons should pay keen attention to these postoperative retinal structures. For the detection ability reason, spectral domain OCT should be used if available.

27-Gauge Vitrectomy System

Surgical outcomes of macular hole surgery with microincision vitrectomy surgery have mostly been reported in studies performed with 23- or 25-gauge systems. Sakaguchi et al. [36] first reported that nonvitrectomizing epiretinal membrane removal surgery can be successfully performed with the newly developed smaller 27-gauge system. Later they also demonstrated that most retinal diseases from macular holes extending to more complex cases like proliferative diabetic retinopathy accompanied by tractional retinal detachment can also be managed with similar surgical outcomes and less invasiveness [37]. At the author's institution, most vitrectomy surgery for macular diseases are currently

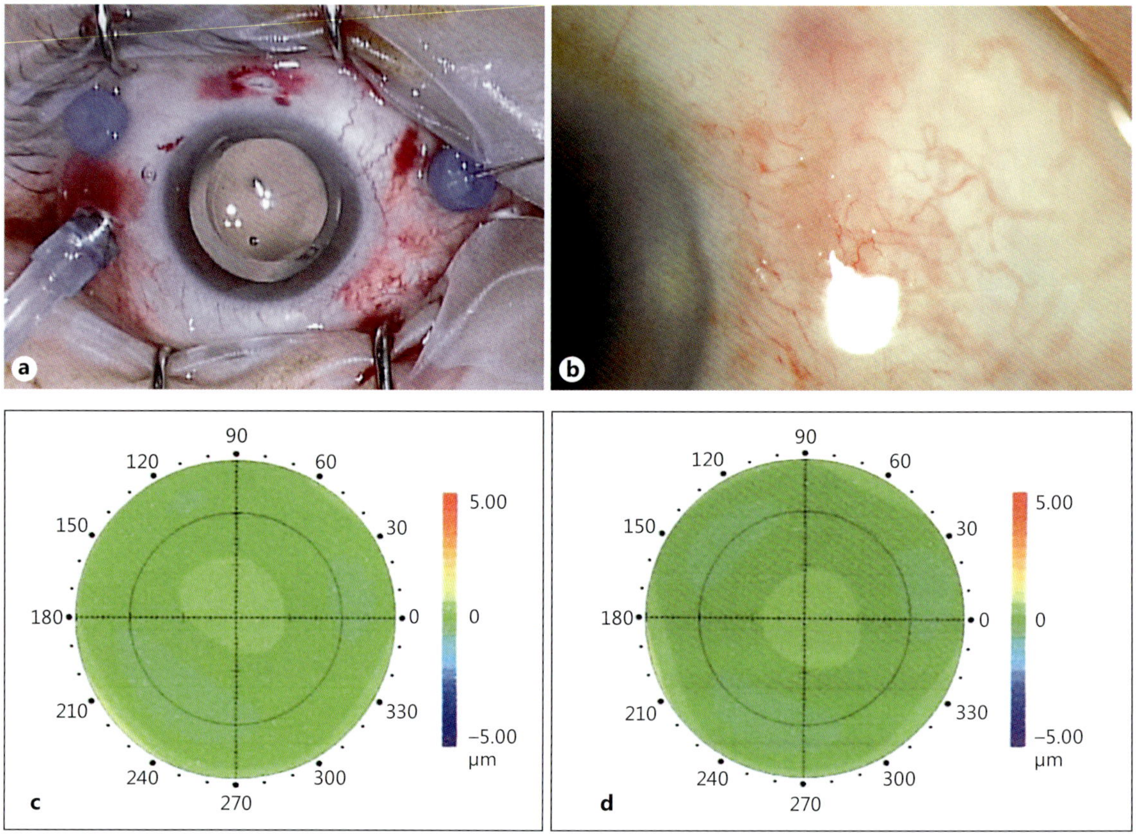

Fig. 6. 27-gauge vitrectomy. **a** Three ports with 27-gauge trocars inserted in place. For the infusion, a high-flow tube is used to sufficiently assure the irrigation volume. **b** The scleral wound is hardly visible even on the next day after surgery and with high magnification. **c, d** Corneal topography images showing preoperative (**c**) and 1 month postoperative (**d**) corneal higher order aberration. Note there is no remarkable change even shortly after surgery.

performed with the 27-gauge system, and observed as well the features mentioned above (fig. 6).

Ocriplasmin

Ocriplasmin is a truncated form of human plasmin and has proteolytic activity for components of the vitreoretinal interface including fibronectin and laminin. Recent preclinical and clinical studies have shown that cleaving the bonds between the vitreous and the retina actually has a substantial effect [38–42]. In multicenter, randomized, double-blind, phase III trials, a single intravitreal injection of ocriplasmin (125 μg) significantly showed a better resolution of macular adhesion (26.5 vs. 10.1% in the placebo group) as well as an increased rate of nonsurgical macular hole closure (40.6 vs. 10.6% in the placebo group) [42]. The preoperative factors reported to contribute to better surgical outcomes are absence of epiretinal membrane, adhesion diameter ≤1,500 μm, age <65 years, and phakic lens status [43]. Regarding ocular adverse events, however, vitreous floaters and photopsia were reported to happen more often in the ocriplasmin-injected group as compared with the placebo group [42]. The incidence of severe adverse events like macular hole formation and retinal detachment were similar. Although this drug has been demonstrated to be an attractive treatment modality for nonsurgical therapy, since only less than a half of the cases fulfilled the primary endpoint, the surgical option will still stay indispensable for this retinal pathology.

Surgical Complications

Complications that may occur from macular hole surgery include iatrogenic retinal breaks and retinal detachment, vitreous hemorrhage, ocular hypotony, and endophthalmitis. Ocular hypertension can also occur due to postoperative gas expansion, ocular inflammation, and the residual steroid used for intraoperative visualization of the vitreous. A dissociated optic nerve fiber layer appearance is a postoperative retinal defect observed after surgery that includes ILM peeling first reported by Tadayoni et al. [44]. Although it has been shown to not directly correlate with visual acuity prognosis so far, a recent report has shown it does have an influence on retinal perimetric sensitivity [29]. Hence, special attention is required for the surgical maneuver of ILM peeling.

References

1 Kelly NE, Wendel RT: Vitreous surgery for idiopathic macular holes. Results of a pilot study. Arch Ophthalmol 1991; 109:654–659.
2 Wendel RT, Patel AC, Kelly NE, Salzano TC, Wells JW, Novack GD: Vitreous surgery for macular holes. Ophthalmology 1993;100:1671–1676.
3 Gass JD: Idiopathic senile macular hole. Its early stages and pathogenesis. Arch Ophthalmol 1988;106:629–639.
4 Gass JD: Reappraisal of biomicroscopic classification of stages of development of a macular hole. Am J Ophthalmol 1995;119:752–759.
5 Gaudric A, Haouchine B, Massin P, Paques M, Blain P, Erginay A: Macular hole formation: new data provided by optical coherence tomography. Arch Ophthalmol 1999;117:744–751.
6 Hee MR, Puliafito CA, Wong C, Duker JS, Reichel E, Schuman JS, Swanson EA, Fujimoto JG: Optical coherence tomography of macular holes. Ophthalmology 1995;102:748–756.
7 Uchino E, Uemura A, Doi N, Ohba N: Postsurgical evaluation of idiopathic vitreomacular traction syndrome by optical coherence tomography. Am J Ophthalmol 2001;132:122–123.
8 Kishi S, Takahashi H: Three-dimensional observations of developing macular holes. Am J Ophthalmol 2000;130:65–75.
9 Duker JS, Kaiser PK, Binder S, de Smet MD, Gaudric A, Reichel E, Sadda SR, Sebag J, Spaide RF, Stalmans P: The International Vitreomacular Traction Study Group classification of vitreomacular adhesion, traction, and macular hole. Ophthalmology 2013;120:2611–2619.
10 Ullrich S, Haritoglou C, Gass C, Schaumberger M, Ulbig MW, Kampik A: Macular hole size as a prognostic factor in macular hole surgery. Br J Ophthalmol 2002;86:390–393.
11 Kusuhara S, Teraoka Escano MF, Fujii S, Nakanishi Y, Tamura Y, Nagai A, Yamamoto H, Tsukahara Y, Negi A: Prediction of postoperative visual outcome based on hole configuration by optical coherence tomography in eyes with idiopathic macular holes. Am J Ophthalmol 2004;138:709–716.
12 Taban M, Sharma S, Ventura AA, Kaiser PK: Evaluation of wound closure in oblique 23-gauge sutureless sclerotomies with visante optical coherence tomography. Am J Ophthalmol 2009;147: 101–107.e1.
13 Taban M, Ventura AA, Sharma S, Kaiser PK: Dynamic evaluation of sutureless vitrectomy wounds: an optical coherence tomography and histopathology study. Ophthalmology 2008;115:2221–2228.
14 Hu AY, Bourges JL, Shah SP, Gupta A, Gonzales CR, Oliver SC, Schwartz SD: Endophthalmitis after pars plana vitrectomy a 20- and 25-gauge comparison. Ophthalmology 2009;116:1360–1365.
15 Oshima Y, Kadonosono K, Yamaji H, Inoue M, Yoshida M, Kimura H, Ohji M, Shiraga F, Hamasaki T: Japan Microincision Vitrectomy Surgery Study G: Multicenter survey with a systematic overview of acute-onset endophthalmitis after transconjunctival microincision vitrectomy surgery. Am J Ophthalmol 2010;150:716–725.e1.
16 Shimada H, Nakashizuka H, Hattori T, Mori R, Mizutani Y, Yuzawa M: Incidence of endophthalmitis after 20- and 25-gauge vitrectomy causes and prevention. Ophthalmology 2008;115:2215–2220.
17 Chen D, Lian Y, Cui L, Lu F, Ke Z, Song Z: Sutureless vitrectomy incision architecture in the immediate postoperative period evaluated in vivo using optical coherence tomography. Ophthalmology 2010;117:2003–2009.
18 Olsen TW, Sternberg P Jr, Capone A Jr, Martin DF, Lim JI, Grossniklaus HE, Aaberg TM Sr: Macular hole surgery using thrombin-activated fibrinogen and selective removal of the internal limiting membrane. Retina 1998;18: 322–329.

19 Park DW, Sipperley JO, Sneed SR, Dugel PU, Jacobsen J: Macular hole surgery with internal-limiting membrane peeling and intravitreous air. Ophthalmology 1999;106:1392–1397, discussion 1397–1398.
20 Da Mata AP, Burk SE, Foster RE, Riemann CD, Petersen MR, Nehemy M, Augsburger JJ: Long-term follow-up of indocyanine green-assisted peeling of the retinal internal limiting membrane during vitrectomy surgery for idiopathic macular hole repair. Ophthalmology 2004;111:2246–2253.
21 Spiteri Cornish K, Lois N, Scott N, Burr J, Cook J, Boachie C, Tadayoni R, la Cour M, Christensen U, Kwok A: Vitrectomy with internal limiting membrane (ILM) peeling versus vitrectomy with no peeling for idiopathic full-thickness macular hole (FTMH). Cochrane Database Syst Rev 2013;6:CD009306.
22 Kadonosono K, Itoh N, Uchio E, Nakamura S, Ohno S: Staining of internal limiting membrane in macular hole surgery. Arch Ophthalmol 2000;118:1116–1118.
23 Kimura H, Kuroda S, Nagata M: Triamcinolone acetonide-assisted peeling of the internal limiting membrane. Am J Ophthalmol 2004;137:172–173.
24 Enaida H, Hisatomi T, Hata Y, Ueno A, Goto Y, Yamada T, Kubota T, Ishibashi T: Brilliant blue G selectively stains the internal limiting membrane/brilliant blue G-assisted membrane peeling. Retina 2006;26:631–636.
25 Schumann RG, Gandorfer A, Priglinger SG, Kampik A, Haritoglou C: Vital dyes for macular surgery: a comparative electron microscopy study of the internal limiting membrane. Retina 2009;29: 669–676.
26 Enaida H, Sakamoto T, Hisatomi T, Goto Y, Ishibashi T: Morphological and functional damage of the retina caused by intravitreous indocyanine green in rat eyes. Graefes Arch Clin Exp Ophthalmol 2002;240:209–213.
27 Kawahara S, Hata Y, Miura M, Kita T, Sengoku A, Nakao S, Mochizuki Y, Enaida H, Ueno A, Hafezi-Moghadam A, Ishibashi T: Intracellular events in retinal glial cells exposed to ICG and BBG. Invest Ophthalmol Vis Sci 2007;48: 4426–4432.
28 Ueno A, Hisatomi T, Enaida H, Kagimoto T, Mochizuki Y, Goto Y, Kubota T, Hata Y, Ishibashi T: Biocompatibility of brilliant blue G in a rat model of subretinal injection. Retina 2007;27:499–504.
29 Nukada K, Hangai M, Ooto S, Yoshikawa M, Yoshimura N: Tomographic features of macula after successful macular hole surgery. Invest Ophthalmol Vis Sci 2013;54:2417–2428.
30 Yamashita T, Yamashita T, Kawano H, Sonoda Y, Yamakiri K, Sakamoto T: Early imaging of macular hole closure: a diagnostic technique and its quality for gas-filled eyes with spectral domain optical coherence tomography. Ophthalmologica 2013;229:43–49.
31 Ip MS, Baker BJ, Duker JS, Reichel E, Baumal CR, Gangnon R, Puliafito CA: Anatomical outcomes of surgery for idiopathic macular hole as determined by optical coherence tomography. Arch Ophthalmol 2002;120:29–35.
32 Michalewska Z, Michalewski J, Adelman RA, Nawrocki J: Inverted internal limiting membrane flap technique for large macular holes. Ophthalmology 2010; 117:2018–2025.
33 Kuriyama S, Hayashi H, Jingami Y, Kuramoto N, Akita J, Matsumoto M: Efficacy of inverted internal limiting membrane flap technique for the treatment of macular hole in high myopia. Am J Ophthalmol 2013;156:125–131.e1.
34 Wakabayashi T, Fujiwara M, Sakaguchi H, Kusaka S, Oshima Y: Foveal microstructure and visual acuity in surgically closed macular holes: spectral-domain optical coherence tomographic analysis. Ophthalmology 2010;117:1815–1824.
35 Christensen UC, Kroyer K, Sander B, Larsen M, la Cour M: Prognostic significance of delayed structural recovery after macular hole surgery. Ophthalmology 2009;116:2430–2436.
36 Sakaguchi H, Oshima Y, Tano Y: 27-gauge transconjunctival nonvitrectomizing vitreous surgery for epiretinal membrane removal. Retina 2007;27: 1302–1304.
37 Oshima Y, Wakabayashi T, Sato T, Ohji M, Tano Y: A 27-gauge instrument system for transconjunctival sutureless microincision vitrectomy surgery. Ophthalmology 2010;117:93–102.e2.
38 de Smet MD, Gandorfer A, Stalmans P, Veckeneer M, Feron E, Pakola S, Kampik A: Microplasmin intravitreal administration in patients with vitreomacular traction scheduled for vitrectomy: the MIVI I trial. Ophthalmology 2009;116:1349–1355, 1355.e1–e2.
39 de Smet MD, Valmaggia C, Zarranz-Ventura J, Willekens B: Microplasmin: Ex vivo characterization of its activity in porcine vitreous. Invest Ophthalmol Vis Sci 2009;50:814–819.
40 Gandorfer A, Rohleder M, Sethi C, Eckle D, Welge-Lussen U, Kampik A, Luthert P, Charteris D: Posterior vitreous detachment induced by microplasmin. Invest Ophthalmol Vis Sci 2004;45:641–647.
41 Stalmans P, Delaey C, de Smet MD, van Dijkman E, Pakola S: Intravitreal injection of microplasmin for treatment of vitreomacular adhesion: results of a prospective, randomized, sham-controlled phase II trial (the MIVI-IIT trial). Retina 2010;30:1122–1127.
42 Stalmans P, Benz MS, Gandorfer A, Kampik A, Girach A, Pakola S, Haller JA, Group M-TS: Enzymatic vitreolysis with ocriplasmin for vitreomacular traction and macular holes. N Engl J Med 2012;367:606–615.
43 Singh RP, Li A, Bedi R, Srivastava S, Sears JE, Ehlers JP, Schachat AP, Kaiser PK: Anatomical and visual outcomes following ocriplasmin treatment for symptomatic vitreomacular traction syndrome. Br J Ophthalmol 2014;98: 356–360.
44 Tadayoni R, Paques M, Massin P, Mouki-Benani S, Mikol J, Gaudric A: Dissociated optic nerve fiber layer appearance of the fundus after idiopathic epiretinal membrane removal. Ophthalmology 2001;108:2279–2283.

Hideyasu Oh, MD, PhD
Hyogo Prefectural Amagasaki Hospital
Higashidaimotsu-cho 1-1-1
Amagasaki 660-0828 (Japan)
E-Mail hideyasu@kuhp.kyoto-u.ac.jp

Oh H, Oshima Y (eds): Microincision Vitrectomy Surgery. Emerging Techniques and Technology.
Dev Ophthalmol. Basel, Karger, 2014, vol 54, pp 159–163 (DOI: 10.1159/000360462)

Macular Diseases: Epiretinal Membrane

Maiko Inoue · Kazuaki Kadonosono

Department of Ophthalmology, Yokohama City University Medical Center, Yokohama, Japan

Abstract

Epiretinal membrane (ERM) is a relatively common macular disease, which forms along the surface of the internal limiting membrane of the retina. Currently, microincision vitrectomy surgery (MIVS) has been confirmed as a minimally invasive and very safe modality of treatment that is useful for improving vision. However, some cases have shown poor visual recovery even after complete removal of the ERM. Since the introduction of spectral domain optical coherence tomography (SD-OCT) was demonstrated to be useful for the noninvasive diagnosis and monitoring of macular diseases, the appearance of the photoreceptor layer on SD-OCT images has been found to be an important prognostic factor for visual recovery and postoperative best-corrected visual acuity after MIVS. Although deciding when to perform a vitrectomy can be difficult, it might be better to schedule vitrectomy surgery while the photoreceptor inner segment/outer segment (IS/OS) junction remains intact. If the preoperative IS/OS junction has already been disrupted, the surgery should be scheduled as early as possible to avoid further disturbances of visual improvement.

Epiretinal membrane (ERM) is a relatively common macular disease that forms along the surface of the internal limiting membrane (ILM) of the retina. Its forms range from translucent wrinkling to an extensive periretinal cellular proliferation. ERM is mainly classified into two types. Secondary ERM is associated with a variety of ocular diseases, such as ocular inflammatory diseases, retinal vascular disease, and retinal detachments. However, in the majority of cases, ERM develops in an eye with no history of ocular disease, and is called 'idiopathic'. The prevalence of ERM ranges from 4.0 to 6.2% and increases with age [1–3]. The progression of ERM, however, is very slow and only some patients complain of visual acuity and distortion which requires treatment. In the Blue Mountains Eye Study, which examined the natural history of ERM, most ERM cases showed no progression for more than 5 years [4]. Concerning ERM treatment, surgical correction of ERM, first reported by Machemer [5] in the mid-1970s, is useful for improving vision. Since then, vitrectomy has been performed for more than 30 years. Currently, due to the development of instrumentation and technique, microincision vitrectomy surgery (MIVS) has been confirmed as a minimally invasive and very safe modality of treatment [6–8].

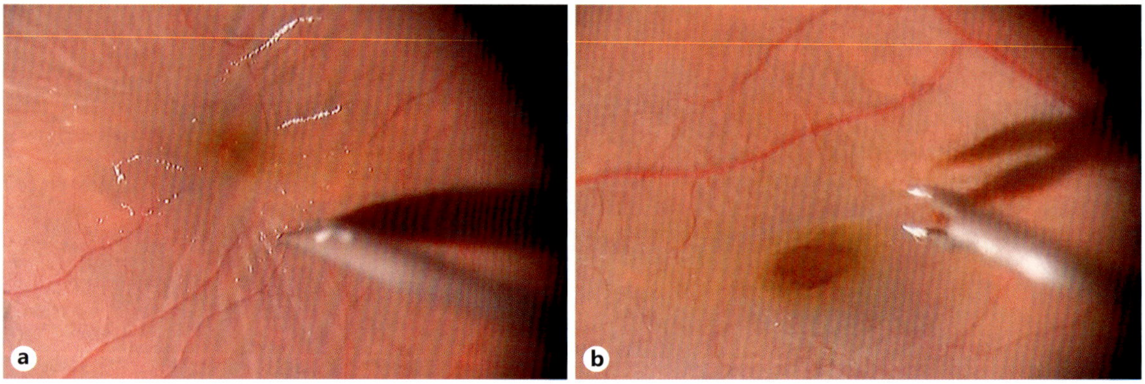

Fig. 1. Picture of ERM removal. **a** The 25-gauge needle is used to create the initial flap of the membrane. **b** Asymmetrical forceps are useful to observe and remove the membrane.

Surgical Procedure

Indication

Surgical indications for ERM are not defined. However, surgical treatment is recommended in cases with (1) decreasing visual acuity or (2) strong distortion even when visual acuity is relatively good.

Removal of the Vitreous

Either a three- or four-port vitrectomy system utilizing chandelier illumination is usually performed. A sharp-edged trocar should be inserted obliquely in an angled manner to achieve a self-sealing sclerotomy postoperatively. It is very important to shave the vitreous around the scleral port in order to prevent the occurrence of iatrogenic breaks at the ora serrata adjacent to the site of cannula when inserting or removing the instruments. Chandelier illumination allows adequate visualization of the retinal fundus during surgery due to its wide range of lighting.

Removal of Epiretinal Membrane

First, the starting point of the peeling should be identified. The edge of the membrane, the thickest part of which is set up as a guide, should be gently lifted off the retinal surface with a 25-gauge needle. Another technique is to directly initiate peeling the ERM with forceps. Subsequently, the edge of the ERM should be lifted softly so as not to pull on the underlying retina (fig. 1).

Internal Limiting Membrane Peeling

The removal of the ILM prevents the proliferation of the residual cellular component on the ILM, which potentially reduces the risk of recurrences of ERM. Adjuvants such as indocyanine green [9] and brilliant blue G [10] should be used before the removal of the ILM. Dyes that stain the ILM help to assist in ILM peeling. When starting ILM peeling, surgeons should begin with temporal raphe to minimize damage of the papillomacular bundle. However, the ILM is frequently attached to the ERM at the time of ERM peeling.

Postoperative Management

The main intra- and postoperative complications are macular holes (created during peeling of the ILM or ERM), iatrogenic rhegmatogenous

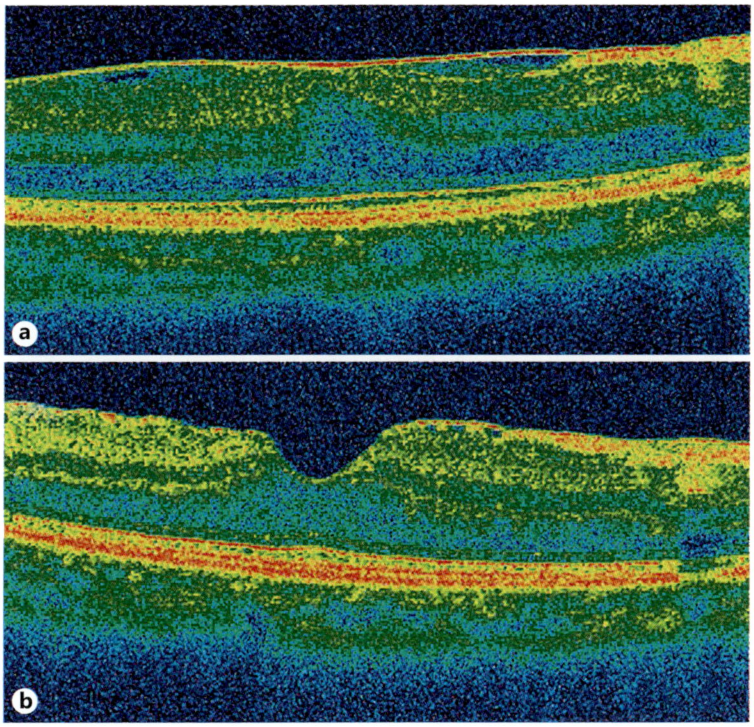

Fig. 2. a SD-OCT at baseline shows ERM with a continuous and hyper-reflective line corresponding to the IS/OS junction, which was judged as an intact IS/OS junction. Visual acuity was 20/50 in the left eye. **b** SD-OCT at 12 months after surgery. ERM is removed and an OCT image shows normal foveal contour. Visual acuity had improved to 20/16.

retinal tear, retinal detachment, and recurrence of ERM due to reproliferation. Intraocular gas tamponade and face-down positioning should be performed in case of a macular hole or retinal break. Cataract progression is also a downside of vitrectomy. However, combined surgery for ERM and cataracts may potentially be as effective as membrane peeling alone with respect to visual and anatomical outcomes [11]. Acute-onset endophthalmitis, although a rare complication of MIVS with an incidence rate of 0.030–0.070%, is a serious and major clinical concern [12–14]. To minimize the risk of MIVS-related endophthalmitis, consistency of sterilization, use of disposable products, prevention of postoperative hypotony, scleral wound closure, patient education, and use of topical antibiotics are encouraged. If surgeons think that self-sealing wounds are incomplete, the scleral wound should be sutured.

Surgical Outcome and Prognostic Factors

Previous reports comparing MIVS and conventional 20-gauge vitrectomy systems have shown that MIVS has advantages such as a reduced operating time and a lower degree of postoperative intraocular inflammation [8]. Furthermore, 25-gauge vitrectomy reportedly enables earlier postoperative visual recovery, compared with 20-gauge vitrectomy, in patients with idiopathic ERM [15]. Most patients with ERM have sufficient visual recovery after MIVS. However, some cases show poor visual recovery even after complete removal of the ERM [16, 17]. Several factors, such as preoperative visual acuity [17], duration of symptoms before the surgery [16], and cystoid macular edema [18] have been suggested as prognostic factors influencing postoperative visual acuity. However, since the introduction of spectral domain optical coherence tomography (SD-

OCT) has been demonstrated to be useful for the noninvasive diagnosis and monitoring of macular diseases, including ERM, the appearance of the photoreceptor layer on SD-OCT images has been found to be an important prognostic factor for visual recovery and postoperative best-corrected visual acuity (BCVA) after ERM surgery [19, 20].

In regard to postoperative BCVA, we reported that a preoperative intact photoreceptor inner segment/outer segment (IS/OS) junction seems to be strongly associated with better postoperative visual acuity and better visual recovery than a disrupted or irregular IS/OS junction [21]. Therefore, preoperative assessment of the IS/OS junction may be an important procedure for predicting surgical outcomes (fig. 2). Furthermore, other recent reports have described the photoreceptor cone outer segment tips to be highly associated with BCVA [22, 23]. Assessing photoreceptor structures by SD-OCT may help in predicting macular function after ERM surgery.

When to Perform Microincision Vitrectomy Surgery

Deciding when to perform a vitrectomy can be difficult. In our study, even if the IS/OS junction is intact or disrupted, MIVS significantly improved the postoperative BCVA as compared with the preoperative visual acuity [19, 20]. Furthermore, patients with disrupted IS/OS junctions after MIVS could achieve anatomic and functional improvement even after 1 year postoperatively, although their visual acuity were still inferior to those with preoperative intact IS/OS junctions [24]. Therefore, it might be better to schedule MIVS while the IS/OS junction remains intact. If the preoperative IS/OS junction has already been disrupted, vitrectomy should be planned as early as possible since formation of a lamellar macular hole and longer diffuse traction induced by ERM might delay IS/OS junction recovery or produce permanent impairment of the photoreceptor layer, resulting in further disturbances of visual improvement.

References

1 Mitchell P, Smith W, Chey T, Wang JJ, Chang A: Prevalence and associations of epiretinal membranes. The Blue Mountains Eye Study, Australia. Ophthalmology 1997;104:1033–1040.

2 Miyazaki M, Nakamura H, Kubo M, et al: Prevalence and risk factors for epiretinal membranes in a Japanese population: the Hisayama study. Graefes Arch Clin Exp Ophthalmol 2003;241:642–646.

3 McCarty DJ, Mukesh BN, Chikani V, et al: Prevalence and associations of epiretinal membranes in the visual impairment project. Am J Ophthalmol 2005;140:288–294.

4 Fraser-Bell S, Guzowski M, Rochtchina E, Wang JJ, Mitchell P: Five-year cumulative incidence and progression of epiretinal membranes: the Blue Mountains Eye Study. Ophthalmology 2003;110:34–40.

5 Machemer R: The surgical removal of epiretinal macular membranes (macular puckers) (author's transl) (in German). Klin Monatsbl Augenheilkd 1978;173:36–42.

6 Fujii GY, De Juan E Jr, Humayun MS, et al: Initial experience using the transconjunctival sutureless vitrectomy system for vitreoretinal surgery. Ophthalmology 2002;109:1814–1820.

7 Fujii GY, De Juan E Jr, Humayun MS, et al: A new 25-gauge instrument system for transconjunctival sutureless vitrectomy surgery. Ophthalmology 2002;109:1807–1812.

8 Rizzo S, Genovesi-Ebert F, Murri S, et al: 25-gauge, sutureless vitrectomy and standard 20-gauge pars plana vitrectomy in idiopathic epiretinal membrane surgery: a comparative pilot study. Graefes Arch Clin Exp Ophthalmol 2006;244:472–479.

9 Kadonosono K, Itoh N, Uchio E, Nakamura S, Ohno S: Staining of internal limiting membrane in macular hole surgery. Arch Ophthalmol 2000;118:1116–1118.

10 Enaida H, Hisatomi T, Goto Y, et al: Preclinical investigation of internal limiting membrane staining and peeling using intravitreal brilliant blue G. Retina 2006;26:623–630.

11 Yiu G, Marra KV, Wagley S, et al: Surgical outcomes after epiretinal membrane peeling combined with cataract surgery. Br J Ophthalmol 2013;97:1197–1201.

12 Shimada H, Nakashizuka H, Hattori T, Mori R, Mizutani Y, Yuzawa M: Incidence of endophthalmitis after 20- and 25-gauge vitrectomy causes and prevention. Ophthalmology 2008;115:2215–2212.

13 Hu AY, Bourges JL, Shah SP, et al: Endophthalmitis after pars plana vitrectomy a 20- and 25-gauge comparison. Ophthalmology 2009;116:1360–1365.
14 Oshima Y, Kadonosono K, Yamaji H, et al: Multicenter survey with a systematic overview of acute-onset endophthalmitis after transconjunctival microincision vitrectomy surgery. Am J Ophthalmol 2010;150:716–725.e1.
15 Kadonosono K, Yamakawa T, Uchio E, Yanagi Y, Tamaki Y, Araie M: Comparison of visual function after epiretinal membrane removal by 20-gauge and 25-gauge vitrectomy. Am J Ophthalmol 2006;142:513–515.
16 Rice TA, De Bustros S, Michels RG, Thompson JT, Debanne SM, Rowland DY: Prognostic factors in vitrectomy for epiretinal membranes of the macula. Ophthalmology 1986;93:602–610.
17 Wong JG, Sachdev N, Beaumont PE, Chang AA: Visual outcomes following vitrectomy and peeling of epiretinal membrane. Clin Experiment Ophthalmol 2005;33:373–378.
18 Trese MT, Chandler DB, Machemer R: Macular pucker. I. Prognostic criteria. Graefes Arch Clin Exp Ophthalmol 1983;221:12–15.
19 Mitamura Y, Hirano K, Baba T, Yamamoto S: Correlation of visual recovery with presence of photoreceptor inner/outer segment junction in optical coherence images after epiretinal membrane surgery. Br J Ophthalmol 2009;93:171–175.
20 Inoue M, Morita S, Watanabe Y, et al: Inner segment/outer segment junction assessed by spectral-domain optical coherence tomography in patients with idiopathic epiretinal membrane. Am J Ophthalmol 2010;150:834–839.
21 Inoue M, Morita S, Watanabe Y, et al: Preoperative inner segment/outer segment junction in spectral-domain optical coherence tomography as a prognostic factor in epiretinal membrane surgery. Retina 2011;31:1366–1372.
22 Shimozono M, Oishi A, Hata M, et al: The significance of cone outer segment tips as a prognostic factor in epiretinal membrane surgery. Am J Ophthalmol 2012;153:698–704.
23 Watanabe K, Tsunoda K, Mizuno Y, Akiyama K, Noda T: Outer retinal morphology and visual function in patients with idiopathic epiretinal membrane. JAMA Ophthalmol 2013;131:172–177.
24 Inoue M, Arakawa A, Yamane S, Kadonosono K: Long-term outcome of preoperative disrupted inner/outer segment junctions assessed using spectral-domain optical coherence tomography in patients with idiopathic epiretinal membrane. Ophthalmologica 2012;228:222–228.

Maiko Inoue, MD
Department of Ophthalmology, Yokohama City University Medical Center
4-57 Urafune-cho, Minami-ku
Yokohama, Kanagawa 232-0024 (Japan)
E-Mail maicoo@urahp.yokohama-cu.ac.jp

Oh H, Oshima Y (eds): Microincision Vitrectomy Surgery. Emerging Techniques and Technology.
Dev Ophthalmol. Basel, Karger, 2014, vol 54, pp 164–173 (DOI: 10.1159/000360463)

Diabetic Macular Edema

Fabio Patelli[a] · Paolo Radice[b] · Enrico Giacomotti[a]

[a]Vitreoretina Surgery, Department of Ophthalmology, Igea Clinic, and [b]Department of Vitreoretina Surgery, Fatebenefratelli Ophthalmic Hospital, Milan, Italy

Abstract

Diabetic macular edema (DME) is one of the most common causes of visual loss in patients with diabetes mellitus. Many patients continue to lose vision despite laser photocoagulation and medical therapies. The two major categories of medications currently used to treat DME are corticosteroids and anti-VEGF agents. The vitreous has been implicated as a cause of macular edema in people with diabetes via several mechanical and physiologic mechanisms, all of which are postulated to lead to increased vascular permeability. Vitrectomy can release the mechanical traction on the macula and increase oxygenation with subsequent reduction in DME. Early vitrectomy even in nontractional DME results in significant macular thinning and may lead to rapid improvement in vision with long-term stabilization. Unfortunately, a randomized trial pitting vitrectomy against the methods currently employed has not yet been performed.

Diabetic macular edema (DME) is one of the most common causes of visual loss in patients with diabetes mellitus [1]. The pathophysiology of DME involves dilated capillaries, retinal microaneurysms, and loss of pericytes, with eventual impairment of the blood-retinal barrier [2]. Breakdown of the blood-retinal barrier results in fluid leakage into the extracellular space, which disrupts macular structure and function on a cellular level [3, 4].

The pathogenesis of DME is at this time poorly defined, but is believed to involve angiogenesis, inflammation, and oxidative stress [5]. Hyperglycemia is reported to lead to capillary endothelial damage and alterations in leukocyte function [6]. In addition, hyperglycemia has been reported to activate oxidative stress agents, such as advanced glycation end-products and the protein kinase C pathway [7]. Various inflammatory mediators appear to play a role in promoting DME, including vascular endothelial growth factor (VEGF) [8], placental growth factor [9], and hepatocyte factor [10].

Diabetic Macular Edema Classification

The Early Treatment Diabetic Retinopathy Study Research Group (ETDRS) defined clinically significant DME as any one of the following:

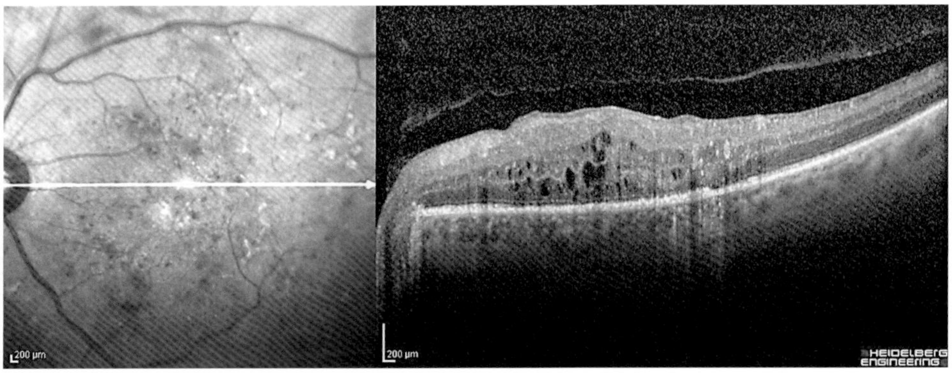

Fig. 1. OCT demonstrating diffuse retinal thickening. Diffuse retinal thickening appears as increased retinal thickness with areas of reduced intraretinal reflectivity.

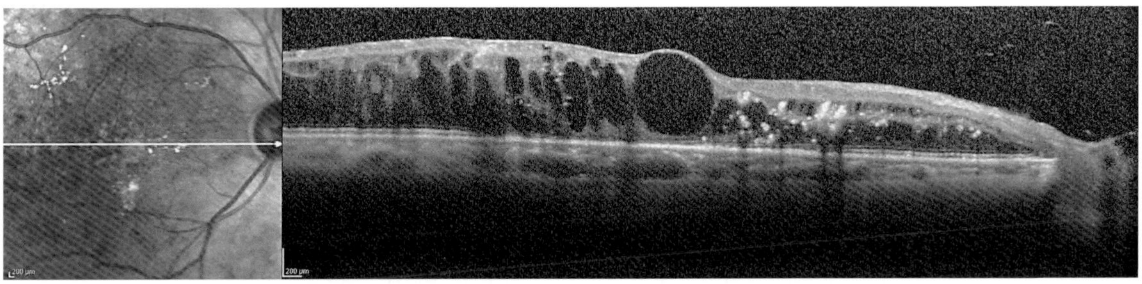

Fig. 2. OCT demonstrating diabetic cystoid macular edema. The scan highlights the large, ovoid areas of low reflectivity, separated by highly reflective septae that represent intraretinal cystoid-like cavities.

- Retinal edema located at or within 500 μm of the center of the macula
- Hard exudates at or within 500 μm of the center, associated with thickening of adjacent retina
- A zone of thickening larger than one disc area if located within 1 disc diameter of the center of the macula

Optical coherence tomography (OCT) has also been shown to be effective in both the qualitative and quantitative description of DME [11–14]. The widely accepted classification was proposed by Kim et al. [15] who described and classified five patterns of DME according to OCT:

- Diffuse retinal thickening (fig. 1)
- Cystoid macular edema (fig. 2)
- Serous retinal detachment without posterior hyaloidal traction (PHT; fig. 3)
- PHT without traction retinal detachment (TRD; fig. 4)
- PHT with TRD (fig. 5)

Medical Therapies for Diabetic Macular Edema

Focal/grid photocoagulation has demonstrated efficacy in a large, prospective, randomized clinical trial [16]. Nevertheless, many patients con-

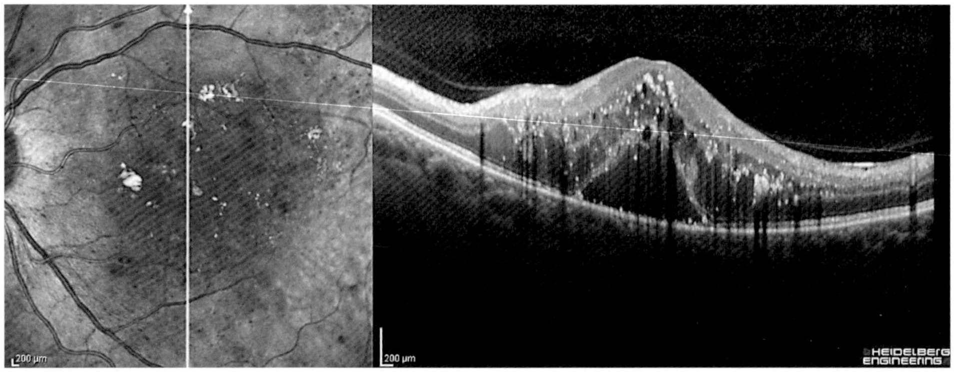

Fig. 3. OCT of a serous retinal detachment not associated with PHT. A dark accumulation of sub-retinal fluid is seen beneath the highly reflective and dome-like elevation of detached retina.

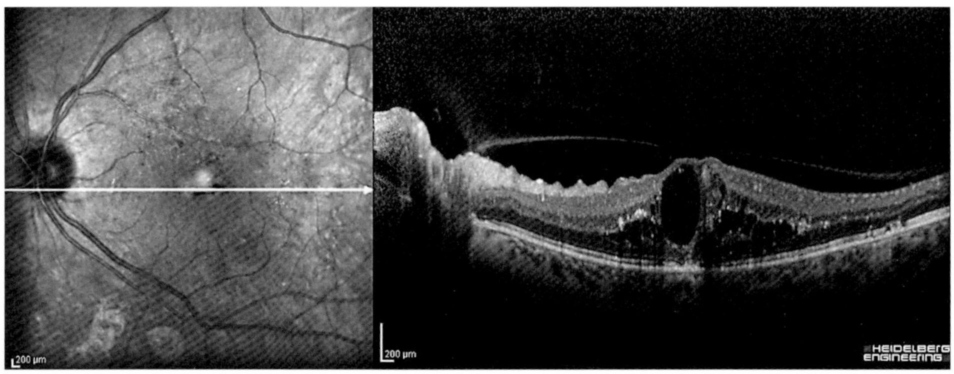

Fig. 4. OCT demonstrating PHT. Tangential traction exerted by the PHT is identified on OCT as a highly reflective band over the retinal surface.

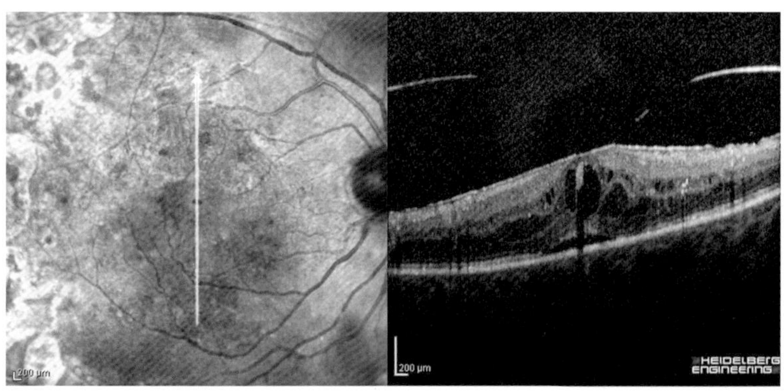

Fig. 5. OCT demonstrating PHT and TRD. PHT is seen as the highly reflective signal arising from the inner retinal surface. The TRD is identified as the area of low signal underlying the highly reflective border of detached retina.

tinue to lose vision despite these interventions [17], which has led to the investigation of pharmacologic therapies for DME [18]. The two major categories of medications currently used to treat DME are corticosteroids and anti-VEGF agents.

The two most commonly used anti-VEGF agents are bevacizumab (Avastin; Genentech, South San Francisco, Calif., USA) and ranibizumab (Lucentis, Genentech). Off-label intravitreal bevacizumab has been reported to have short-term efficacy in the treatment of DME in multiple randomized clinical trials [19, 20]. Ranibizumab has been approved by the FDA for the intravitreal treatment of exudative age-related macular degeneration [21, 22], macular edema secondary to retinal vein occlusion at a 0.5-mg dose [23, 24], and DME at a 0.3-mg dose [25, 26].

Corticosteroids may have multiple mechanisms of action in the treatment of DME. In addition to their anti-inflammatory properties, corticosteroids have been reported to reduce the activity of VEGF [27]. Intravitreal triamcinolone acetonide has been reported as being effective in the treatment of DME [28].

The dexamethasone drug delivery system (Ozurdex; Allergan, Irvine, Calif., USA) is a biodegradable, sustained-release device approved by the FDA for the treatment of macular edema associated with retinal vein occlusion and noninfectious posterior segment uveitis. A phase 2 randomized clinical trial in patients with persistent macular edema, secondary to various etiologies, including DME, showed that the dexamethasone drug delivery system produced improvements in visual acuity, macular thickness, and fluorescein leakage that were sustained for up to 6 months [29]. A more recent study reported that the dexamethasone drug delivery system improved visual acuity and macular edema in previously vitrectomized eyes with diffuse DME [30].

Several randomized clinical trials have shown the efficacy of ranibizumab in the treatment of DME. The Ranibizumab for Edema of the Macula in Diabetes (READ-2) study randomized 126 eyes with DME to three groups: ranibizumab only (injection at baseline and months 1, 3, and 5), photocoagulation (at baseline and at 3 months if needed), and combined ranibizumab and photocoagulation (photocoagulation and ranibizumab at baseline, and ranibizumab at 3 months if needed) [31]. Patients randomized to ranibizumab only showed a significantly better visual outcome at 6 months compared with the other two groups. At 24 months, the study reported that intravitreal ranibizumab provided persistent treatment benefits [26]. Two-year visual outcomes were similar to 1-year results and reinforced the conclusion that ranibizumab with prompt or deferred photocoagulation should be considered for patients with vision impairment worse than 20/32 secondary to DME [32].

The RESTORE phase 3 study reported that ranibizumab monotherapy or combined with laser photocoagulation provided superior visual acuity gain over standard photocoagulation in the treatment of DME [33].

In contrast to intravitreal corticosteroids, cataract progression associated with intravitreal VEGF antagonists has not been identified. Some patients do have sustained intraocular pressure elevation following repeated injections of VEGF antagonists [34], but this effect does not appear to be as strong as that associated with intravitreal corticosteroids.

Aflibercept, or VEGF trap-eye (Eylea, Regeneron, Tarrytown, N.Y., USA), is a recombinant fusion protein with activity against all VEGF-A isoforms and placental growth factor that is approved by the FDA for the treatment of neovascular age-related macular degeneration and has been shown to have short-term efficacy in the treatment of DME [35]. The DA VINCI study assessed the efficacy and safety of intravitreal aflibercept versus laser photocoagulation in the treatment of DME. In this study population, intravitreal aflibercept produced significant improvements in visual acuity and retinal thickness, as compared to laser photocoagulation at both 24 and 52 weeks. Presently, aflibercept has not been approved by the FDA or EU for the treatment of DME.

The Role of the Vitreous and Vitrectomy in Diabetic Macular Edema

The vitreous has been implicated as a cause of macular edema in people with diabetes via several mechanical and physiologic mechanisms, all of which are postulated to lead to increased vascular permeability [36–45]. Suggested mechanisms include the following:

- Destabilization of the vitreous by abnormal glycation and cross-linking of vitreal collagen, leading to traction on the macula
- Accumulation and concentration of factors causing vasopermeability in the premacular vitreous gel
- Accumulation of chemoattractant factors in the vitreous, leading to the cellular migration to the posterior hyaloid, contraction, and macular traction [37–39, 42, 44]

The observation that release of mechanical traction on the macula with subsequent reduction in DME, either by spontaneous posterior vitreous detachment or with vitrectomy, lends support to this line of reasoning [38, 40, 41, 43, 45]. Furthermore, the evidence that increased oxygenation can reduce DME [46] suggests an additional physiologic advantage, potentially conferred by vitrectomy.

Increased oxygen tension counteracts the diabetes-induced retinal hypoxia responsible for VEGF upregulation and blood-retinal barrier breakdown, decreasing exudation from the retinal capillaries and resolving DME. Vitrectomy increases the oxygen concentration at the inner retinal surface by improving bulk flow of oxygen-rich aqueous from the highly vascularized iris and ciliary body to the posterior pole [47]. Hence, improved oxygen tension in the inner retina is a potent way to decrease macular edema by downregulating VEGF production [48].

The perifoveal microcirculation in eyes with diabetic cystoid macula edema was significantly increased after vitrectomy, as compared with that before surgery, and a significant correlation was found between the increase in perifoveal microcirculation and the improvement in visual acuity [49].

Kim et al. [15] noticed a significant association between decreased visual acuity and the presence of PHT without TRD. The traction produced by the vitreomacular interface alone has been postulated to play a role in the development of DME. This vitreomacular interface has been thought to cause tangential traction, which could lead to macular edema. However, it is impossible to determine whether the premacular vitreous changes cause the macular traction and edema, or whether the diabetic retinopathy leads to the vitreous changes and, thus, the macular traction and edema. Whatever the cause, identifying the structural changes in patients with DME using OCT may allow more effective management of these patients.

Surgical Procedure

In patients affected by diabetic macula edema, the following surgical procedure is employed:

(1) Cataract surgery in phakic patients is performed at the same time as vitrectomy.
(2) A three-port pars plana vitrectomy using a 25-gauge system is carried out. After removal of the anterior and central vitreous, a vitreous detachment is performed, when not present, using the vitrectome probe aspiration only. If the vitreous is not easily visible or it is not sure that all the vitreous has been removed,

triamcinolone acetonide is injected to better visualize the residual vitreous. All the peripheral vitreous is removed without base shaving, only a small residual vitreous skirt is left.

(3) Once all of the posterior hyaloid has been removed, the internal limiting membrane (ILM) is stained. Different dyes can be used, typically blue dyes like triphenylmethane or green dyes like indocyanine green. The blue dye is injected under balanced salt solution (better with the infusion closed and washed out after 2 min). Diluted indocyanine green at a concentration of 0.1% is injected over the macula under balanced salt solution and immediately washed out in order to avoid dye toxicity. Usually, indocyanine green staining of the ILM is more visible than blue dye staining. ILM staining is more important in diabetic patients whose ILM is often more difficult to remove completely because it breaks and is strongly adherent to the retina. When possible, ILM should be removed throughout the macula.

(4) After ILM peeling, the peripheral retina is checked in order to see if retinal breaks are present.

(5) Panretinal photocoagulation is performed when necessary, and once the trocar's cannulas are removed dexamethasone (2 mg) is injected subconjunctivally.

Vitrectomy: When?

It is well accepted that in the presence of an evident traction over the macula (detected biomicroscopically and/or by the OCT), vitrectomy is considered the first therapeutic approach. In eyes with traction to the macula, the mechanical removal of the traction by pars plana vitrectomy seems to be effective [37, 42, 50, 51].

Removal of the ILM at time of vitrectomy has been associated with somewhat greater reduction in retinal thickness, but no association has been found with visual acuity improvement.

Few previous reports in the literature have evaluated factors associated with visual acuity or anatomic outcomes after vitrectomy for DME. In a retrospective study of 486 eyes that underwent vitrectomy and lensectomy for diffuse nontractional DME, Kumagai et al. [52] found that visual outcomes with ILM peeling were better than those associated with preservation of the ILM in a univariate analysis.

In diffuse DME, the ILM is thickened and a variety of cellular elements, especially numerous kinds of inflammatory cells, adhere to the inner surface of the ILM. To attenuate diffuse DME, vitrectomy combined with ILM peeling to remove the inflammatory cells and the physical barrier might be effective.

Several papers have underlined the advantages of ILM removal in these eyes, but the main problem of these studies is that it is very difficult to standardize preoperative DME characteristics because some eyes had been subject to prior laser treatments, treatment with various steroids, or anti-VEGF injections.

The role of vitrectomy compared with other approaches in the management of DME remains uncertain because the potential benefits and risks have not been clearly defined in the context of long-term, adequately sized, randomized clinical trials.

Several studies have shown limited efficacy in vitrectomy for diffuse DME without evident traction [53, 54]. Other clinical studies have, however, shown that vitrectomy for diffuse DME without evident traction leads to visual improvement of two or more lines in 38–100% of eyes. In a larger series (>50 cases) [34, 40, 55–60], visual improvement in approximately 50% of the cases was described.

Proposed reasons for poor visual acuity after complete resolution of DME were macular ischemia [61, 62], photoreceptor dysfunction [54, 63], and accumulated subfoveal hard exudates

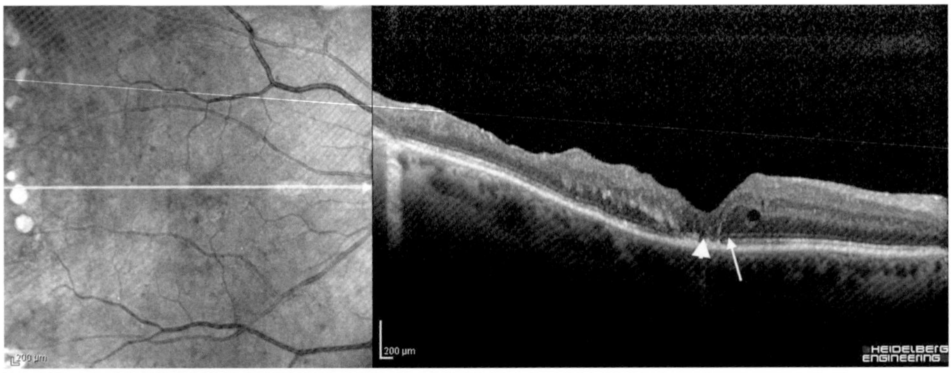

Fig. 6. OCT after vitrectomy for DME. The edema is not present. The ELM is well evident near the fovea as a hyperreflective layer (arrow), but is not evident in the fovea area (arrowhead).

[64]. Improvements in photoreceptor layer visualization, as assessed by spectral domain OCT, may provide a better opportunity to understand poor visual outcome. In particular, the integrity of the external limiting membrane (ELM) and the inner and outer segments of the photoreceptor junction seems to correlate with good visual acuity in patients with DME.

Recently, several studies have shown that ELM interruptions visible on spectral domain OCT are associated with lower visual acuity outcome in patients with clinically significant DME [65–68] (fig. 6). This is possibly because the integrity of the ELM has a critical role in restoration of the photoreceptor microstructures and alignment. Earlier reported approaches [69–71] relied on manual tracing of the corresponding surface or on detecting ELM on 2D B-scans. However, such studies rely on manual interpretation of the state of the ELM, and high intra- and interobserver variabilities are likely. Automated 3D analysis of the ELM is of great interest because of its potential to elucidate structural abnormalities with minimal variability and to possibly predict visual outcomes in DME.

Conclusions

The goal of vitrectomy in DME patients should be to dry the retina as quickly and completely as possible. The posterior hyaloid should be removed as completely as possible, and the ILM should be peeled with the assistance of staining substances to prevent postsurgical proliferation of ERMs, to minimize preretinal sequestration of VEGF, and to maximize diffusion of oxygen into the retina. Accurate spectral domain OCT evaluation of the ELM and the inner and outer segment layer should be performed before and after surgery to predict visual acuity in these patients, even if further studies are required to better define their role. Early vitrectomy results in significant macular thinning and may lead to rapid improvement in vision with long-term stabilization. Unfortunately, a randomized trial pitting vitrectomy against the methods currently employed has not yet been performed. As medical budgets become tighter and alternative therapies, including anti-VEGF injections, become more expensive, vitrectomy may emerge as the preferred low-cost, longer-duration therapy.

References

1 Klein R, Knudtson MD, Lee KE, Gangnon R, Klein BE: The Wisconsin Epidemiologic Study of Diabetic Retinopathy XXIII: the twenty-five-year incidence of macular edema in persons with type I diabetes. Ophthalmology 2009;116:497–503.

2 Ciulla TA, Amador AG, Zinman B: Diabetic retinopathy and diabetic macular edema: pathophysiology, screening, and novel therapies. Diabetes Care 2003;26:2653–2664.

3 Knudsen ST, Bek T, Poulsen PL, Hove MN, Rehling M, Mogensen CE: Macular edema reflects generalized vascular hyperpermeability in type 2 diabetic patients with retinopathy. Diabetes Care 2002;25:2328–2334.

4 Rotsos TG, Moschos MM: Cystoid macular edema. J Clin Ophthalmol 2008;2:919–930.

5 Ehrlich R, Harris A, Ciulla TA, Kheradiya N, Winston DM, Wirostko B: Diabetic macular oedema: physical, physiological and molecular factors contribute to this pathological process. Acta Ophthalmol 2010;88:279–291.

6 Morigi M, Angioletti S, Imberti B, et al: Leukocyte-endothelial interaction is augmented by high glucose concentrations and hyperglycemia in a NF-kB-dependent fashion. J Clin Invest 1998;101:1905–1915.

7 Brownlee M: The pathobiology of diabetic complications: a unifying mechanism. Diabetes 2005;54:1615–1625.

8 Shams N, Ianchulev T: Role of vascular endothelial growth factor in ocular angiogenesis. Ophthalmol Clin North Am 2006;19:335–344.

9 Miyamoto N, de Kozak Y, Jeanny JC, et al: Placental growth factor-1 and epithelial haemato-retinal barrier breakdown: potential implication in the pathogenesis of diabetic retinopathy. Diabetologia 2007;50:461–470.

10 Cai W, Rook SL, Jiang ZY, Takahara N, Aiello LP: Mechanisms of hepatocyte growth factor-induced retinal endothelial cell migration and growth. Invest Ophthalmol Vis Sci 2000;41:1885–1893.

11 Puliafito CA, Hee MR, Lin CP, et al: Imaging of macular disease with optical coherence tomography. Ophthalmology 1995;102:217–229.

12 Otani T, Kishi S, Maruyama Y: Patterns of diabetic macular edema with optical coherence tomography. Am J Ophthalmol 1999;127:688–693.

13 Yamamoto S, Yamamoto T, Hayashi M, et al: Morphological and functional analysis of diabetic macular edema by optical coherence tomography and multifocal electroretinograms. Graefes Arch Clin Ophthalmol 2001;239:96–101.

14 Sanchez-Tocino H, Alvarez-Vidal A, Maldonado MJ, et al: Retinal thickness study with optical coherence tomography in patients with diabetes. Invest Ophthalmol Vis Sci 2002;43:1588–1594.

15 Kim BY, Smith SD, Kaiser PK: Optical coherence tomography patterns of diabetic macular edema. Am J Ophthalmol 2006;142:405–412.

16 Photocoagulation for diabetic macular edema: Early Treatment Diabetic Retinopathy Study report number 1. Early Treatment Diabetic Retinopathy Study research group. Arch Ophthalmol 1985;103:1796–1806.

17 Lee C, Olk R: Modified grid laser photocoagulation for diffuse diabetic macular edema: long-term visual results. Ophthalmology 1991;98:1594–1602.

18 Javey G, Schwartz SG, Flynn HW Jr: Emerging pharmacotherapies for diabetic macular edema. Exp Diabetes Res 2012;2102:548732.

19 Diabetic retinopathy clinical research network, Scott IU, Edwards AR, et al: A phase II randomized clinical trial of intravitreal bevacizumab for diabetic macular edema. Ophthalmology 2007;114:1860–1867.

20 Michaelides M, Kaines A, Hamilton RD, et al: A prospective randomized trial of intravitreal bevacizumab or laser therapy in the management of diabetic macular edema (BOLT study): 12-month data. Report 2. Ophthalmology 2010;117:1078–1086.

21 Rosenfeld PR, Brown DM, Heier JS, et al: Ranibizumab for neovascular age-related macular degeneration. N Engl J Med 2006;335:1419–1431.

22 Brown DM, Kaiser PK, Michels M, et al: Ranibizumab versus verteporfin for neovascular age-related macular degeneration. N Engl J Med 2006;335:1432–1444.

23 Campochiaro PA, Heier JS, Feiner L, et al: Ranibizumab for macular edema following branch retinal vein occlusion: six-month primary end point results of a phase III study. Ophthalmology 2010;117:1102–1112.

24 Brown DM, Campochiaro PA, Singh RP, et al: Ranibizumab for macular edema following central retina vein occlusion: six-month primary end point results of a phase III study. Ophthalmology 2010;117:1124–1133.

25 Massin P, Bandello F, Garweg JG, et al: Safety and efficacy of ranibizumab in diabetic macular edema (RESOLVE study): a 12-month, randomized, controlled, double-masked, multicenter phase II study. Diabetes Care 2010;33:2399–2405.

26 Nguyen QD, Shah SM, Khwaja AA, et al: Two-year outcomes of ranibizumab for edema of the macula in diabetes (READ-2) study. Ophthalmology 2010;117:2146–2151.

27 Nauck M, Roth M, Tamm M, et al: Induction of vascular endothelial growth factor by platelet-activating factor and platelet-derived growth factor is downregulated by corticosteroids. Am J Respir Cell Mol Biol 1997;16:398–406.

28 Patelli F, Fasolino G, Radice P, et al: Time course of changes in retinal thickness and visual acuity after intravitreal triamcinolone acetonide for diffuse diabetic macula edema with and without previous macular laser treatment. Retina 2005;25:840–845.

29 Kuppermann BD, Blumenkranz MS, Haller JA, et al: Randomized controlled study of an intravitreous dexamethasone drug delivery system in patients with persistent macular edema. Arch Ophthalmol 2007;125:309–317.

30 Boyer DS, Faber D, Gupta S, et al: Dexamethasone intravitreal implant for treatment of diabetic macular edema in vitrectomized patients. Retina 2011;31:915–923.

31 Nguyen QD, Shah SM, Heier JS, et al: Primary end point (six months) results of the ranibizumab for edema of the macula in diabetes (READ-2) study. Ophthalmology 2009;116:2175–2181.

32 Elman MJ, Bressler NM, Qin H, et al: Expanded 2-year follow-up of ranibizumab plus prompt or deferred laser or triamcinolone plus prompt laser for diabetic macular edema. Ophthalmology 2011;118:609–614.
33 Mitchell P, Bandello F, Schmidt-Erfurth U, et al: The RESTORE study: ranibizumab monotherapy or combined with laser versus laser monotherapy for diabetic macular edema. Ophthalmology 2011;118:615–625.
34 Good TJ, Kimura AE, Mandava N, Kahook MY: Sustained elevation of intraocular pressure after intravitreal injections of anti-VEGF agents. Br J Ophthalmol 2011;95:1111–1114.
35 Do DV, Nguyen QD, Shah SM, et al: An exploratory study of the safety, tolerability and bioactivity of a single intravitreal injection of vascular endothelial growth factor trap-eye in patients with diabetic macular oedema. Br J Ophthalmol 2009; 93:144–149.
36 Dillinger P, Mester U: Vitrectomy with removal of the internal limiting membrane in chronic diabetic macular oedema. Graefes Arch Clin Exp Ophthalmol 2004;242:630–637.
37 Figueroa MS, Contreras I, Noval S: Surgical and anatomical outcomes of pars plana vitrectomy of diffuse nontractional diabetic macular edema. Retina 2008; 28:420–426.
38 Ikeda T, Sato K, Katano T, Hayashi Y: Vitrectomy for cystoid macular edema with attached posterior hyaloid membrane in patients with diabetes. Br J Ophthalmol 1999;83:12–14.
39 La Heij EC, Hendrikse F, Kessels AGH, Derhaag PJFM: Vitrectomy results in diabetic macular oedema without evident vitreomacular traction. Graefes Arch Clin Exp Ophthalmol 2001;239: 264–270.
40 Lewis H, Abrams GW, Blumenkranz MS, Campo RV: Vitrectomy for diabetic macular traction and edema associated with posterior hyaloidal traction. Ophthalmology 1992;99:753–759.
41 Nasrallah FP, Jalkh AE, Van Coppenolle F, et al: The role of the vitreous in diabetic macular edema. Ophthalmology 1988;95:1335–1339.
42 Otani T, Kishi S: A controlled study of vitrectomy for diabetic macular edema. Am J Ophthalmol 2002;134:214–219.
43 Pendergast SD, Hassan TS, Williams GA, et al: Vitrectomy for diffuse diabetic macular edema associated with a taut premacular posterior hyaloid. Am J Ophthalmol 2000;130:178–186.
44 Stefansson E, Landers MB 3rd, Wolbarsht ML: Increased retinal oxygen supply following pan-retinal photocoagulation and vitrectomy and lensectomy. Trans Am Ophthalmol Soc 1981;79: 307–334.
45 Yamamoto T, Akabane N, Takeuchi S: Vitrectomy for diabetic macular edema: the role of posterior vitreous detachment and epimacular membrane. Am J Ophthalmol 2001;132:369–377.
46 Nguyen QD, Shah SM, Van Anden E, et al: Supplemental oxygen improves diabetic macular edema: a pilot study. Invest Ophthalmol Vis Sci 2004;45:617–624.
47 Stefansson E, Landers MB 3rd, Wolbarsht ML: Vitrectomy, lensectomy, and ocular oxygenation. Retina 1982;2: 159–166.
48 Hosford GE, Olson DM: Effects of hyperoxia on VEGF, its receptors, and HIF-2alpha in the newborn rat lung. Am J Physiol Lung Cell Physiol 2003; 285:L161–L168.
49 Kadonosono K, Itoh N, Ohno S: Perifoveal microcirculation before and after vitrectomy for diabetic cystoid macular edema. Am J Ophthalmol 2000;130: 740–744.
50 Van Effenterre G, Guyot-Argenton C, Guiberteau B, Hany I, Lacotte JL: Macular edema caused by contraction of the posterior hyaloid in diabetic retinopathy. Surgical treatment of a series of 22 cases (in French). J Fr Ophthalmol 1993; 16:602–610.
51 Massin P, Duguid G, Erginay A, Haouchine B, Gaudric A: Optical coherence tomography for evaluating diabetic macular edema before and after vitrectomy. Am J Ophthalmol 2003;135:169–177.
52 Kumagai K, Furukawa M, Ogino N, Larson E, Iwaky M, Tachi N: Long-term follow-up of vitrectomy for diffuse nontractional diabetic macular edema. Retina 2009;29:464–472.
53 Thomas D, Bunce C, Moorman C, Laidlaw DA: A randomized controlled feasibility trial of vitrectomy versus laser for diabetic macular oedema. Br J Ophthalmol 2005;89:81–86.
54 Shah SP, Patel M, Thomas D, Aldington S, Laidlaw DA: Factors predicting outcome of vitrectomy for diabetic macular oedema: results of a prospective study. Br J Ophthalmol 2006;90:33–36.
55 Kojima T, Terasaki H, Nomura H, et al: Vitrectomy for diabetic macular edema: effect of glycemic control (HbA(1c)), renal fuction (creatinine) and other local factors. Ophthalmic Res 2003;35:192–198.
56 Stefaniotou M, Aspiotis M, Kalogeropoulos C, et al: Vitrectomy results for diffuse diabetic macular edema with and without inner limiting membrane removal. Eur J Ophthalmol 2004;14;137–143.
57 Parolini B, Panozzo G, Gusson E, et al: Diode laser, vitrectomy and intravitreal trimcinolone. A comparative study for the treatment of diffuse non-tractional diabetic macular edema. Semin Ophthalmol 2004;19:1–12.
58 Kralinger MT, Pedri M, Kralinger F, Troger J, Kieselbach GF: Long-term outcome after vitrectomy for diabetic macular edema. Ophthalnologica 2006;220: 147–152.
59 Yamamoto T, Takeuchi S, Sato Y, Yamashita H: Long-term follow-up results of pars plana vitrectomy for diabetic macular edema. Jpn J Ophthalmol 2007; 51:285–291.
60 Shimonagano Y, Makiuchi R, Miyazaki M, Doi N, Uemura A, Sakamoto T: Results of visual acuity and foveal thickness in diabetic macular edema after vitrectomy. Jpn J Ophthalmol 2007;51: 204–209.
61 Goebel W, Kretzchmar-Gross T: Retinal thickness in diabetic retinopathy: a study using optical coherence tomography (OCT). Retina 2002;22:759–767.
62 Klein R, Klein BE, Moss SE, Linton KL: The Beaver Dam Eye Study. Retinopathy in adults with newly discovered and previously diagnosed diabetes mellitus. Ophthalmology 1992;99:58–62.
63 Otani T, Kishi S: A controlled study of vitrectomy for diabetic macular edema. Am J Ophthalmol 2002;134:214–219.
64 Otani T, Kishi S: Tomographic findings of foveal hard exudates in diabetic macular edema. Am J Ophthalmol 2001;131: 50–54.

65 Wakabayashi T, Fujiwara M, Sakaguchi H, Kusaka S, Oshima Y: Foveal microstructure and visual acuity in surgically closed macular holes: spectral-domain optical coherence tomographic analysis. Ophthalmology 2010;117:1815–1824.
66 Sakamoto A, Nishijima K, Kita M, Oh H, Tsujikawa A, Yoshimura N: Association between foveal photoreceptor status and visual acuity after resolution of diabetic macular edema by pars plana vitrectomy. Graefes Arch Clin Exp Ophthalmol 2009;247:1325–1330.
67 Costa RA, Calucci D, Skaf M, et al: Optical coherence tomography 3: automatic delineation of the outer neural retinal boundary and its influence on retinal thickness measurements. Invest Ophthalmol Vis Sci 2004;45:2399–2406.
68 Otani T, Yamaguchi Y, Kishi S: Correlation between visual acuity and foveal microstructural changes in diabetic macular edema. Retina 2010;30:774–780.
69 Fernández EJ, Povazay B, Hermann B, et al: Three-dimensional adaptive optics ultrahigh-resolution optical coherence tomography using a liquid crystal spatial light modulator. Vision Res 2005;45:3432–3444.
70 Schmitz-Valckenberg S, Fleckenstein M, Göbel AP, Hohman TC, Holz FG: Optical coherence tomography and autofluorescence findings in areas with geographic atrophy due to age-related macular degeneration. Invest Ophthalmol Vis Sci 2011;52:1–6.
71 Cho M, Witmer MT, Favarone G, Chan RP, D'Amico DJ, Kiss S: Optical coherence tomography predicts visual outcome in macula-involving rhegmatogenous retinal detachment. Clin Ophthalmol 2012;6:91–96.

Fabio Patelli, MD
Head Vitreoretina Service Igea Clinic, Director Milano Retina Center
Carones Ophthalmology Center
Via Pietro Mascagni 20
IT–20122 Milan (Italy)
E-Mail fabio@patelli.it

Oh H, Oshima Y (eds): Microincision Vitrectomy Surgery. Emerging Techniques and Technology.
Dev Ophthalmol. Basel, Karger, 2014, vol 54, pp 174–181 (DOI: 10.1159/000360464)

Vitrectomy Surgery for Primary Retinal Detachment

Renaud Duval[a, b] · Kourous A. Rezaei[c, d]

[a]Department of Ophthalmology, University of Montréal, and [b]Maisonneuve-Rosemont Hospital, Montréal, Qué., Canada; [c]Department of Ophthalmology, Rush University Medical Center, and [d]Illinois Retina Associates, Chicago, Ill., USA

Abstract

Small-gauge pars plana vitrectomy has emerged as one of the leading approaches to the management of primary retinal detachment in recent years. Developments in technology and instrumentation have improved this procedure and given surgeons a wide variety of tools to tackle this pathology. In this chapter, the techniques utilized in the management of primary retinal detachments are discussed.

Surgical management of primary rhegmatogenous retinal detachment has changed drastically over the years, and the incremental improvements in the repair of retinal detachment have led to progressively higher success rates. Jules Gonin's [1] first operation using thermocautery to coagulate both the choroid and retina at the location of the retinal break achieved retinal reattachment in 30–40% of cases. Rosengren [2] demonstrated that internal tamponade of the retinal break with air following external diathermy achieved retinal reattachment in 76% of cases. Custodis [3] introduced scleral indentation in 1949 and brought the success rate up to 84%. In the early 1970s, Machemer et al. [4] introduced vitrectomy causing a paradigm shift in the management of retinal detachment. 20-gauge instrumentation was widely used until the advent of small-gauge surgery with the 25-gauge system by Fujii et al. [5], the 23-gauge system by Eckardt [6], and finally the 27-gauge system by Oshima et al. [7]. Following such advances in technology, the use of pars plana vitrectomy (PPV) for the repair of rhegmatogenous retinal detachment increased dramatically. Medicare data for fees in the USA shows a 72% increase in the use of PPV for rhegmatogenous retinal detachment from 1997 to 2007 [8]. A number of factors are responsible for such a gain in popularity: improved cutters and fluidics, wide-angle visualization, availability of heavy liquids, and improved retinopexy techniques. Successful outcomes of small-gauge PPV for the repair of rhegmatogenous retinal detachment has been shown to be high in most series, with primary success rates reaching up to 95.7% [9]. In this chapter some of the techniques developed by retina surgeons from around the world that we have utilized in the repair of primary retinal detachment using small-gauge PPV surgery are discussed.

Surgical Techniques

Instrumentation

Vitrectomy with either 23- or 25-gauge cannulated trocar systems has many advantages such as decreased rate of scelrotomy suturing with less trauma to the conjunctiva and subsequent dry eye symptoms, reduced postoperative suture-induced astigmatism, improved patient comfort in the postoperative period with faster recovery, more efficient surgical time, reduced rate of sclerotomy-related retinal breaks, and reduced air jet toxicity [10–17].

The use of valved trocars has further improved the fluidics in vitrectomy surgery, offering a closed system. This reduces the potential for retinal incarceration, limits the formation of bubbles at the fluid-heavy liquid interface when exchanging instruments, and reduces the risk of intraoperative suprachoroidal hemorrhage due to intraoperative hypotony.

Illumination during vitrectomy surgery has significantly improved in recent years, especially with the advent and improvements in small-gauge chandelier light illumination, lighted and curved laser probes allowing surgeon-assisted scleral depression, and endolaser treatment close to the ora serrata in phakic patients without the need for an endoilluminator [18].

Wide-angle visualization provided by either a contact or a noncontact system is another major advancement in PPV surgery for retinal detachment repair. New-generation viewing systems offer excellent viewing angles even through small pupils, often without needing a skilled assistant.

Anesthesia, Prepping, and Draping

Anesthesia for small-gauge PPV consists of either local or general anesthesia. The type of anesthesia selected should be tailored to the patient. General anesthesia can be delivered either in the form of endotracheal intubation or laryngeal mask anesthesia. In the hands of an experienced anesthetist, laryngeal mask anesthesia is a very safe and efficient procedure with the added benefit of increased postoperative comfort for the patients. It also diminishes the risk of having the patient cough or 'buck' on the endotracheal tube during or after extubation, which has been associated with massive suprachoroidal hemorrhage [19]. General anesthesia eliminates patient movement during surgery and the discomfort associated with scleral depression. In appropriate patients, local anesthesia alone is safe and effective, offering excellent analgesia and akinesia for the duration of even the longest of cases: approximately 5.0 ml of a 50/50 mixture of 2% xylocaine (AstraZeneca, Wilmington, Del., USA) and 0.5% bupivacaine (AstraZeneca) injected into the retrobulbar space by inserting a 25-gauge Atkinson needle (BD Visitec, Franklin Lanes, N.J., USA) connected to a 10-ml syringe into the lower eyelid, at the junction between the lateral and middle third. Supplemental retrobulbar anesthesia during the case can be delivered by making a conjunctival snip in the inferior fornix and passing a curved retrobulbar cannula into the sub-Tenon space. Optimal anesthesia is essential since vitrectomy for repair of primary retinal detachment may involve manipulation of the globe with scleral depression.

Care is taken in positioning the patient's head to assure that the patient's chin is positioned in a horizontal plane (not angled) to ensure adequate exposure of the entire retina throughout the surgery, especially in patients with prominent brows or small palpebral fissures. Prepping the skin around the eye and the eye lashes with 10% povidone-iodine solution (Rougier, Mirabel, Que., Canada) and the conjunctiva with 5% povidone-iodine solution following the draping is done in a sterile fashion.

Preservative-free lubricant (Genteal; Alcon, Fort Worth, Tex., USA) is applied on the surface of the cornea. Attention is given throughout the surgery to avoid corneal drying and to minimize the need for epithelial debridement

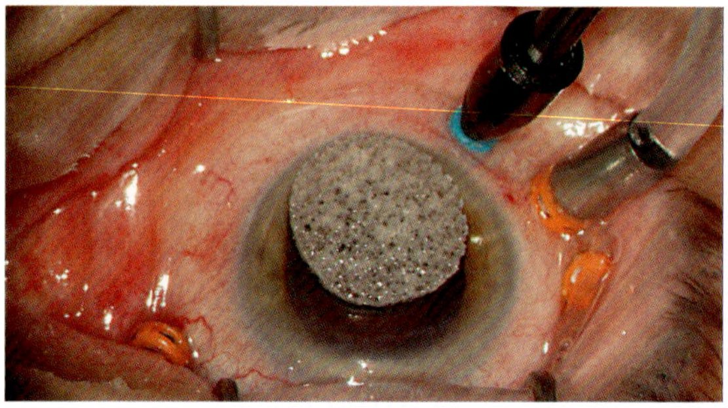

Fig. 1. The location of valved trochars (Alcon MIVS) and chandelier light (Alcon) during vitrectomy surgery for retinal detachment. A corneal protector is used to avoid microscope light toxicity during trochar insertion. The chandelier light is inserted inferotemporally below the infusion light for maximum inferior illumination.

during surgery [20]. Further, a corneal protector is placed on the surface of the cornea when no intravitreal procedures are performed, i.e. during trocar insertion and removal at the beginning and end of surgery to reduce retinal light exposure.

Vitrectomy Procedure

The location of the sclerotomies is measured with callipers. Generally, in phakic eyes, the sclerotomies are measured at 4 mm posterior to the limbus to limit the possibility of accidental lens touch during surgery. In pseudophakic and aphakic patients, the sclerotomies are placed between 3 and 3.5 mm posterior to the limbus. The eye is stabilized with toothed forceps and the trocars are inserted in a bevelled fashion. An angle of around 20° is used for trocar insertion and kept throughout the creation of the sclerotomy to generate an oblique scleral tunnel, which is likely to be self-sealing at the conclusion of the surgery. The inferotemporal infusion cannula is placed in the usual manner at the meridian of the inferior border of the lateral rectus muscle and its tip is visualized prior to turning on the infusion. The superotemporal and superonasal sclerotomies may be placed around the meridians of the upper borders of the lateral and medial recti muscles to ensure maximum range of movement, making sure to avoid injuring the ciliary arteries and nerves. A chandelier light (25-gauge Alcon Chandelier Lighting System; Alcon, Fort Worth, Tex., USA) is used in vitrectomies for repairing primary retinal detachment. The trocar for the chandelier light is inserted inferotemporally, just inferior to the infusion cannula (fig. 1). During peripheral scleral depressed vitreous shaving, this localization ensures superior visualization and shaving of the inferior peripheral vitreous (without the need of an endoilluminator), which is the most frequent site of proliferative vitreoretinopathy and recurrent retinal detachment [21]. The incision is not bevelled to avoid the angling of the chandelier light during surgery, and may need to be sutured at the conclusion of the operation.

The chandelier light is inserted perpendicular to the sclera to prevent lenticular glare during surgery in phakic patients. Furthermore, care is taken to turn off the chandelier light when not needed and to avoid shining the chandelier light directly on the macula.

The fluidic parameters of the vitrectomy machine are set to proportional vacuum with the highest constant cut rate available (Alcon). The maximum vacuum can be set at 650 mm Hg and is controlled with the foot pedal. The cut rate is currently set at 5,000 cuts/min and is not changed throughout the surgery. During peripheral vitreous shaving, the vacuum is kept at around 100–150 mm Hg to prevent peripheral iatrogenic breaks. For efficient vitrectomy, the vitrectomy probe engages the vitreous at all times (by moving it towards the vitreous).

Illumination intensity is kept as low as necessary for visualization throughout the surgery to minimize any light toxicity. This is especially true for the chandelier light which is often immobile throughout the surgery. The chandelier light does not need to be kept on throughout the surgery and should be turned on only when needed.

Removing the Vitreous

Vitrectomy is begun by inserting the instruments in the vitreous cavity. The first step is to verify the perfusion of the optic nerve. The pulsation of the central retinal artery and/or the sudden pallor of the optic nerve may indicate a mismatch between pressure of the infusion line inside the eye and the patient's diastolic blood pressure. Keeping the infusion pressure around 25 mm Hg and avoiding a diastolic blood pressure below 60 mm Hg usually allows adequate optic nerve and retinal perfusion during surgery with valved trocar systems.

The next step is induction of posterior vitreous detachment (PVD). Although most patients with retinal detachment already have PVD, many times they may only have partial PVD. Young and highly myopic patients usually do not have PVD upon presentation.

PVD is induced by positioning the cutter just above the optic nerve, turning off the cutting function of the vitreous cutter, and applying almost full aspiration. Attention should be given to avoid ocular hypotony and retinal incarceration into the tip of the vitrectomy probe during this step. Once the posterior hyaloid (or Weiss ring) is engaged, the posterior hyaloid is elevated in an anterior-posterior direction while monitoring the status of the detached retina using wide-angle visualization. In case the retina is partially detached, the port of the cutter is kept away from the detached area throughout this maneuver to prevent incarceration of the retina into the vitrectomy probe. In total retinal detachment, the light pipe can be used to shield the port of the vitrectomy from a very mobile retina. In case the retina is very mobile, the amount of vacuum may need to be adjusted. In very bullous retinal detachment, the subretinal fluid may be drained through the peripheral break prior to induction of PVD. In these scenarios, a localized vitrectomy is performed around the break followed by drainage of the subretinal fluid through the same break. This generally leads to a dramatic flattening of the detached retina, making the induction of the PVD and vitrectomy easier and safer.

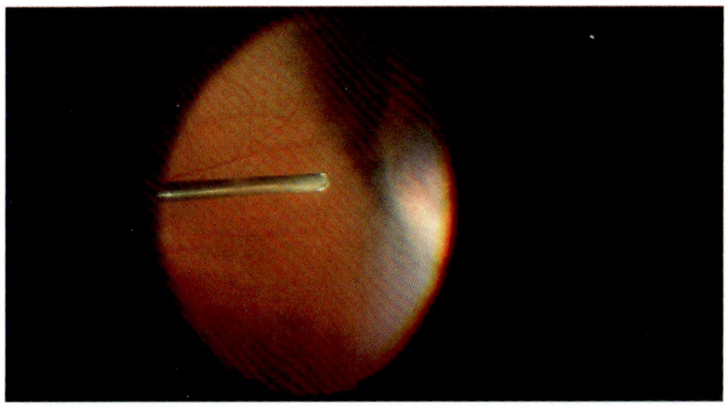

Fig. 2. Scleral depressed vitrectomy by the surgeon in a phakic patient. Illumination is provided by chandelier light. The cutter shaft is almost parallel to the surface of the retina. Lower suction and the maximum cut rate is used during peripheral shaving. The cutter should never be anterior to the ora in a phakic patient.

The separation of the hyaloid should be extended as far anteriorly as possible and deemed safe. Once the posterior hyaloid/Weiss ring is engaged, attention should be given to the peripheral retina using the wide-angle viewing system. The appearance of peripheral retinal hemorrhages, which are generally the precursors of iatrogenic peripheral retinal breaks during this maneuver, is a reliable sign that the posterior edge of the anterior vitreous base has been reached and that further hyaloid separation is not possible and should not be attempted.

Following the induction of PVD, core vitrectomy is performed followed by peripheral vitrectomy. A thorough shaving of the vitreous base over 360° may reduce the potential for recurrence of the retinal detachment from vitreous traction. Scleral depression is utilized to adequately visualize the peripheral vitreous (fig. 2). Although a skilled assistant could provide the required support for this task, greater control and independence is achieved with the use of chandelier illumination. The vitreous base is meticulously shaved over 360° with the help of scleral depression. The infusion pressure may be reduced to

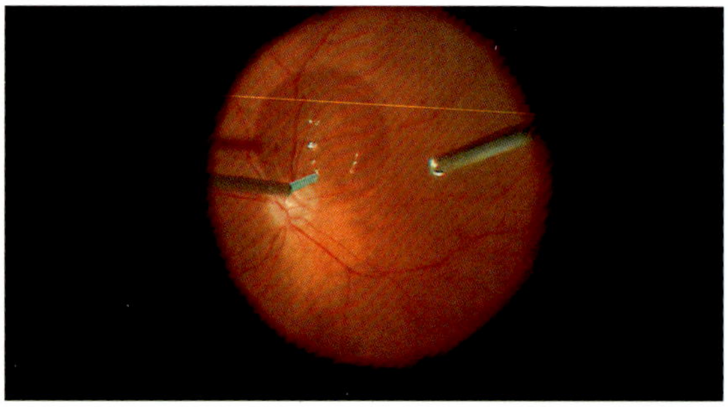

Fig. 3. Perfluoron injection in a patient with valved trochars. The injections are done slowly and optic nerve perfusion is monitored during the injection. For egression of the fluid during injection, one may either use the vent supplied with the trochars or suction of the cutter as shown in this figure. Illumination is provided through chandelier light.

15–20 mm Hg to ease scleral indentation. The scleral depression is performed gently by applying constant pressure. Sudden changes in depression pressure including extreme depression of the sclera or letting go of the depression should be avoided during this procedure. In phakic patients, the shaft of the cutter needs to be almost parallel to the retina (and not angled) to avoid touching the lens. Further, peripheral vitreous shaving should never be attempted anterior to the ora in phakic patients since it would lead to iatrogenic cataract formation.

During peripheral vitreous shaving, vitreous traction is relieved around all the breaks, including amputating the flap of horseshoe tears. Following peripheral vitreous shaving, the peripheral retina is examined with a scleral depressor and endoilluminator over 360°. All retinal breaks are identified and marked with either endodiathermy or endolaser. Shifting the fluid away from under the break with scleral depression and using the endolaser on a higher duration and power is generally enough to mark the breaks and often avoids the need for using endodiathermy. It is important to mark the breaks prior to the use of any tamponade agent since they can make the recognition of the breaks difficult.

Flattening the Retina

Drainage of subretinal fluid and flattening of the retina is performed in one of two approaches depending on the location of the retinal breaks and the conformation of the retinal detachment. For posteriorly located breaks and small detachments, a fluid-air exchange can be performed while the subretinal fluid is aspirated through the retinal break with the soft-tip endodrainage cannula. Caution must be observed when performing this maneuver in macula on retinal detachments to avoid the expansion of subretinal fluid under the macula. For anteriorly located breaks and large detachments, we prefer the use of heavy liquids such as Perfluoron (Alcon) to expel the subretinal fluid through the peripheral break [22]. When using valved trocars, care must be taken to prevent the increase of intraocular pressure while injecting heavy liquids into the eye since it is a closed system. This can be achieved in several ways:

- Using a dual-bore cannula (MedOne Surgical Inc., Sarasota, Fla., USA)
- Placing a vent (Alcon) in one of the valved trocars and using the chandelier light for illumination
- Aspirating fluid with the vitrector while injecting the heavy liquid and using chandelier light for illumination (preferred technique)
- Removing the chandelier light from its cannula (25-gauge EDGEPLUS trocar/cannula; Alcon, Fort Worth, Tex., USA) and leaving the trocar (which is not valved) open temporarily

The heavy liquid is injected slowly over the optic nerve while monitoring the perfusion of the optic nerve. The tip of the cannula is kept inside the heavy liquid bubble throughout the injection process (fig. 3). The eye may be tilted away from the retinal break (prior to the heavy liquid reaching it) to optimize the displacement of subretinal fluid through the peripheral break. The retina is usually almost completely reattached under heavy liquid following this step.

In cases of midperipheral breaks or fairly large breaks, the heavy liquid may be injected up to the posterior edge of the retinal break, and then a partial air-fluid exchange is performed to displace the anterior subretinal fluid through the break. This approach may minimize the possibility of heavy liquid migration into the subretinal space.

Retinopexy
Retinopexy is applied once the retina is flattened under air or heavy liquid. A curved illuminated laser probe is ideal for this task. It provides excellent illumination during scleral depressed anterior photocoagulation in phakic patients (fig. 4a). Alternatively, a curved nonilluminated laser probe can be used together with chandelier light illumination. In pseudophakic or aphakic patients, a straight laser probe may be used. Initial settings for the endolaser can be at 200 ms for duration and 160 mW for power and then titrated to obtain a moderate intensity laser burn (fig. 4b). Endolaser is first applied around the breaks and then one may perform 360° scleral depressed photocoagulation on the peripheral vitreous base up to the ora serrata. The laser burns are more confluent in the area of retinal detachment and less confluent in attached retina. One must avoid laser burns at the 3-o'clock and 9-o'clock meridians (posterior ciliary nerves).

During scleral depressed peripheral endolaser photocoagulation, it is important to release scleral depression slowly while working under heavy liquids to prevent the formation of bubbles at the heavy liquid-fluid interface.

Heavy Liquid Removal
Once retinopexy is completed, the heavy liquid is removed during a fluid-air exchange. At the beginning of the exchange, the soft-tip cannula is kept in the fluid phase above the heavy liquid to transform the vitreous cavity into a two-phase system: air and heavy liquid [23]. The soft-tip cannula on the extrusion line is then kept on the break to aspirate any anterior subretinal fluid that is being displaced posteriorly by the enlarging air bubble [24]. It is paramount not to release aspiration during this process since heavy liquid may reflux from the cannula and enter the subretinal space due to gravitational forces. Once all anterior fluid has been drained and the level of the heavy liquid is past the most posterior of retinal breaks, the soft-tip cannula is placed above the optic nerve and the heavy liquid is completely removed from the eye. The heavy liquid is then washed off of the extrusion line by aspirating a small quantity of balanced salt solution (Bausch & Lomb, Rochester, N.Y., USA) from a plastic cup. A few drops of balanced salt solution are then squirted on the retinal surface with a 30-gauge needle on a 1-ml syringe to gather and help remove small residual heavy liquid droplets [25]. The anterior retina is reexamined one final time under air to assure all the breaks are well surrounded, and if necessary supplemental photocoagulation is added.

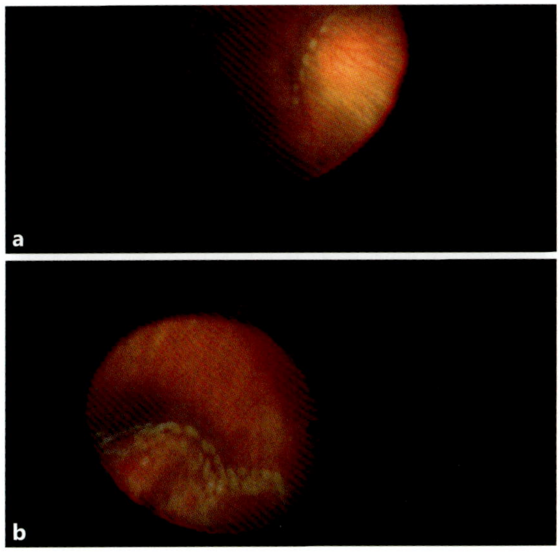

Fig. 4. a Scleral depressed peripheral endolaser treatment in a phakic patient. This maneuver is performed with the curved lighted laser probe (Alcon). Background illumination is provided through the chandelier light at a lower setting (generally 10% illumination). **b** Laser spots during scleral depressed peripheral endolaser treatment.

Sclerotomy Closure and Gas Injection

Preservative free lubricant (Genteal, Alcon) is applied to the surface of the cornea and a corneal protector is placed on the cornea. The chandelier cannula is removed and the sclerotomy is sutured with 8-0 Vicryl (Ethicon, Somerville, N.J., USA) since it does not have a bevelled insertion. All the trocars are removed. Brief compression of the sclerotomy site with a cotton-tip is performed to assure they are water tight. In case of sclerotomy leakage, a transconjunctival 8-0 Vicryl suture is passed through the leaking sclerotomy. Air is replaced with a nonexpansile concentration of long-acting gas (usually 14% C_3F_8; Sonomed Escalon, Lake Success, N.Y., USA) through a chimney technique. The desired concentration and type of gas is prepared inside a 60-ml syringe connected to a 30-gauge needle. A chimney is prepared by removing the plunger of a 3-ml syringe connected to a 25-gauge needle. Both needles are inserted into the vitreous cavity through the pars plana superiorly around 11 o'clock and 1 o'clock, and the air-gas exchange is performed by having an assistant inject the gas. Attention must be given to assure that the tip of the needle is inside the vitreous cavity. After injecting about 50 ml of the gas volume, the chimney is removed and the intraocular pressure is measured with the Barraquer tonometer (Ocular Instruments, Bellevue, Wash., USA). Additional gas is injected as needed to achieve a target intraocular pressure of around 10–15 mm Hg. Subconjunctival injection of steroids and antibiotics is given followed by application of topical cycloplegic drops and antibiotic ointment. The eye is patched and a shield is placed over the eye.

Postoperatively

All patients are positioned face down at the conclusion of surgery. Patients are routinely evaluated on postoperative day 1.

A Few Pearls for the Safe, Efficient, and Successful Repair of Primary Retinal Detachment

- Chandelier light illumination allows scleral depressed vitreous shaving without the need for a skilled assistant
- Decrease retinal light exposure by turning off the chandelier light when not in use and adjust its light intensity to the minimal amount needed
- Lowering the infusion pressure during the scleral depressed vitrectomy reduces the amount of force needed to indent the sclera
- During 360° laser photocoagulation, avoid burns, 3- and 9-o'clock meridians, and apply less confluent laser to the attached retina.
- Gentle release of scleral depression while indenting under heavy liquid minimizes bubble creation
- In a very bullous detachment, reducing the height of the detachment by draining the subretinal fluid at the beginning of the case may simplify the subsequent maneuvers
- While lasering under air for an extended period of time, consider reducing the air pressure to around 25 mm Hg (with valved trocars) and place a few drops of balanced salt solution on the posterior pole to prevent the drying of the macula and its associated toxic effects [26]

References

1 Gonin J: Le traitement du décollement rétinien. Ann Ocul 1921;158:175–194.

2 Rosengren B: Über die Behandlung der Netzhaut-Ablösung mittelst Diathermie und Luftinjektionen in den Glaskörper. Acta Ophthalmol 1938;16:3–42.

3 Custodis E: Bedeutet die Plombeaufnahung auf die Sklera einen Fortschritt in der operativen Behandlung der Netzhaut-Ablösung? Ber Dtsch Ophthalm Ges 1953;58:102.

4 Machemer R, Buettner H, Norton EW, Parel JM: Vitrectomy: a pars plana approach. Trans Am Acad Ophthalmol Otolaryngol 1971;75:813.

5 Fujii GY, de Juan E Jr, Humayun MS, Pieramici DJ, Chang TS, Awh C, Ng E, Barnes A, Wu SL, Sommerville DN: A new 25-gauge instrument system for transconjunctival sutureless vitrectomy surgery. Ophthalmology 2002;109:1807–1812.
6 Eckardt C: Transconjunctival sutureless 23-gauge vitrectomy. Retina 2005;25:208–211.
7 Oshima Y, Wakabayashi T, Sato T, Ohji M, Tano Y: A 27-gauge instrument system for transconjunctival sutureless microincision vitrectomy surgery. Ophthalmology 2010;117:93–102.
8 Ramulu PY, Do DV, Corcoran KJ, Corcoran SL, Robin AL: Use of retinal procedures in Medicare beneficiaries from 1997 to 2007. Arch Ophthalmol 2010;128:1335–1340.
9 Schneider EW, Geraets RL, Johnson MW: Pars plana vitrectomy without adjuvant procedures for repair of primary rhegmatogenous retinal detachment. Retina 2012;32:213–219.
10 Fujii GY, De Juan E Jr, Humayun MS, et al: Initial experience using the transconjunctival sutureless vitrectomy system for vitreoretinal surgery. Ophthalmology 2002;109:1814–1820.
11 Lakhanpal RR, Humayun MS, de Juan E Jr, et al: Outcomes of 140 consecutive cases of 25-gauge transconjunctival surgery for posterior segment disease. Ophthalmology 2005;112:817–824.
12 Gosse E, Newsom R, Lochhead J: The incidence and distribution of iatrogenic retinal tears in 20-gauge and 23-gauge vitrectomy. Eye (Lond) 2012;26:140–143.
13 Nakano T, Uemura A, Sakamoto T: Incidence of iatrogenic peripheral retinal breaks in 23-gauge vitrectomy for macular diseases. Retina 2011;31:1997–2001.
14 Issa SA, Connor A, Habib M, Steel DH: Comparison of retinal breaks observed during 23 gauge transconjunctival vitrectomy versus conventional 20 gauge surgery for proliferative diabetic retinopathy. Clin Ophthalmol 2011;5:109–114.
15 Scartozzi R, Bessa AS, Gupta OP, Regillo CD: Intraoperative sclerotomy-related retinal breaks for macular surgery, 20- vs. 25-gauge vitrectomy systems. Am J Ophthalmol 2007;143:155–156.
16 Hirata A, Yonemura N, Hasumura T, Murata Y, Negi A: Effect of infusion air pressure on visual field defects after macular hole surgery. Am J Ophthalmol 2000;130:611–616.
17 Duval R, Hui JM, Rezaei KA: Rate of sclerotomy suturing in 23-gauge primary vitrectomy. Retina 2014;34:679–683.
18 Eckardt C: Twin lights: a new chandelier illumination for bimanual surgery. Retina 2003;23:893–894.
19 Pollack AL, McDonald HR, Ai E, Johnson RN, Dugel PU, Folk J, Grand MG, Lambert HM, Schwartz S, Miller RD: Massive suprachoroidal hemorrhage during pars plana vitrectomy associated with Valsalva maneuver. Am J Ophthalmol 2001;132:383–387.
20 Garcia-Valenzuela E, Abdelsalam A, Eliott D, Pons M, Iezzi R, Puklin JE, McDermott ML, Abrams GW: Reduced need for corneal epithelial debridement during vitreo-retinal surgery using two different viscous surface lubricants. Am J Ophthalmol 2003;136:1062–1066.
21 Sternberg P Jr, Meredith T: Management of recurrent retinal detachment after silicone oil injection. Arch Ophthalmol 1987;105:27–28.
22 Coll GE, Chang S, Sun J, Wieland MR, Berrocal MH: Perfluorocarbon liquid in the management of retinal detachment with proliferative vitreoretinopathy. Ophthalmology 1995;102:630–638.
23 Chang S, Lincoff H, Zimmerman NJ, Fuchs W: Giant retinal tears. Surgical techniques and results using perfluorocarbon liquids. Arch Ophthalmol 1989;107:761–766.
24 Kirchhof B, Wong D: Essentials in Ophthalmology: Vitreo-Retinal Surgery. Berlin, Springer, 2007.
25 Garcia-Valenzuela E, Ito Y, Abrams GW: Risk factors for retention of subretinal perfluorocarbon liquid in vitreoretinal surgery. Retina 2004;24:746–752.
26 Winter M, Eberhardt W, Scholz C, Reichenbach A: Failure of potassium siphoning by Müller cells: a new hypothesis of perfluorocarbon liquid-induced retinopathy. Invest Ophthalmol Vis Sci 2000;41:256–261.

Kourous A. Rezaei, MD
Illinois Retina Associates, Ingalls Hospital Professional Building
71 West 156th Street, Suite 400
Harvey, IL 60426 (USA)
E-Mail karezaei@yahoo.com

Oh H, Oshima Y (eds): Microincision Vitrectomy Surgery. Emerging Techniques and Technology.
Dev Ophthalmol. Basel, Karger, 2014, vol 54, pp 182–187 (DOI: 10.1159/000360465)

Management of Giant Retinal Tears Using Microincision Vitrectomy Surgery

Hiroshi Kunikata

Department of Ophthalmology, Tohoku University Graduate School of Medicine, Sendai, Japan

Abstract

Giant retinal tears (GRTs; ≥90°) are rare and difficult to treat successfully for even experienced vitreous surgeons. Using microincision vitrectomy surgery (MIVS) to treat GRTs has been an important advancement. Here we describe the surgical technique and its complications. ***Surgical Technique:*** Initially, the eye is carefully vitrectomized with MIVS using a modern wide-viewing system and chandelier illumination. Perfluorocarbon liquid (PFCL) is then gently injected. After endophotocoagulation, the PFCL is exchanged for silicone oil (SO) for a 2-week course of intraocular tamponade. Complete retinal reattachment and visual recovery are achieved after the SO is removed. ***Complications:*** Postoperative complications in the retina include macular pucker, subretinal PFCL, retinal folds, cystoid macular edema, and redetachment due to proliferative vitreoretinopathy. All complications can be resolved with medication or surgery. ***Conclusions:*** The techniques for MIVS offer a feasible new approach for treating eyes with GRTs. In combination with intraoperative use of PFCL and a 2-week course of SO tamponade, MIVS is highly recommended to all vitreous surgeons seeking an excellent rate of reattachment.

Giant retinal tears (GRTs; ≥90°) are difficult to treat successfully (fig. 1) even for experienced vitreous surgeons due to the condition's rarity and the technical difficulty involved. Various treatments have been used for GRTs including scleral buckling, pneumatic retinopexy, pars planar vitrectomy with gas tamponade, and vitrectomy with silicone oil (SO) tamponade. Temporary intraoperative tamponade with perfluorocarbon liquid (PFCL) has been found to increase the successful reattachment rate from about 20 to 90% [1–7].

Techniques for microincision vitrectomy surgery (MIVS) using 25- and 23-gauge instruments

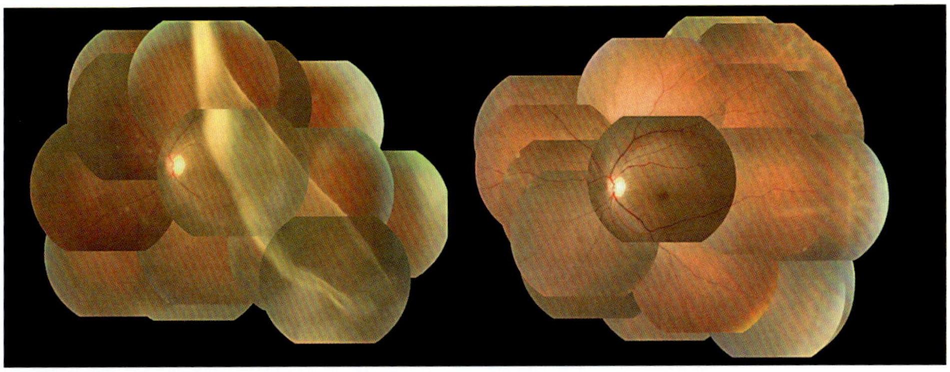

Fig. 1. Representative eye with a 180° GRT. Preoperative (left) and postoperative (right) fundus photographs of the eye of an adult man with a GRT-induced retinal detachment.

were first reported in 2002 and 2005, respectively [8, 9]. These techniques have become part of common practice throughout the world. The popularity of MIVS has been enhanced by clinical studies demonstrating that in comparison with other techniques, it leads to significantly less need for conjunctival injection as well as less postoperative corneal astigmatism and discomfort.

This section reports surgical techniques and complications of MIVS for GRTs.

Surgical Technique

Surgery for GRTs should be performed under retrobulbar anesthesia and does not require conjunctival peritomy. In all cases, 25- and 23-gauge MIVS are better choices than 20-gauge pars planar vitrectomy because MIVS uses a trocar cannula which can protect the sclerotomy port and reduce the occurrence of intraoperative iatrogenic retinal breaks. Phacoemulsification and aspiration and intraocular lens implantation should be performed unless the patient has no lens opacity and is under 50 years of age. In order to completely remove the peripheral vitreous, MIVS instrumentation with a wide-viewing system and chandelier illumination should be used (fig. 2). After resecting the vitreal core, the peripheral vitreous is shaved. It is important to shave as much as possible without causing retinal injury with the vitreous cutter. After shaving, PFCL is injected on the disc under low infusion pressure, and the vitreous cavity is filled with PFCL. Caution is advised due to the high risk of causing subretinal PFCL in eyes with a GRT. Next, endophotocoagulation is performed in double lines along the margins of the GRT. Finally, the PFCL is directly exchanged for SO for the recommended 2-week course of intraocular tamponade. Postoperatively, antibiotics and corticosteroids are injected subconjunctivally.

After the 2-week course of SO tamponade, the SO is removed from the vitreous cavity as the endophotocoagulation scarring process should be complete. Intraocular SO can lead to postoperative complications such as glaucoma or proliferative vitreoretinopathy (PVR); thus, this technique requires two vitreous surgeries. In the first, the retina is reattached and the SO tamponade is injected. In the second, the SO is removed. The use of an adjunctive encircling buckle has been debated [7, 10–12]; however, we believe that, in principle, initial MIVS for GRTs does not need to be combined with an encircling

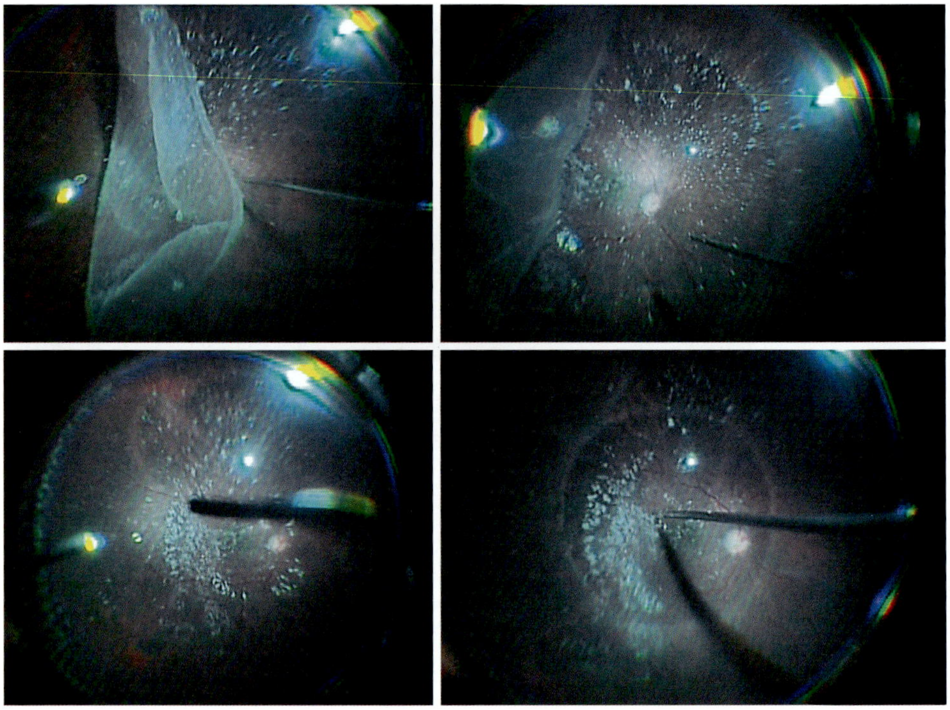

2

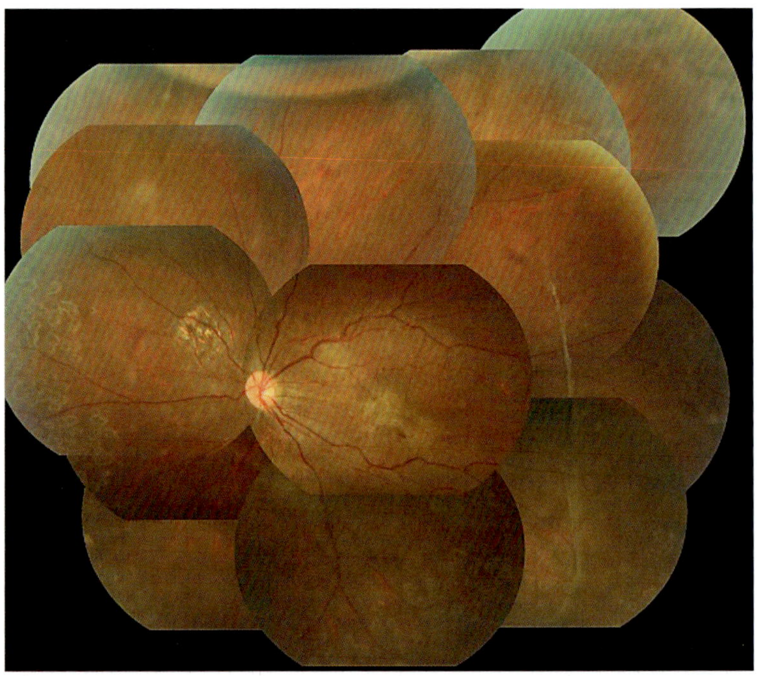

3

Fig. 2. Upper left: intraoperative photograph of the fundus showing a 150° GRT. Upper right: intraoperative photograph of the fundus showing reattachment of the retina with the use of PFCL. Lower left: intraoperative photograph of the fundus taken just after endophotocoagulation of the GRT. Lower right: PFCL being directly exchanged with SO for a 2-week course of intraocular tamponade.

Fig. 3. Photograph of macular pucker that developed after 25-gauge vitrectomy for a GRT. It was treated with membrane peeling.

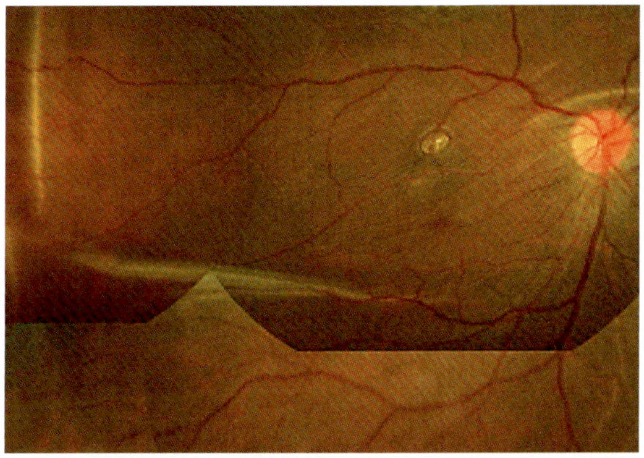

Fig. 4. Photograph of retained subretinal PFCL and retinal folds after 25-gauge vitrectomy for a GRT. It is impossible to correct retinal folds, but the retained subretinal PFCL located in the posterior pole should be removed.

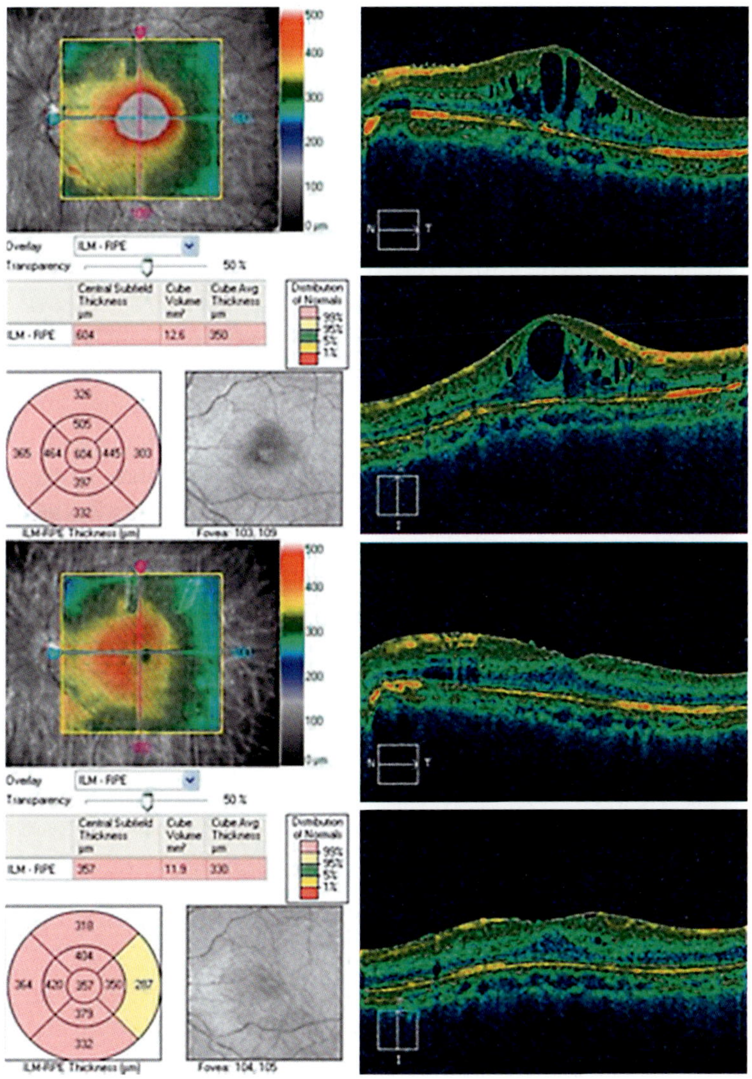

Fig. 5. Upper: image of eye with postoperative CME that was treated with a posterior sub-Tenon steroid injection. Lower: the CME in this case was resolved after two injections of steroids.

buckle. All patients should receive a complete ophthalmological examination ≥6 months after surgery.

Complications

The rate of surgical complications after MIVS for GRTs is 40–50%; complications include postoperative macular pucker (fig. 3), retention of subretinal PFCL (fig. 4), retinal folds (fig. 4), cystoid macular edema (CME; fig. 5), and redetachment of the retina due to PVR [7]. If PFCL-SO exchange is omitted, there is also a very high risk of postoperative retinal slippage and retinal folds, which are difficult or impossible to treat postoperatively. Therefore, SO should be used in all cases of GRTs, even when the GRT is relatively small, i.e. ≤180°, to avoid such irreversible retinal complications and promote complete retinal attachment. Moreover, recent advances in MIVS techniques have made it possible to use SO in all cases, as they have allowed the injection of SO even through a 25-gauge cannula. Additionally, it is important to remove the SO two weeks after the initial vitrectomy to prevent secondary glaucoma and promote rapid visual improvement. A longer tamponade period is only advisable in cases of PVR or atopic retinal detachment.

Macular pucker is simple to remove completely with surgery several months after the initial operation. In cases of retention of subretinal PFCL, treatment is only necessary if the PFCL is located in the posterior pole. The subretinal PFCL should be completely removed at the time of the second vitrectomy to remove the SO. After cutting the retinal surface with a microvitreal blade, the PFCL should be gently aspirated with a soft-tip microneedle. Cases of postoperative CME should be treated with a posterior sub-Tenon steroid injection (fig. 5). Multiple injections may be needed to resolve recurrent CME, but treatment should succeed as long as there is no retinal pucker. Eyes with retinal redetachment require immediate surgical treatment. In such cases, it is advisable to perform vitrectomy accompanied with scleral encircling or a longer course of SO tamponade, as previous research on 20-gauge pars planar vitrectomy has shown that omitting the encircling scleral buckle was significantly associated with redetachment [10, 11]. When MIVS is used to treat GRTs in patients with conditions such as PVR or severe atopic dermatitis, it is also advisable to use an encircling buckle.

Conclusions

To date, surgical treatment for GRTs remains difficult and the rate of surgical complications is high. However, new techniques for MIVS such as a wide-viewing system and chandelier illumination offer a feasible new approach for treating eyes with GRTs. In combination with intraoperative use of PFCL and a 2-week course of SO tamponade, MIVS is highly recommended to all vitreous surgeons seeking an excellent rate of reattachment.

References

1 Schepens CL, Freeman HM: Current management of giant retinal breaks. Trans Am Acad Ophthalmol Otolaryngol 1967;71:474–487.

2 Norton EW, Aaberg T, Fung W, Curtin VT: Giant retinal tears. I. Clinical management with intravitreal air. Am J Ophthalmol 1969;68:1011–1021.

3 Machemer R, Allen AW: Retinal tears 180 degrees and greater. Management with vitrectomy and intravitreal gas. Arch Ophthalmol 1976;94:1340–1346.

4 Chang S, Lincoff H, Zimmerman NJ, Fuchs W: Giant retinal tears. Surgical techniques and results using perfluorocarbon liquids. Arch Ophthalmol 1989; 107:761–766.
5 Scott IU, Murray TG, Flynn HW Jr, Feuer WJ, Schiffman JC: Outcomes and complications associated with giant retinal tear management using perfluoro-n-octane. Ophthalmology 2002;109:1828–1833.
6 Lee SY, Ong SG, Wong DW, Ang CL: Giant retinal tear management: an Asian experience. Eye (Lond) 2009;23:601–605.
7 Kunikata H, Abe T, Nishida K: Successful outcomes of 25- and 23-gauge vitrectomies for giant retinal tear detachments. Ophthalmic Surg Lasers Imaging 2011;42:487–492.
8 Fujii GY, De Juan E Jr, Humayun MS, et al: A new 25-gauge instrument system for transconjunctival sutureless vitrectomy surgery. Ophthalmology 2002;109:1807–1812, discussion 1813.
9 Eckardt C: Transconjunctival sutureless 23-gauge vitrectomy. Retina 2005;25:208–211.
10 Al-Khairi AM, Al-Kahtani E, Kangave D, Abu El-Asrar AM: Prognostic factors associated with outcomes after giant retinal tear management using perfluorocarbon liquids. Eur J Ophthalmol 2008;18:270–277.
11 Goezinne F, La Heij EC, Berendschot TT, et al: Low redetachment rate due to encircling scleral buckle in giant retinal tears treated with vitrectomy and silicone oil. Retina 2008;28:485–492.
12 Shunmugam M, Ang GS, Lois N: Giant retinal tears. Surv Ophthalmol 2014;59:192–216.

Hiroshi Kunikata, MD, PhD
Associate Professor and Vice Chairman, Department of Ophthalmology
Tohoku University Graduate School of Medicine
1-1 Seiryo-machi, Aoba-ku
Sendai 980-8574 (Japan)
E-Mail kunikata@oph.med.tohoku.ac.jp

Oh H, Oshima Y (eds): Microincision Vitrectomy Surgery. Emerging Techniques and Technology.
Dev Ophthalmol. Basel, Karger, 2014, vol 54, pp 188–195 (DOI: 10.1159/000360466)

Proliferative Vitreoretinopathy

Carl Claes • Anna Paula Lafetá

Claes Retina Clinic, Antwerp, Belgium

Abstract

Proliferative vitreoretinopathy is a sophisticated disease that complicates vitreoretinal pathologies like retinal detachments. Since its first description in the 1960s, we have learned a lot about this pathological entity; however, despite a large number of promising laboratory and clinical pharmacological research projects, we are still unable to stop proliferation and are certainly not able to prevent this terrible complication. As a result, vitreoretinal surgeons still have to fight membrane formation in complicated and long vitreoretinal procedures. Fortunately, a revolution has taken place in equipment for these procedures. This chapter will examine the pathophysiology, classification, and pharmacotherapy, and describe the strategy and rationale of how to deal with this recurrent condition and to limit and contain its sequelae.

Proliferative vitreoretinopathy (PVR) is the most common cause of rhegmatogenous retinal detachment (RRD) surgery failure [1–5]. Accounting for approximately 75% of all primary surgical failures, PVR complicates 5–10% of all retinal detachment repairs. It occurs after primary RRD repair surgery or in long-standing primary detachments.

Etiology, Pathophysiology, and Natural History

PVR originates at the time of retinal break or trauma, followed by the migration of retinal pigment epithelial (RPE) cells from their normal location at Bruch's membrane to the vitreous cavity. There, proliferation and epithelial-mesenchymal transformation takes place as well as transformation into fibroblast-like cells. These events in concert with an activation of glial cells, hyalocytes, and immune cells are key cellular events in the onset of the disease. The interplay between the cellular events and various growth factors, cytokines, and matrix proteins thereby drives the undesirable development of PVR, characterized by the formation of scar-like fibrovascular membranes that give rise to redetachment as they contract. The whole process is somehow analogous to a wound-healing process, including inflammation, proliferation, and scar modulation that can follow a normal healing path with tissue remodeling and repair, or can take the abnormal path with protracted healing [6, 7].

RRD causes a breakdown in the blood-retinal barrier, triggering cell migration and proliferation, involving especially RPE cells, fibrous astrocytes, fibroblasts, myofibroblasts, and macrophages [7], and also causing chemotaxis of other inflammatory cells involved in the healing process [8]. Different signals have been found to play a role in migration and proliferation of RPE cells, including loss of contact, signaling from photoreceptors, and response to factors present in the vitreous, in addition to other signals secreted by inflammatory cells.

First, loss of contact for RPE cells and loss of communication from adjacent cells induces their proliferation and dedifferentiation to repair the defect [9, 10]. This migration, proliferation, and differentiation inside the vitreous is influenced by the growth factors and cytokines present in the vitreous or that access the eye from the circulation. Growth factors identified that are likely involved in regulation of cell growth include platelet-derived growth factor (PDGF), TGF-β, epidermal growth factor, TNF-α, TNF-β, fibroblast growth factor, and others. Cytokines like IL-1, IL-6, IL-8, IL-10, and INF-γ have also been identified. These growth stimuli are believed to contribute to cell-growth regulation in PVR [11].

Schepens [12] described the natural course of PVR in 3 stages: pre-PVR, early PVR, and well-established PVR. In the pre-PRV stage, examination reveals extensive liquefaction of the vitreous gel producing an optically empty zone between the thickened posterior cortical layer of the vitreous and the shrunken anterior vitreous. PVR can have an acute onset and may develop overnight with recurrent RRD. It is usually preceded by a generalized haziness in the vitreous gel, which is caused by an outpouring of serum protein in the gel. Slit-lamp examination reveals fibrous condensation of the gel; intravitreal membranes, cellular particles, and blood clots in the vitreous gel; partial or absent posterior vitreous detachment, and a dull reflex on the retinal surface due to an extensive preretinal membrane. These findings are present prior to the development of PVR [12, 13].

One of the first ophthalmoscopically detectable signs of the early PVR stage is a grayish color of the fundus reflex and a hazy image of the fundus as a consequence of vitreous organization [12]. Retinal vessels may have a dilated and tortuous appearance and equatorial intraretinal hemorrhages may be present. Retinal breaks previously closed by surgery reopen and new breaks can develop. Detached retina shows fixed folds and does not flatten with bed rest. Preretinal membranes cause a loss of transparency and give the detached retina a grayish hue [13].

Vitreous examination reveals an intense flare due to an increase of proteinaceous deposits and a generalized condensation and contraction of the gel contribute to its hazy appearance. Despite this phenomenon, posterior vitreous detachment is rarely observed and, if present, is usually partial and atypical [13]. This finding presents with a strong vitreoretinal adhesion and, as a result of the further contraction of the vitreous towards its base, the detached retina is dragged anteriorly, eventually causing a detachment of the ora serrata and epithelium of the pars plana ciliaris. Progression of the PVR process leads to a funnel-shaped retinal detachment. In the early stages, the funnel is wide anteriorly and narrow posteriorly. With progression of the process, the funnel gradually becomes narrow towards the anterior part until it is completely closed.

PVR usually becomes well established several weeks after onset. The retina is completely detached and fixed retinal folds develop. Further evolution is characterized by shrinkage of a strong preretinal membrane resulting in narrowing of the cone into a funnel. In this stage, contraction of the preretinal membranes results in formation of fixed retinal folds. Three types of retinal folds have been observed:

(1) Radial retinal folds with a triangular form and with rounded apices and that are narrower near the optic disc than near the

equator; these are radially oriented and, in advanced cases, their overlapping edges obscure the disc

(2) Equatorial retinal folds seen parallel to the equator are often associated with intraretinal hemorrhages and vitreous membranes originating from them

(3) Star-shaped folds converging toward a central point can be seen over all quadrants of the fundus [14, 15]

In well-established PVR the vitreous cavity is clearer than in earlier-stage PVR because most of the protein-rich material in the gel is resolved. Brownish particles persist and numerous membranes are present.

Subretinal membranes have been reported in about 3% of retinal detachments [16], and their incidence is related to the duration of the detachment. Multiple subretinal white dots are the first ophthalmoscopic sign of the development of a subretinal membrane. The membranes start growing as sheets, but break up into bands as the cells contract, with the stronger parts remaining intact [17].

Risk Factors

All RRD go through the healing process, but only a few develop PVR by production and persistence of the hyperplastic fibrotic tissue. A suitable environment needs to be created for the development of PVR, such as a disturbance of the anatomic integrity of the retina and a partial posterior vitreous detachment which permits cell dispersion and membrane formation [18]. In general, any process that changes vascular permeability, breaks down the blood-retinal barrier, or damages the retinal integrity increases the probability of PVR formation.

Specific risk factors that have been identified include: uveitis; large, giant or multiple tears; vitreous hemorrhage; large RRD (>2 quadrants); pre- or postoperative choroidal detachment; preoperative PVR; aphakia; multiple previous surgeries; use of vitrectomy to repair RD; cryopexy or endolaser application, and intravitreal use of SF_6, sodium iodate, or epinephrine [19–22].

Classification

The term 'proliferative vitreoretinopathy' was introduced in 1983 by the Retina Society Terminology Committee [1] to describe a condition which was formerly called massive vitreous retraction [25–27], massive preretinal retraction [28], and massive preretinal proliferation [29]. A classification of PVR seemed indispensable to describe the different degrees of PVR and the impact on treatment on various stages.

According to the Retina Society classification, PVR was a classified as: grade A (minimal); grade B (moderate); grade C (marked) which was subdivided in C-1, -2, or -3 according to the number of quadrants involved, and grade D (massive), subdivided in D1, -2, or -3 according to the state of the opening of the funnel shape.

Later on, in 1989 the Silicone Oil Study Group amended the classification which was again modified in 1991 to the one currently in use: grade A = limited to the presence of vitreous cells or haze, grade B = presence of rolled or irregular edges of a tear or inner retinal surface wrinkling denoting subclinical contraction, and grade C = presence of preretinal or subretinal membranes. Grade C was divided in anterior (Ca) or posterior (Cp) and from 1 to 12 depending of the number of clock hours involved [30] (fig. 1, 2).

Management

Surgery has been the standard treatment for PVR. The goal of surgery is to reattach the retina and restore the normal anatomy and function by identifying all the breaks and relieving

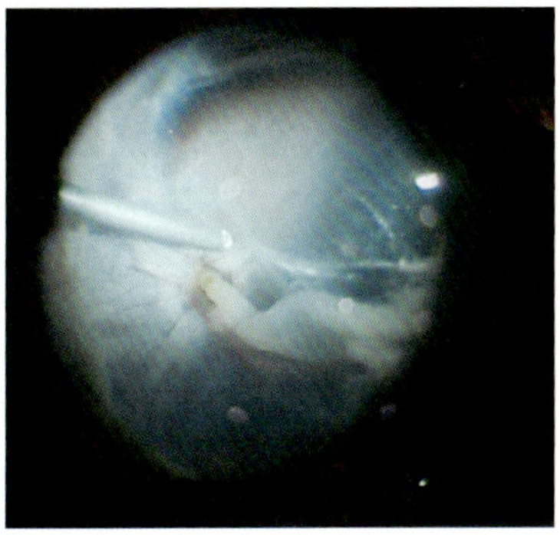

Fig. 1. Advanced PVR with fixed posterior circular fibrosis forming a 'napkin ring'.

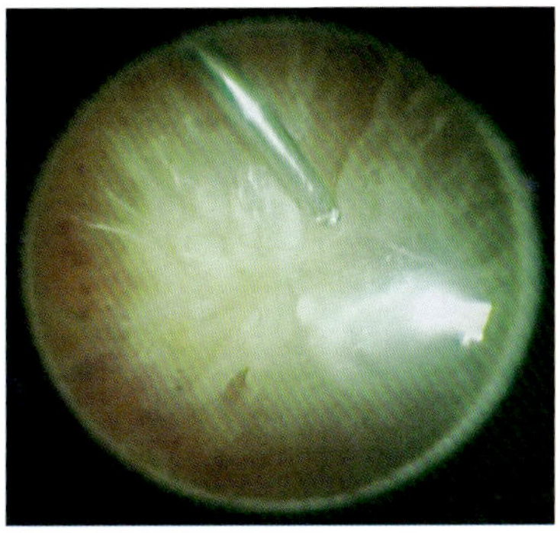

Fig. 2. Advanced PVR (Ca12, Cp12), posterior hyaloid removal.

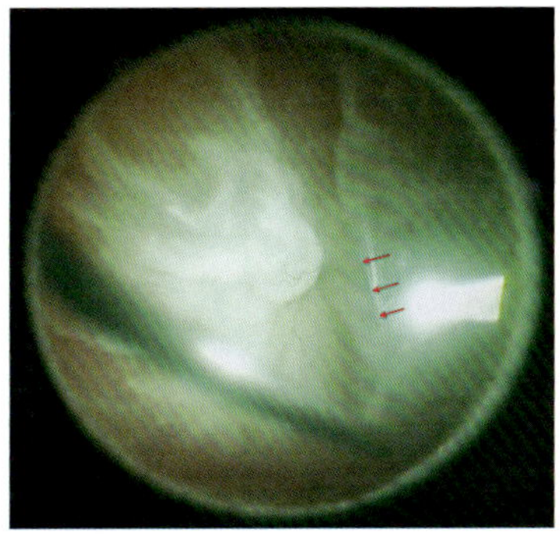

Fig. 3. Bimanual delamination of posterior hyaloid with 20-gauge illuminated spatula.

4

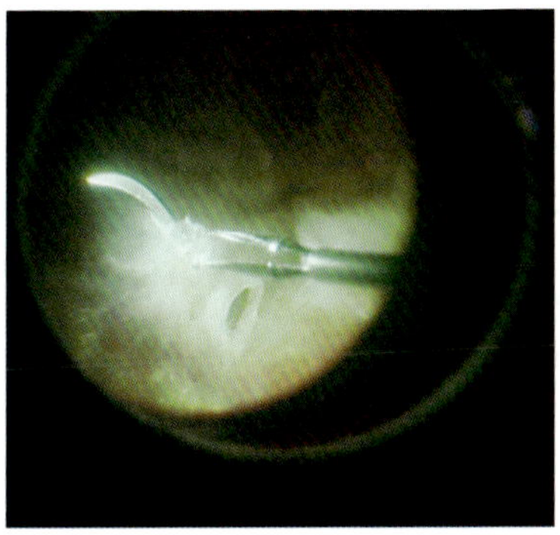

5

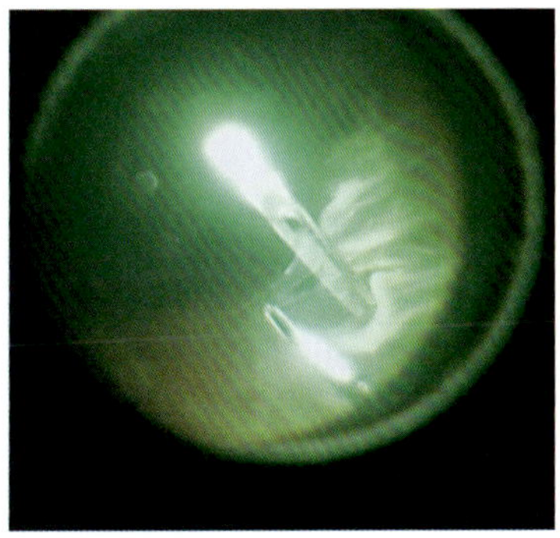

Fig. 4. Bimanual delamination of posterior hyaloid with illuminated fork.
Fig. 5. Bimanual surgery using 23-gauge illuminated spatula and forceps.

all significant vitreoretinal traction. There have been tremendous advances in surgical techniques and technology for managing vitreoretinal diseases.

There are different approaches to PVR surgery. The one we have found to be most beneficial is based on the techniques that were developed by Zivojnovic et al. [31], which can deal with advanced cases of PVR, trauma, and PDR. The idea is to remove all traction, extrinsic as well as intrinsic contraction. Bimanual surgical maneuvers are indispensable in the treatment of this pathology. The use of silicone oil is combined with judiciously executed manipulations and retinotomies. Today we have the choice of a chandelier light, fixed in the pars plana, or illuminated instrumentation. Chandelier lights allow bimanual peeling and provide good illumination during vitreous base shaving and peripheral laser, but sometimes need some positioning adaptation.

My favorite instrument for dissection is an illuminated spatula, for which I have developed several designs with different companies. The last edition from Alcon is available gauges of 23 and 25 and hopefully soon in 27 gauge. The spatula contains a thin, rounded tip and its shape allows for blunt dissection without perforating the underlying retina. These instruments provide wide-field illumination without blinding reflexes (fig. 3–5).

Nowadays, the use of encircling bands is less popular. Personally, I rarely use encircling

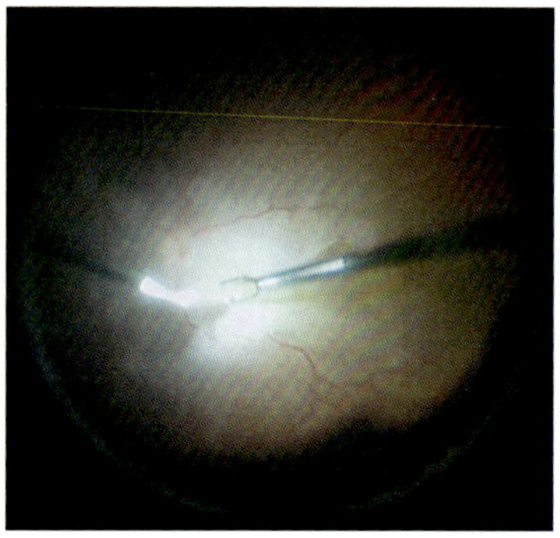

Fig. 6. Posterior vitreous detachment (arrows).

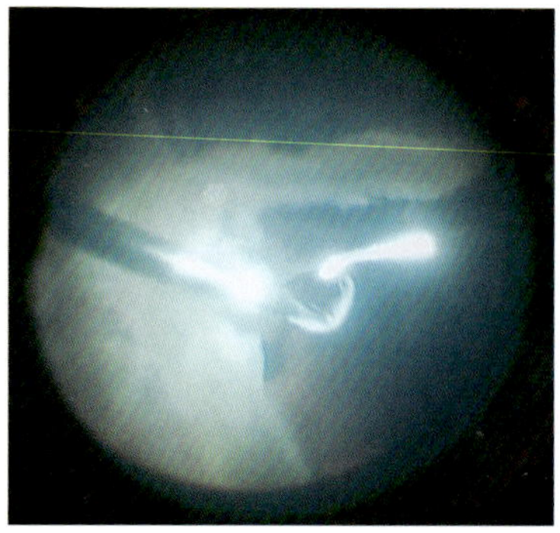

Fig. 7. Removal of subretinal PVR.

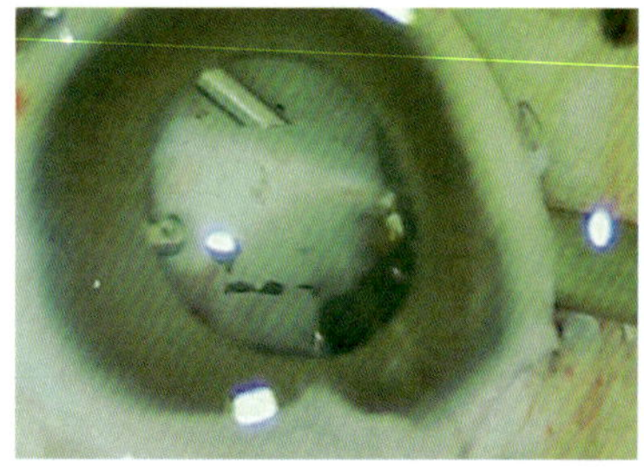

Fig. 8. Incarcerated retina at sclerotomy.

bands in PVR in combination with silicone oil. An indication might be a case that demonstrates a contracted vitreous base to avoid retinotomies.

Basic Surgical Techniques (Preventing/Limiting Proliferative Vitreoretinopathy)

Release the Traction from the Posterior Hyaloid Membrane

Too many times we encounter a totally attached posterior hyaloid in recurrent retinal detachments. This is particularly true in children and myopes. We advise the use of intraoperative Triescense in primary cases to decrease the chances of redetachment. Often bimanual hyaloid delamination techniques are necessary to eliminate this traction (fig. 2–4, 6).

Remove All Membranes

The best chance to obtain anatomic reconstruction is usually to peel as many membranes as possible, epiretinal and mostly subretinal membranes (fig. 7). If this is not sufficient to relax the traction or contraction of the retina, gentle retinal massage is applied to flatten the retina.

Nowadays, I try to avoid retinotomies as much as possible.

A common mistake that we encounter in reinterventions after failed surgeries are central and large retinotomies that can trigger very aggressively recurrent PVR which can endanger the future survival of the functional eye.

Removal of the ILM from the posterior pole might be defended in cases with a high risk of recurrences in order to reduce the effect of the PVR membranes by eliminating the scaffold.

Extensive Peripheral Cleaning

In advanced PVR cases, the periphery often requires more attention than the posterior pole of the eye. Inadequate peripheral vitrectomy is often the cause of recurrent retinal detachment, providing a nice scaffold for reproliferation.

Vitreous base contraction, peripheral trough formation in anterior PVR, and vitreous and/or retina incarceration in the sclerotomies (fig. 8) are some of the classical challenges for the PVR surgeon.

Injecting silicone oil or long-standing gases in eyes with large remnants of vitreous or membranes and concurrent traction creates a time bomb that will detonate days to weeks after the surgery.

Use Silicone Oil Judiciously, with Timely Removal

Silicone oil is not a treatment for PVR. We prefer to use it in PVR cases to be able to time a reintervention appropriately when recurrent mem-

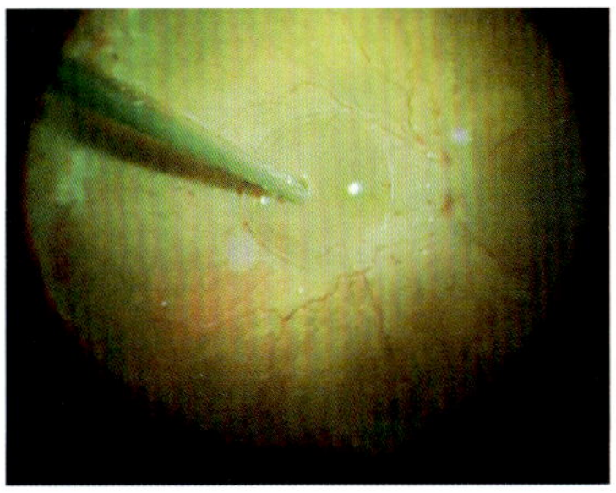

Fig. 9. Perfluorocarbon-silicone oil exchange.

branes are mature enough to be peeled completely, before redetachment and damage to the retina is too extensive. It limits postoperative inflammation and allows immediate visual recovery without positioning. These characteristics are well appreciated by the patients (fig. 9).

Silicone oil provides a long-lasting tamponade effect, but it should be removed timely. A good time to extract the oil is when the reproliferation process is burned out and the retina is nicely attached. Of course, this represents a wide variation depending on underlying pathology. Some extreme forms of hypotony will not allow silicone removal.

Pharmacological Treatment

Medical treatment has been directed toward preventing one or more of the involved pathologies, including anti-inflammatory, antiproliferative, antineoplastic, antigrowth factor, and antioxidant agents. Different drugs and drug delivery systems have been tested for PVR treatment. Medications may be useful in the management of patients undergoing surgical repair of a RD associated with PVR [32].

Steroids (topical subconjunctival/posterior sub-Tenon's/oral prednisone) have been found to be effective in reducing postoperative reproliferation: different animal experimental studies have shown a benefit with intra- or periocular use of steroids [33–35]. However, human studies have demonstrated different results, i.e. minimal difference in PVR formation, a decrease (but with short follow-up), or beneficial in preventing PVR formation [36–40].

Minocycline (a neuroprotective agent and glial cell inhibitor) has been found to inhibit photoreceptor apoptosis and glial cell proliferation in an animal model of RD (recommended dosage: 100 mg 1 tablet PO b.i.d. for 2 weeks (start 1 week prior to surgery and continue for 1 week after surgery).

Low-molecular-weight heparin infusion and 5-fluorouracil have shown good results in reducing PVR formation [41, 42], and daunorubicin (a topoisomerase inhibitor that inhibits DNA and RNA) has also showed promising results [43, 44].

Densiron (Medicel, Boston) heavy silicone oil is an effective heavier-than-water endotamponade agent that prevents fluid accumulation under the inferior retina and may limit the rate of redetachment from inferior retinectomy [45].

Other drugs studied include [46]:

- VitrenAse (Vit 100), an antiproliferative agent that halts growth of PVR membranes by stopping the formation of proteins necessary to make new scar tissue
- Taxol stabilizing and colchicine inhibiting microtubul formation can inhibit RPE and fibroblast migration and proliferation
- Retinoic acid promotes growth factor arrest of RPE cells in vitro
- Glucosamine, an inhibitor of N-linked oligosaccharide biosyntesis and processing is reported to inhibit growth of various cell types
- DNA-RNA chimeric ribozymes, a cell-cycle-controlling gene that inhibits cell division
- Etoposide and tacrolimus
- Kinase inhibitors like hypericin and alkylphosphocholine, protein kinase C

inhibitors, herbimycin A (tyrosine kinase inhibitor), or PDGF receptor kinase inhibitor AG1295
- Tranlisat, an inhibitor of TGF-β
- Suramin, an antiparasitic that affects growth factor binding
- Prinomastat, a matrix metalloprotease inhibitor
- N-acetylcysteine, an antioxidant that has indirect PDGF receptor activation, blocking the vitreous-driven activation of PDGF receptor-α

References

1 The Retina Society Terminology Committee: The classification of retinal detachment with proliferative vitreoretinopathy. Ophthalmology 1983;90: 121–125.

2 Rachal WF, Burton TC: Changing concepts of failure after retinal detachment surgery. Arch Ophthalmol 1979;97:480–483.

3 Hilton GF: Subretinal pigment migration. Effects of cryosurgical reattachment. Arch Ophthalmol 1974;91:445.

4 Charles S: Vitrectomy for retinal detachment. Trans Ophthalmol Soc UK 1990; 100:542–549.

5 The Silicone Study Group: Proliferative vitreoretinopathy. Am J Ophthalmol 1985;99:593–595.

6 Wilkins RB, Kulwin DR, Wendell L: Hughes Lecture. Wound healing. Ophthalmology 1979;86:507–510.

7 Vinores SA, Campochiaro PA, Conway BP: Ultrastructural and electron immunocytochemycal characterization of cells in epiretinal membranes. Invest Ophthalmol Vis Sci 1990;31:14–28.

8 Wiedemann P: Growth factors in retinal diseases: proliferative vitreoretinopathy, proliferative diabetic retinopathy, and retinal degeneration. Surv Ophthalmol 1992;35:373–384.

9 Heriot WJ, Machmer R: Pigment epithelial repair. Graefes Arch Clin Exp Ophthalmol 1992;230:91–100.

10 Anderson DH, Stern WH, Fisher SK, Erickson PA, Borgula GA: The onset of pigment epithelial proliferations after retinal detachment. Invest Ophthalmol Vis Sci 1991;21:10–16.

11 Lei H, Rheaume MA, Kaslaukas A: Recent developments in our understanding of how platelet derived growth factor (PDGF) and its receptors contribute to proliferative vitreoretinopathy. Exp Eye Res 2010;90:376–381.

12 Schepens CL: Retinal detachment and allied diseases. Philadelphia, WB Saunders, 1983, p 197.

13 Tolentino FI, Schepens CL, Freeman HM: Vitreoretina Disordors: Diagnostic and Management. Philadelphia, WB Saunders, 1976, p 480.

14 Hirose T, Schepens CL, Lopansri C: Subtotal open sky vitrectomy for severe retinal detachment occurring as a late complication of ocular trauma. Ophthalmology 1981;88:1–9.

15 Claes C, Freeman HM, Tolentino FI: PVR: An overview; in: Proliferative Vitreoretinopathy (PVR). New York, Springer, 1988, pp 3–11.

16 Wallyn RH, Hilton GF: Subretinal fibrosis in retinal detachment. Arch Ophthalmol 1979;97:2128–2129.

17 Stenberg P, Machemer R: Subretinal proliferation. Am J Ophthalmol 1984;98: 456–462.

18 Wiedemann P, Heimann K: Proliferative retinopathy. Pathogenesis and possibilities for treatment with cytostatic drugs (in German). Klin Monatsbl Augenheilkd 1986;188:559–564.

19 Bonnet M: Clinical findings associated with the development of postoperative PVR in primary rhegmatogenous retinal detachment; in Heimann K, Wiedemann P (eds): Proliferative Vitreoretinopathy. Heidelberg, Kaden, 1989, pp 8–20.

20 Aguirrebeña A, Saornil MA, Giraldo A, Pastor JC: Incidencia da vitreorretinopatia proliferante (VRP) en el desprendimento de retina regmatógeno. Arch Soc Esp Oftalmol 1986;51:229–234.

21 Bonnet M: Clinical factors predisposing to massive proliferative vitreoretinopathy in rhegmatogenous retinal detachment. Ophthalmologica 1984;188:148–152.

22 Cowley M, Conway BP, Campochiaro PA, et al: Clinical risk factors for proliferative vitreoretinopathy. Arch Ophthalmol 1989;107:1147–1151.

23 Kampik A, Green WR, Michels RG, Rice TA: Epiretinale Membranen nach Photokoagulation (postkoagulative Maculopathie). Ber Dtsch Ophthalmol Ges 1981;78:593–598.

24 Campochiaro PA, Bryan JA, Conway BP, Jaccoma EH: Intravitreous chemotactic and mitogenic activity. Implication of blood-retinal barrier breakdown. Arch Ophthalmol 1986;104:1685–1687.

25 Hruby K: Massive vitreous retraction (in German). Doc Ophthalmol 1969;26: 555–565.

26 Scott JD: The treatment of massive vitreous retraction. Trans Ophathalmol Soc UK 1973;93:417–423.

27 Havener WH: Massive vitreous retraction. Int Ophthalmol Clin 1976;16:135–155.

28 Cibis PA: Recent methods in the surgical treatment of retinal detachment: intravitreal procedures. Trans Ophthalmol Soc UK 1965;85:111–127.

29 Tolentino FI, Schepens CL, Freeman HM: Massive preretinal proliferation: a biomicroscopic study. Arch Ophthalmol 1967;78:16.

30 Machemer R, Aaberg TM, Freeman HM, Irvine AR, Lean JS, Michels RM: An update classification retinal detachment with proliferative vitreoretinopathy. Am J Ophathalmol 1991;112:159–165.

31 Zivojnovic R, et al: Treatment of traumatic traction detachment in eyes with PVR and severe damage to the anterior segment; in: Proliferative Vitreoretinopathy (PVR). New York, Springer, 1988, pp 76–80.

32 Sun JK, Arroyo JG: Adjunctive therapies for proliferative vitreoretinopathy. Int Clin Ophthalmol 2004;44:1–10.

33 Hui YN, Liang HC, Cai YS, Kirchhof B, Heimann K: Corticosteroids and daunomycin in the prevention of experimental proliferative vitreoretinopathy induced by macrophages. Graefes Arch Clin Exp Ophthalmol 1993;231:109–114.
34 Tano Y, Chandler D, Machemer R: Treatment of intraocular proliferation with intravitreal injection of triamcinolone acetonide. Am J Ophthalmol 1980; 90:810–816.
35 Rubsamen PE, Cousins SW: Therapeutic effect of periocular corticosteroids in experimental proliferative vitreoretinopathy. Retina 1997;17:44–50.
36 Koerner F, Merz A, Gloor B, Wagner E: Postoperative retinal fibrosis – a controlled clinical study of systemic steroid therapy. Graefes Arch Clin Exp Ophthalmol 1982;219:268–271.
37 Hui YN, Hu D: Prevention of experimental proliferative vitreoretinopathy with daunomycin and triamcinolone based on the time course of the disease. Graefes Arch Clin Ophthalmol 1999;237: 601–605.
38 Jonas JB, Hayler JK, Panda-Jones S: Intravitreal injection of crystalline cortisone as adjunctive treatment of proliferative vitreoretinopathy. Br J Ophthalmol 2000;84:1064–1067.
39 Bali E, Feron EJ, Peperkamp E, Veckeneer M, Mulder PG, van Meurs JC: The effect of a preoperative subconjuctival injection of dexamethasone on blood-retinal barrier breakdown following scleral buckling retinal detachment surgery: a prospective randomized placebo-controled double blind clinical trial. Graefes Arch Clin Exp Ophthalmol 2010;7:957–962.
40 Chen W, Chen H, Hou P, Fok A, Hu Y, Lam DS: Midterm results of low-dose intravitreal triamcinolone as adjunctive treatment for proliferative vitreoretinopathy. Retina 2011;31:1137–1142.
41 Asaria RH, Kon CH, Bunce C, et al: Adjuvant 5-fluoracil and heparin prevents proliferative vitreoretinopathy: results from a randomized, double-blind, controlled clinical trial. Ophthalmology 2001;108:1179–1183.
42 Garcia RA, Sanchez JG, Arevalo JF: Combined 5-fluoracil, low-molecular weight heparin, and silicone oil in the management of complicated retinal detachment with proliferative vitreoretinopathy grade C. Ophthalmic Surg Lasers Imaging 2007;38:276–282.
43 Wiedemann P, Hilgers RD, Bauer P, Heimann K: Adjunctive daunorubicin in the treatment of proliferative vitreoretinopathy: results of a multicenter clinical trial. Daunomycin Study Group. Am J Ophthalmol 1998;126:550–559.
44 Shinohara K, Tanaka M, Sakuma T, Kobayashi Y: Efficacy of daunorubicin encapsulated in liposome for the treatment of proliferative vitreoretinopathy. Ophthalmic Surg Lasers Imaging 2003;34: 299–305.
45 Lim BL, Vote B: Densiron intraocular tamponade: a case series. Clin Experiment Ophthalmol 2008;36:261–264.
46 Sadaka A, Giuliari GP: Proliferative vitreoretinopathy: current and emerging treatments. Clin Ophthalmol 2012;6: 1325–1333.

Carl Claes, MD
Claes Retina Clinic, Antwerp
Speelhofdreef 8
BE–Schilde 2979 (Belgium)
E-Mail claes.md@skynet.be

Oh H, Oshima Y (eds): Microincision Vitrectomy Surgery. Emerging Techniques and Technology.
Dev Ophthalmol. Basel, Karger, 2014, vol 54, pp 196–203 (DOI: 10.1159/000360467)

Surgical Management of Retinal Diseases: Proliferative Diabetic Retinopathy and Traction Retinal Detachment

Yousef J. Cruz-Iñigo · Luis A. Acabá · Maria H. Berrocal

Department of Ophthalmology, University of Puerto Rico, San Juan, Puerto Rico

Abstract

Current indications for pars plana vitrectomy in patients with proliferative diabetic retinopathy (PDR) include vitreous hemorrhage, tractional retinal detachment (TRD), combined tractional and rhegmatogenous retinal detachment (CTRRD), diabetic macular edema associated with posterior hyaloidal traction, and anterior segment neovascularization with media opacities. This chapter will review the indications, surgical objectives, adjunctive pharmacotherapy, microincision surgical techniques, and outcomes of diabetic vitrectomy for PDR, TRD, and CTRRD. With the availability of new microincision vitrectomy technology, wide-angle microscope viewing systems, and pharmacologic agents, vitrectomy can improve visual acuity and achieve long-term anatomic stability in eyes with severe complications from PDR.

Pars plana vitrectomy was initially performed on diabetic patients with nonclearing vitreous hemorrhage. The results obtained were favorable and triggered a strong interest for studying disease pathogenesis as well as improving surgical techniques and technologies in order to maximize outcomes and minimize complications. The Diabetic Retinopathy Treatment Study was pivotal in showing the impact of early diabetic vitrectomy [1–4].

In the past 12 years, 23-, 25-, and 27-gauge transconjunctival sutureless vitrectomy systems have been introduced [5–7] and antiangiogenic molecules have become available as adjuvants in diabetic vitrectomy [8–12]. These technologies have streamlined vitrectomy procedures, expanded the pathologies that can be addressed with vitrectomy, and improved outcomes.

Current objectives of vitrectomy in proliferative diabetic retinopathy (PDR) include removal of vitreous opacities, excision of the posterior hyaloid, release of retinal traction, retinal reattachment, treatment of retinal ischemia, and prevention of fibrovascular proliferation. The most frequent indications for vitrectomy in patients with PDR include: nonclearing vitreous hemorrhage, tractional retinal detachment (TRD), combined tractional and rhegmatogenous retinal detachment (CTRRD), macular traction syndromes, and neovascular glaucoma.

Vitreous Hemorrhage

Vitreous hemorrhage was the most common indication for vitrectomy in patients with PDR. Although with the introduction of panretinal photocoagulation (PRP) the prevalence of severe vitreous hemorrhage has decreased over time, it still remains a common indication worldwide. PRP causes regression of neovascular tissue, thus helping prevent future hemorrhages and retinal detachments.

In the early 1980s it was common to wait for clearing of vitreous hemorrhage since instrumentation was limited, intraoperative photocoagulation was not available, and complications including rebleeding were common [13]. With new technological advances, fewer complications are seen with diabetic vitrectomy. Currently, early vitrectomy is indicated for dense vitreous hemorrhages, while observation is reserved for mild cases that could clear spontaneously. When vitreous hemorrhage obscures a fundus view, B-scan ultrasonography is required to rule out concomitant retinal detachment.

Surgical objectives include removing vitreous opacities caused by bleeding, relieving vitreoretinal traction by removing the posterior hyaloid and epiretinal membranes, and applying endophotocoagulation to achieve regression of proliferative tissue [14].

Surgical management of this condition has been simplified with microincision vitrectomy surgery and wide-angle viewing systems. New vitrectors in 23, 25 and 27 gauge with optimized fluidics and cutting rates of up to 7,500 cuts/min allow for very efficient vitreous removal with minimized traction on the retina. Optimized intraocular pressure control minimizes bleeding during surgery and reduces the need for endocautery. The introduction of curved laser probes allow for complete photocoagulation up to the ora serrata even in phakic eyes. These techniques result in long-term stabilization of vitrectomized eyes.

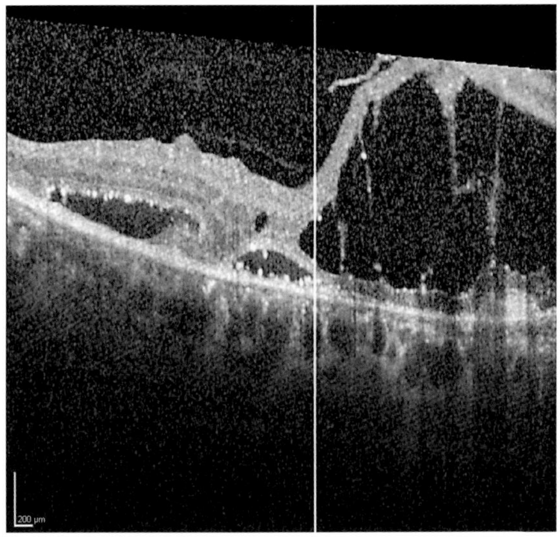

Fig. 1. Optical coherence tomography of an eye with long-standing TRD with severe cystoid degeneration, localized detachment, and membranes on the retinal surface.

Tractional Retinal Detachment and Traction and Rhegmatogenous Retinal Detachment

TRD has been the most frequent indication for vitrectomy in diabetic patients, accounting for 40% of diabetic vitrectomies [15]. TRD results from progressive fibrovascular proliferation and contraction, which pulls the neurosensory retina away from the retinal pigment epithelium. This detachment can involve the macula causing severe visual acuity loss. With progressive fibrovascular contraction in eyes with a TRD and thin ischemic retina, retinal breaks can occur resulting in a TRD with a rhegmatogenous component (CTRRD). These patients present with abrupt and rapidly progressive visual loss.

Fundoscopic findings include a taut, concave, immobile retina without breaks with associated fibrovascular areas of proliferation. Optical coherence tomography is useful in determining the degree of foveal involvement in tractional detachments as well as the concomitant presence of epiretinal membranes (fig. 1). It

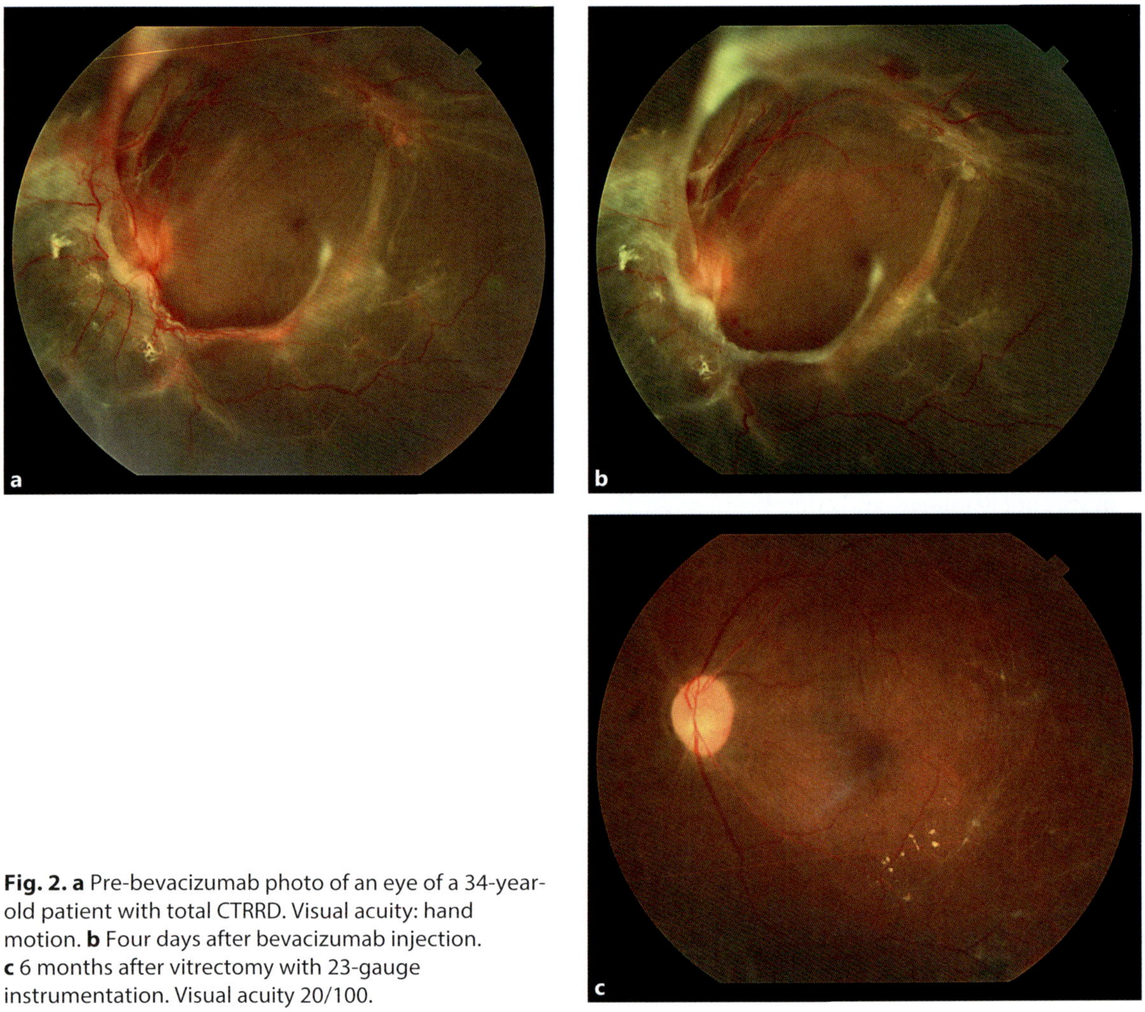

Fig. 2. a Pre-bevacizumab photo of an eye of a 34-year-old patient with total CTRRD. Visual acuity: hand motion. **b** Four days after bevacizumab injection. **c** 6 months after vitrectomy with 23-gauge instrumentation. Visual acuity 20/100.

is not uncommon for eyes with a vitreous hemorrhage to have areas of TRD discovered during surgery.

The objectives of vitrectomy are to relieve retinal traction, detach and remove the posterior hyaloid, reattach the retina, and treat areas of retinal ischemia to prevent vascular endothelial growth factor (VEGF) production and consequent neovascularization. Traditionally, surgery is done for TRDs that threaten or involve the fovea while photocoagulation is indicated for small extrafoveal TRDs, as these can remain stable for years without the need for vitrectomy.

Surgical complexity is very variable, and depends on how strongly the fibrovascular tissue adheres to the retina, degree of vascularity, extension of membranes, and the thinness and degree of ischemia of the retina. Preoperative administration of anti-VEGF for eyes with severe vascular tissue reduces the risk of intraoperative bleeding and facilitates the surgery. Low doses (12.5 mg) of bevacizumab (Avastin) should be injected no more than 5 days prior to surgery to avoid increased fibrovascular contraction and subsequent worsening of the retinal detachment [12, 16, 17] (fig. 2a–c). Despite the fact that microincision probes serve as multifunction instruments, precluding the need for many instruments during the procedure, it is still important to have all the ancillary instrumentation that may be required including hyaluronic acid, scissors, chandelier illuminators, forceps, and diathermy.

The surgical technique involves performing a core vitrectomy, removing all vitreous opacities, and detaching the posterior hyaloid. Areas of fibrovascular proliferation are segmented or dissected with the vitrectomy probe or with scissors or bimanual techniques (fig. 3). The aim is to remove all of the fibrovascular tissue that causes traction. In cases with very adherent tissue, chandeliers for bimanual techniques or hyaluronic acid injection to separate fibrovascular tissue from the retina can be useful. If removal of the fibrovascular tissue is possible without iatrogenic breaks, photocoagulation is then applied. However, air-fluid exchange at the end of the procedure with prone positioning for a few days is indicated when foveal elevation or folds are prominent to reduce postoperative metamorphopsia. Nasal areas of traction that do not threaten to involve the posterior pole do not need to be removed as long as there is no rhegmatogenous component or iatrogenic breaks.

The most serious complication of vitrectomy for TRD is the creation of iatrogenic retinal breaks. When these occur the surgeon should remove all the fibrovascular tissue, drain the subretinal liquid, perform air-fluid exchange, photocoagulate the breaks, and use long-acting intraocular gas or silicone oil tamponade.

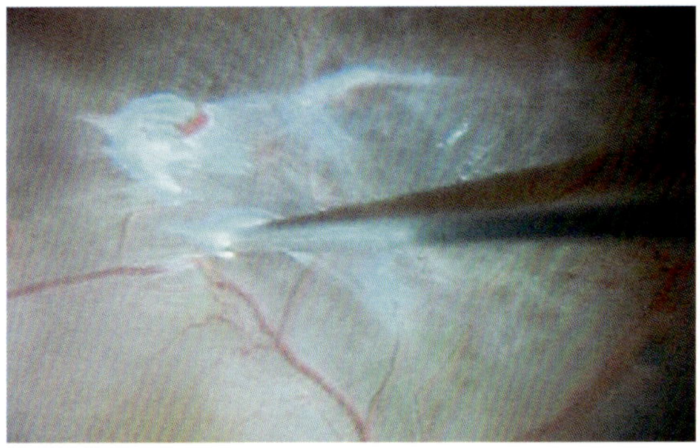

Fig. 3. Membrane dissection with 27-gauge vitrectomy probe in a TRD.

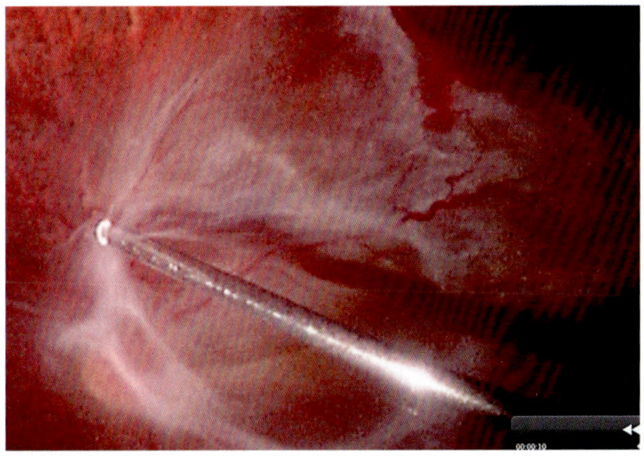

Fig. 4. Blunt dissection of fibrovascular tissue with a 27-gauge vitrectomy probe on CTRRD.

Combined Tractional and Rhegmatogenous Retinal Detachment

Strong vitreoretinal traction produced by fibrovascular tissue can threaten retinal surface integrity. If a retinal break occurs, then liquefied vitreous can penetrate into the subretinal space and separate the overlying retina from the retinal pigment epithelium causing CTRRD. Fundoscopic findings in these combined detachments show a convex retina with bullous or mobile retina in some areas (fig. 4). Retinal breaks are usually localized posterior to the equator and adjacent to areas of fibrovascular proliferation in a thin retina. Symptoms include sudden, progressive, and profound visual loss. In these cases, early vitrectomy is indicated to prevent permanent visual loss [18, 19].

These are the most complex diabetic surgeries as they require difficult techniques for removing fibrovascular tissue from the detached retina, closing retinal breaks, and reattaching the retina. Particularly useful instruments are the 25- and

27-gauge vitreous cutters introduced between the membranes to dissect and shave the fibrovascular tissue. In addition, cutting rates of up to 7,500 cuts/min exert minimal traction over the detached retina and chandelier illuminators, particularly 25- or 29-gauge, and facilitate bimanual fibrovascular tissue dissection (fig. 5a, b). In addition, hyaluronic acid can be used to separate the attached fibrous membranes from the mobile retina. Although the prognosis is reserved, good preoperative prognostic factors include recent onset, visual acuity of 5/200 or better, and absence of rubeosis and of retinal detachment involving the macula [15, 20].

Complications

Complications of vitrectomy for PDR, TRD, and CTRRD include rebleeding or nonclearing residual vitreous hemorrhage. This is more common in cases that have very vascular membranes and in patients with uncontrolled hypertension who are anticoagulated or have hypotony on the first day postoperatively. This can resolve with observation, can be managed with an in-office air-fluid exchange, or with a repeat vitrectomy in the operating room. Other complications include rhegmatogenous retinal detachment from iatrogenic breaks that were either not detected during the surgery or that reopened. In these cases a reoperation with a long-acting tamponade either with gas or silicone oil is required. Rubeosis and neovascular glaucoma are challenging complications. They are seen in very ischemic eyes or eyes that have peripheral detachments, and are managed with anti-VEGF injections, photocoagulation, repair of peripheral detachment if present, and sometimes a silicone oil tamponade.

Severe Fibrovascular Proliferation

Understanding the different types of vitreoretinal adhesions in PDR helps the surgeon to establish the best surgery for each patient. According to the Diabetic Retinopathy Vitrectomy Study Research Group, the most adequate candidates for early vitrectomy are patients with severe fibrovascular proliferation, and those with extensive prior photocoagulation or those with media opacities that prevent photocoagulation [2]. Others have confirmed that despite early and extensive retinal photocoagulation, fibrovascular and neovascular proliferations progress rapidly [21]. Thus, early vitrectomy offers the best results as neovascularization of the optic nerve and posterior pole rarely occurs following surgical excision of the posterior cortical vitreous.

Difficult Diabetic Vitrectomies

Diabetic eyes are more susceptible to cataract formation and corneal edema causing poor visibility during long surgical procedures. Prior to microincision victrectomy surgery, either irrigating glucose solutions or corneal epithelium debridement were used to improve visibility [22]. Microincision victrectomy surgery has shortened surgical time and, consequently, these complications are now seen less frequently.

Microincision surgery has reduced the frequency of iatrogenic breaks in several ways: microcannulas protect the vitreous base when entering and removing instruments such as scissors and forceps, the vitrectomy probe can be used as a multipurpose instrument and cutting rates of up to 7,500 cuts/min allow vitreous removal with minimal traction, and intraocular pressure control helps to prevent intraocular turbulence which can cause vitreous and retinal avulsions during surgery.

The diabetic eye, due to its ischemic state, is more susceptible to neovascularization at the sclerotomy entry sites and vitreous base [23, 24]. Most commonly this is evident for eyes requiring reoperation and with large sclerotomies. Smaller sclerotomies using 25- and 23-gauge systems help reduce inflammation and neovascularization responsible for postoperative bleeding.

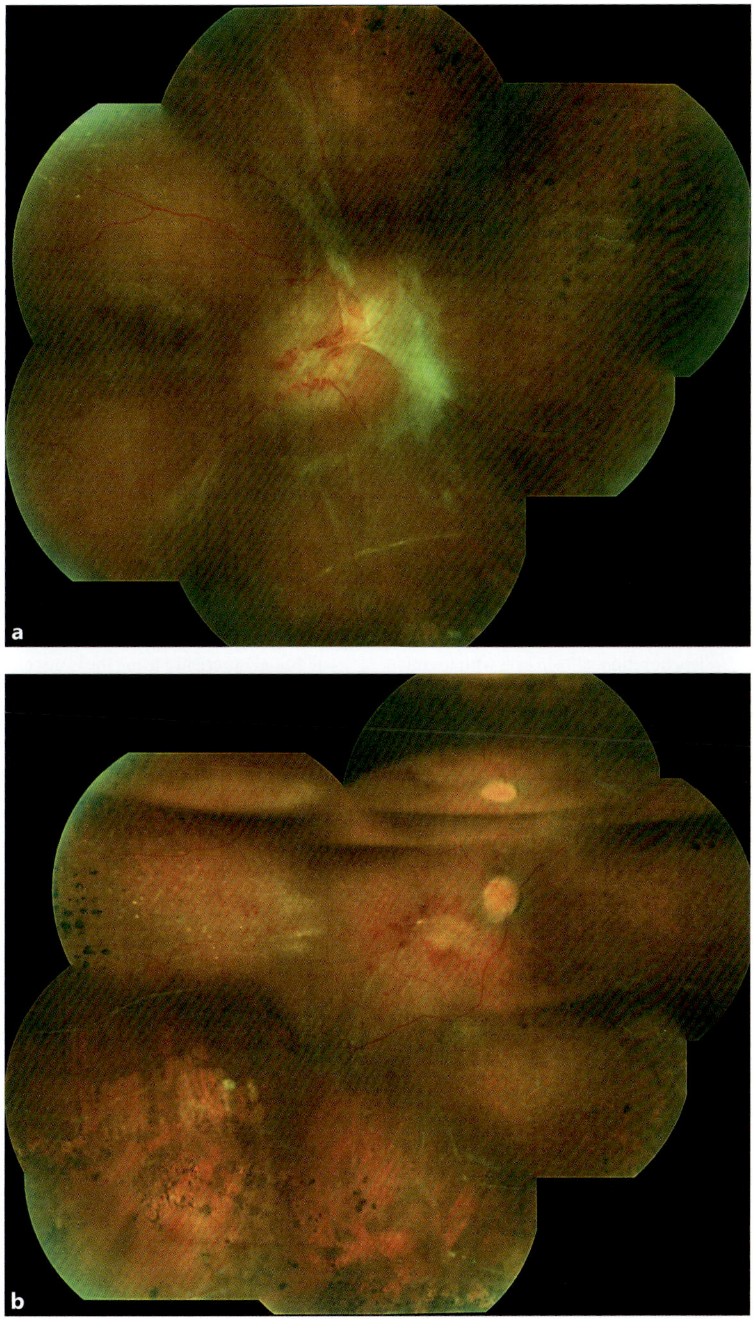

Fig. 5. a Preoperative traction and rhegmatogenous retinal detachment with fibrovascular proliferation and subretinal membranes managed with 25-gauge vitrectomy.
b Postoperative view with an attached retina and 30% residual gas bubble.

Intraoperative bleeding in diabetic eyes is a common problem. If severe, completing the procedure can become very challenging. Bleeding commonly occurs in neovascular areas, particularly when exchanging instruments due to sudden changes in intraocular pressure. However, the new vitrectomy systems, combined with smaller sclerotomies, allow for controlling intraocular pressure during surgery and reduced bleeding. In addition, preoperative treatment with an antiangiogenic agent facilitates dissecting fibrovascular membranes in patients with tractional and/or rhegmatogenous retinal detachments.

Conclusion

Microincision vitrectomy surgery is ideal for late complications of PDR. Small-gauge instrumentation allow for rapid, safe, and elegant removal of fibrovascular tissue. High-speed cutting rates minimize traction. Preoperative application of antiangiogenic therapy, for selected cases, and reduced surgical time have decreased surgical complications and increased positive outcomes. As a result, surgical intervention for complicated diabetic retinopathy can be performed earlier than suggested by the DVS, allowing for better visual and anatomical results.

References

1 Early vitrectomy for severe proliferative diabetic retinopathy in eyes with useful vision. Clinical application of results of a randomized trial – Diabetic Retinopathy Vitrectomy Study Report 4. The Diabetic Retinopathy Vitrectomy Study Research Group. Ophthalmology 1988;95:1321–1334.
2 Early vitrectomy for severe vitreous hemorrhage in diabetic retinopathy. Two-year results of a randomized trial. Diabetic Retinopathy Vitrectomy Study Report 2. The Diabetic Retinopathy Vitrectomy Study Research Group. Arch Ophthalmol 1985;103:1644–1652.
3 Early vitrectomy for severe vitreous hemorrhage in diabetic retinopathy. Four-year results of a randomized trial: Diabetic Retinopathy Vitrectomy Study Report 5. Arch Ophthalmol 1990;108:958–964.
4 Early vitrectomy for severe proliferative diabetic retinopathy in eyes with useful vision. Results of a randomized trial – Diabetic Retinopathy Vitrectomy Study Report 3. The Diabetic Retinopathy Vitrectomy Study Research Group. Ophthalmology 1988;95:1307–1320.
5 Fujii GY, De Juan E Jr, Humayun MS, Pieramici DJ, Chang TS, Awh C, et al: A new 25-gauge instrument system for transconjunctival sutureless vitrectomy surgery. Ophthalmology 2002;109:1807–1812.
6 Fujii GY, De Juan E Jr, Humayun MS, et al: Initial experience using the transconjunctival sutureless vitrectomy system for vitreoretinal surgery. Ophthalmology 2002;109:1814–1820.
7 Eckardt C: Transconjunctival sutureless 23-gauge vitrectomy. Retina 2005;25:208–211.
8 da R Lucena D, Ribeiro JA, Costa RA, et al: Intraoperative bleeding during vitrectomy for diabetic tractional retinal detachment with versus without preoperative intravitreal bevacizumab (IBeTra study). Br J Ophthalmol 2009;93:688–691.
9 Rizzo S, Genovesi-Ebert F, Di Bartolo E, et al: Injection of intravitreal bevacizumab (Avastin) as a preoperative adjunct before vitrectomy surgery in the treatment of severe proliferative diabetic retinopathy (PDR). Graefes Arch Clin Exp Ophthalmol 2008;246:837–842.
10 Yeoh J, Williams C, Allen P, et al: Avastin as an adjunct to vitrectomy in the management of severe proliferative diabetic retinopathy: a prospective case series. Clin Experiment Ophthalmol 2008;36:449–454.
11 Ishikawa K, Honda S, Tsukahara Y, Negi A: Preferable use of intravitreal bevacizumab as a pretreatment of vitrectomy for severe proliferative diabetic retinopathy. Eye (Lond) 2009;23:108–111.
12 Oshima Y, Shima C, Wakabayashi T, et al: Microincision vitrectomy surgery and intravitreal bevacizumab as a surgical adjunct to treat diabetic traction retinal detachment. Ophthalmology 2009;116:927–938.
13 Michels RG, Rice TA, Rice EF: Vitrectomy for diabetic vitreous hemorrhage. Am J Ophthalmol 1983;95:12–21.
14 Chaudhry NA, Lim ES, Saito Y, et al: Early vitrectomy and endolaser photocoagulation in patients with type I diabetes with severe vitreous hemorrhage. Ophthalmology 1995;102:1164–1169.
15 Rice TA, Michels RG, Rice EF: Vitrectomy for diabetic traction retinal detachment involving the macula. Am J Ophthalmol 1983;95:22–33.
16 Arevalo JF, Maia M, Flynn HW Jr, et al: Tractional retinal detachment following intravitreal bevacizumab (Avastin) in patients with severe proliferative diabetic retinopathy. Br J Ophthalmol 2008;92:213–216.
17 Arevalo JF, Sanchez JG, Saldarriaga L, et al: Retinal detachment after bevacizumab. Ophthalmology 2011;118:2304.e3–e7.
18 Thompson JT, de Bustros S, Michels RG, Rice TA: Results and prognostic factors in vitrectomy for diabetic tractionrhegmatogenous retinal detachment. Arch Ophthalmol 1987;105:503–507.

19 Yang CM, Su PY, Yeh PT, Chen MS: Combined rhegmatogenous and traction retinal detachment in proliferative diabetic retinopathy: clinical manifestations and surgical outcome. Can J Ophthalmol 2008;43:192–198.
20 Rice TA, Michels RG, Rice EF: Vitrectomy for diabetic rhegmatogenous retinal detachment. Am J Ophthalmol 1983; 95:34–44.
21 Davis MD: Vitreous contraction in PDR. Arch Ophthalmol 1965;74:741–751.
22 Smiddy WE, Feuer W: Incidence of cataract extraction after diabetic vitrectomy. Retina 2004;24:574–581.
23 Rice TA, Michels RG, Maguire MG, Rice EF: The effect of lensectomy on the incidence of iris neovascularization and neovascular glaucoma after vitrectomy for diabetic retinopathy. Am J Ophthalmol 1983;95:1–11.
24 Jaffe GJ, Lewis H, Han DP, Williams GA, Abrams GW: Treatment of postvitrectomy fibrin pupillary block with tissue plasminogen activator. Am J Ophthalmol 1989;108:170–175.

Yousef J. Cruz-Iñigo
Department of Ophthalmology
University of Puerto Rico
Rio Piedras Medical Center
00909 San Juan (Puerto Rico)
E-Mail yousef.cruz@upr.edu

Oh H, Oshima Y (eds): Microincision Vitrectomy Surgery. Emerging Techniques and Technology.
Dev Ophthalmol. Basel, Karger, 2014, vol 54, pp 204–212 (DOI: 10.1159/000360468)

Myopic Traction Maculopathy

María Gómez-Resa · Anniken Burés-Jelstrup · Carlos Mateo
Instituto de Microcirugía Ocular (IMO), Barcelona, Spain

Abstract
Myopic traction maculopathy is a high myopia-related complication caused by several mechanisms with traction as a common pathway. Macular hole-related retinal detachment is considered to be the final stage of progressive foveoschisis. In this setting, release of all vitreous and epiretinal tractions is essential in order to achieve surgical success. Pars plana vitrectomy has proven useful in the treatment of myopic foveoschisis, with both good visual and anatomical results. However, the surgical technique for the treatment of macular hole-related retinal detachment is still a controversial issue: reoperations are common and the final visual prognosis is limited, especially in those cases with a pronounced posterior staphyloma. We must also bear in mind that a highly myopic eye has some characteristic traits that may complicate vitreoretinal surgery. In these cases, microincision vitrectomy surgery may offer some advantages compared to conventional vitrectomy.

The term 'myopic traction maculopathy' was proposed by Panozzo and Mercanti [1] to encompass various findings by optical coherence tomography (OCT) in highly myopic eyes, all with traction in common. Among these findings, tangential premacular vitreous traction [2–8], stretched retinal vessels [8, 9], the presence of epiretinal membranes [9], an abnormally rigid inner limiting membrane [1, 10, 11], and the posterior staphyloma [2, 3] have been described. Progressive traction of these structures will determine the evolution of myopic traction maculopathy [3]. Myopic foveoschisis (MF) often represents an initial stage of a macular hole retinal detachment (MHRD), especially in cases with associated foveal detachment [12–14].

Myopic Foveoschisis

MF has recently been described [2], thanks to the advances in OCT imaging. Since the introduction of OCT in clinical practice, the incidence of MF has been reported to range between 9 and 34% in highly myopic eyes with a posterior staphyloma [1, 7]. Back in 1958, Phillips [15] was the first to describe a retinal elevation within the posterior pole in the absence of a macular hole (MH), possibly explained by retinal schisis (fig. 1). In some cases, biomicroscopy shows epiretinal membranes or pseudomacular holes [16].

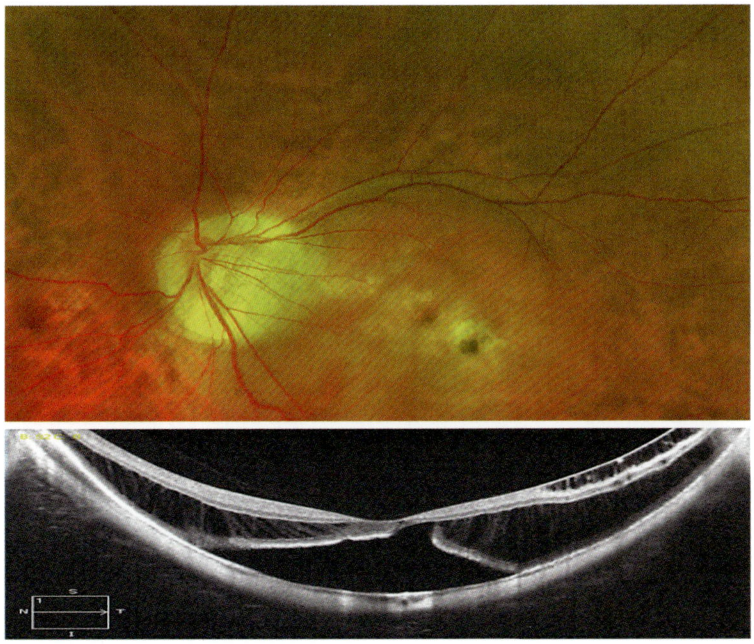

Fig. 1. MF and foveal detachment.

OCT is the gold standard for the diagnosis of MF and allows one to quantify the degree of schisis and its longitudinal progression. Other associated features depicted by OCT are epiretinal tractions, inner and outer retinal defects (lamellar holes), and foveal detachments (fig. 2). A thorough OCT examination of the posterior pole, searching for paravascular or peripapillary retinal breaks, or breaks close to atrophic areas, should be performed before establishing a definite diagnosis of MF [14]. These types of breaks are typically infradiagnosed since they tend to be missed in biomicroscopic examination, which can ultimately lead to surgical failure.

MF tends to remain both anatomically and functionally stable for long periods of time [3, 17], and even sporadic cases of spontaneous resolution have been described [18]. As a general rule, visual acuity tends to decline when the fovea detaches [2, 17], although functional and anatomical status are not always directly correlated [16]. Surgery is usually considered when there is visual loss and/or metamorphopsia attributed to the progression of the disease [19]. A previous history of MHRD in the other eye should also be taken into account [4, 12]. Surgery seems to play a prophylactic role in cases with associated foveal detachment or lamellar MH and helps to prevent progression towards a MH [4], with or without retinal detachment, which has a poorer visual and anatomic prognosis.

Surgical Technique

The principal role of vitrectomy is to remove all intraocular vitreoretinal tractions. Microincision vitrectomy surgery has potential advantages compared to conventional vitrectomy in highly myopic eyes, especially since the thin sclera of these eyes may lead to several intraoperative complications. Microcannulas have shown a reduction of the incidence of iatrogenic peripheral breaks [20]. The valved microcannula systems prevent uncontrolled intraocular pressure changes, which may induce pupil closure or even intraoperative choroidal detachment. Despite the lower range of complications with the small-gauge system, visu-

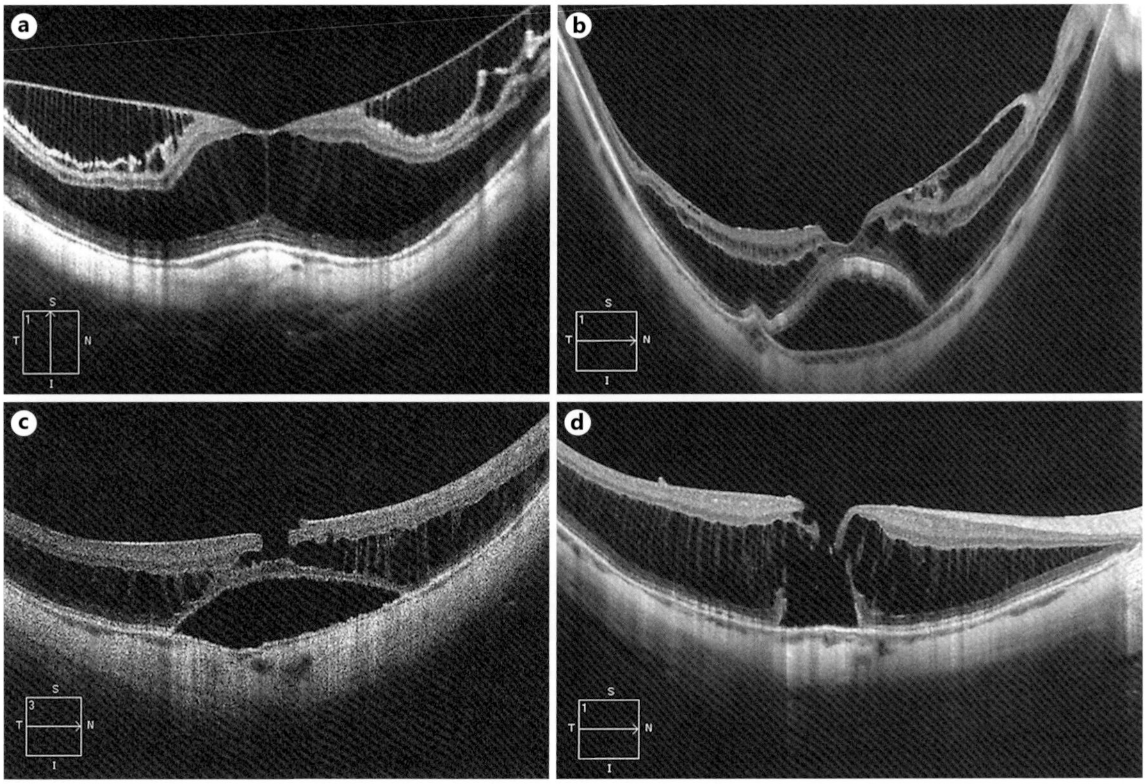

Fig. 2. a Progressive retinoschisis. **b** Retinoschisis and foveal detachment with clear epiretinal traction. **c** Foveal detachment and inner lamellar MH. **d** Full-thickness MH hole with schisis.

al results show no differences with the two techniques [21].

The use of triamcinolone or trypan blue improves visualization of the vitreous during surgery [6, 12] since posterior vitreous schisis and firmly adhered vitreous cortex on the retinal surface [13] are common findings in myopic eyes. Both forceps and the Tano diamond dust scraper are recommended to remove all vitreous remnants. The length of the forceps and other surgical instruments must be chosen carefully since axial lengths of 30 mm or more are not uncommon in these highly myopic eyes [22].

Internal limiting membrane (ILM) peeling is a controversial issue [6]. Some case series of vitrectomy without ILM peeling have reported good anatomical and functional results [8, 19] even in eyes with a pronounced posterior staphyloma [8]. This suggests that ILM peeling is not essential for this purpose. The rationale behind ILM removal is to reduce macular traction causing foveoschisis and foveal detachment [12, 23], and also to confirm removal of all epiretinal tissue [13]. On the other hand, ILM removal favors retinal elongation in order to adapt to the posterior staphyloma, although the absence of ILM results in a more fragile retina [24].

ILM peeling is performed with forceps and is usually previously stained with indocyanine green, trypan blue, or brilliant blue [12, 13] (fig. 3). Due to the inherent traits of highly myopic eyes, it is advisable to stain more than once in

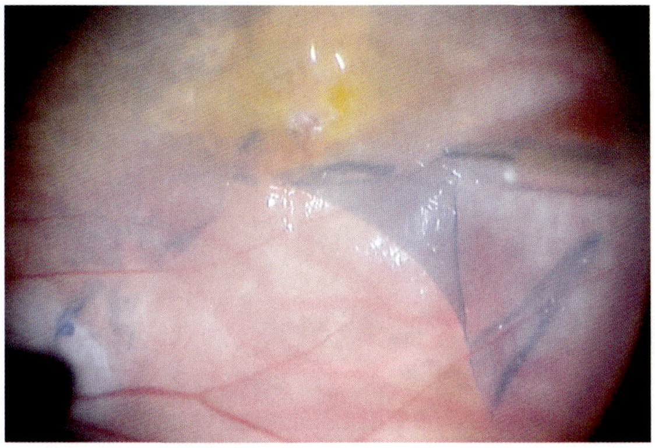

Fig. 3. ILM peeling.

order to confirm a complete removal of the ILM. ILM peeling is difficult and associated with multiple complications in highly myopic eyes. The ILM in myopes is thin, sticky, and tends to break constantly during its removal [25].

The use of gas in these cases remains controversial. Panozzo and Mercanti [13] published a report of 24 cases treated with vitrectomy without gas tamponade, and obtained slow but progressive anatomic resolution. The role of gas tamponade after fluid-air exchange is also uncertain [4, 6] since anatomic resolution usually occurs after the gas has cleared out [8]. The most commonly used gas tamponades are perfluoropropane [6] or sulfur hexafluoride [4] at a nonexpansile concentration. Face-down positioning is required for a period of 24 h to 2 weeks postoperatively [4, 8]. In eyes with foveal detachment, the gas may push the subretinal fluid inside the limited area of the posterior staphyloma and towards the weak point of the fovea, causing the formation of a MH [12]. Hirakata and Hida [12] suggested using silicone oil tamponade in cases with a poor vision in the opposite eye. In 2006, Baba et al. [26] used macular buckling alone to treat cases with foveoschisis and foveal detachment, achieving a visual improvement of two or more lines in 66% of the eyes. Mateo et al. [27, 28] showed similar results in a large series using macular buckling combined with vitrectomy (fig. 4). When associated with a MH, combined vitrectomy and macular buckling achieves a 100% rate of MH closure, and visual improvement in 81% of patients [29].

Results

OCT is a fundamental tool in the postoperative follow-up [4]. Both foveoschisis and foveal detachment tend to improve immediately after surgery and then more gradually over the next 6–12 months [4, 13]. This is the natural course for 75–100% of cases [4, 6, 30], which tend to remain stable once improvement has occurred [12].

Some factors are associated with a worse surgical outcome, such as degenerative myopic fundus alterations [16], a severe posterior staphyloma, and a thin choroid [30]. In some series, up to 70% of patients with associated foveal detachment showed visual improvement compared to only 42% of the patients without associated foveal detachment [31, 32].

Both a postoperative decrease of the central macular thickness and integrity of the inner segment/outer segment junction are associated with a better visual outcome [33]. Kim et al. [31] compared visual outcomes in patients who received a gas tamponade after vitrectomy and ILM peeling with those who did not, and found no statistically significant differences between the two groups in terms of visual gain (55.6 vs. 62.5%) or foveoschisis resolution (88.9 vs. 75%). The only significant difference encountered in their study was faster resolution of the foveoschisis in the patients treated with a gas tamponade (2.25 vs. 4.5 months).

Complications

MH development after vitrectomy is one of the most feared complications in patients with foveoschisis [4, 12]. The incidence of MH development is variable (0–27%) [16, 34], but in all cases visual acuity tends to decline [4, 12]. Foveoschisis cases with associated severe foveal detach-

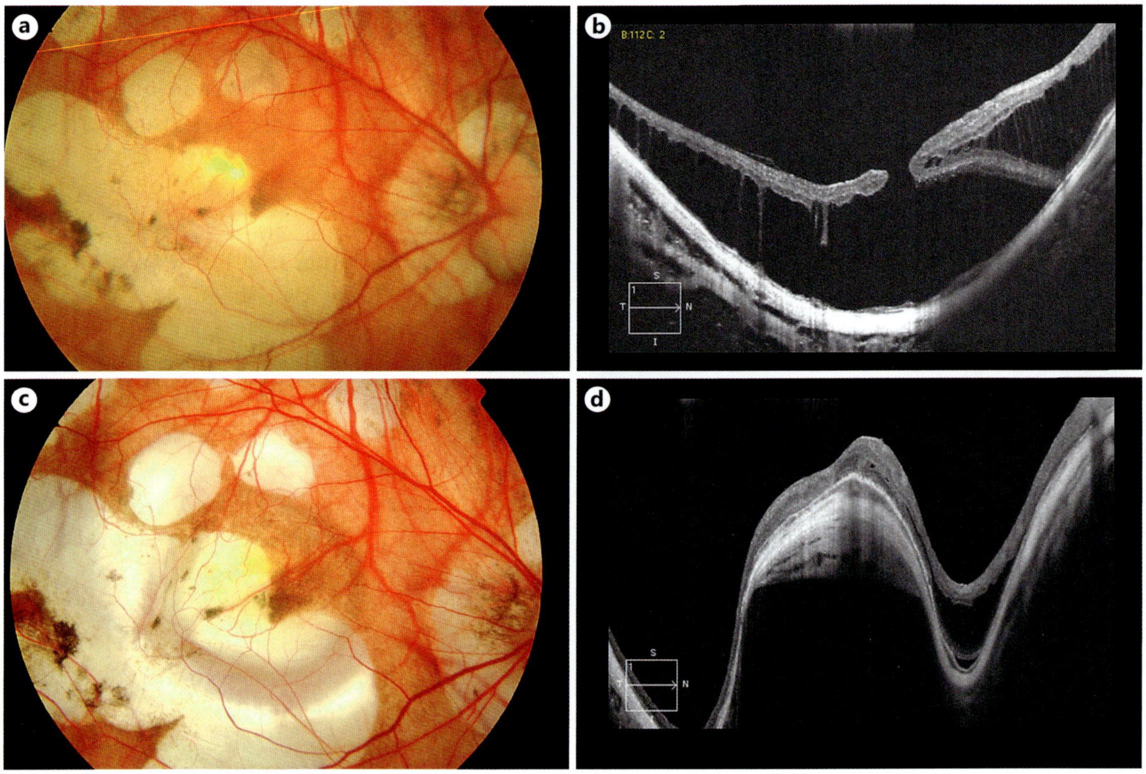

Fig. 4. a High myopia with posterior staphyloma. **b** Full-thickness MH with retinoschisis. **c** Macular buckling. **d** Postoperative spectral domain OCT after combined macular buckling and pars plana vitrectomy.

ment [12] as well as eyes with a preoperative inner segment/outer segment junction defect [35] are more prone to MH development after surgery. Shimada et al. [36] suggested a fovea-sparing ILM peeling technique to avoid iatrogenic MH development (fovea sparing group 0%; complete ILM peeling group 16.7%). Another complication is the recurrence of the foveal detachment, due to an incomplete removal of the vitreoretinal tractions [12]. Cataract progression after vitrectomy is also a known surgical complication. Thus, combined phacoemulsification with intraocular lens implantation and vitrectomy is a widely accepted surgical option to avoid having to perform another surgical procedure [6, 19].

Macular Hole Retinal Detachment

MHRD is a severe retinal complication that almost exclusively occurs in highly myopic eyes with a pronounced posterior staphyloma. Various surgical techniques have been used throughout time, such as diathermy, pneumoretinopexy, scleral shortening, and macular buckling. Gonvers and Machemer [37] were the first to describe the use of vitrectomy with gas-fluid exchange for this purpose in 1982. Since then, several reports have been published describing variations of the vitrectomy technique, using silicone oil tamponade, ILM peeling, inverted ILM flap technique, laser around the MH, or a buckle as adjunctive treatment (encircling or macular buckle) [38, 39] (fig. 5). The overall surgical success rate in MHRD is poorer

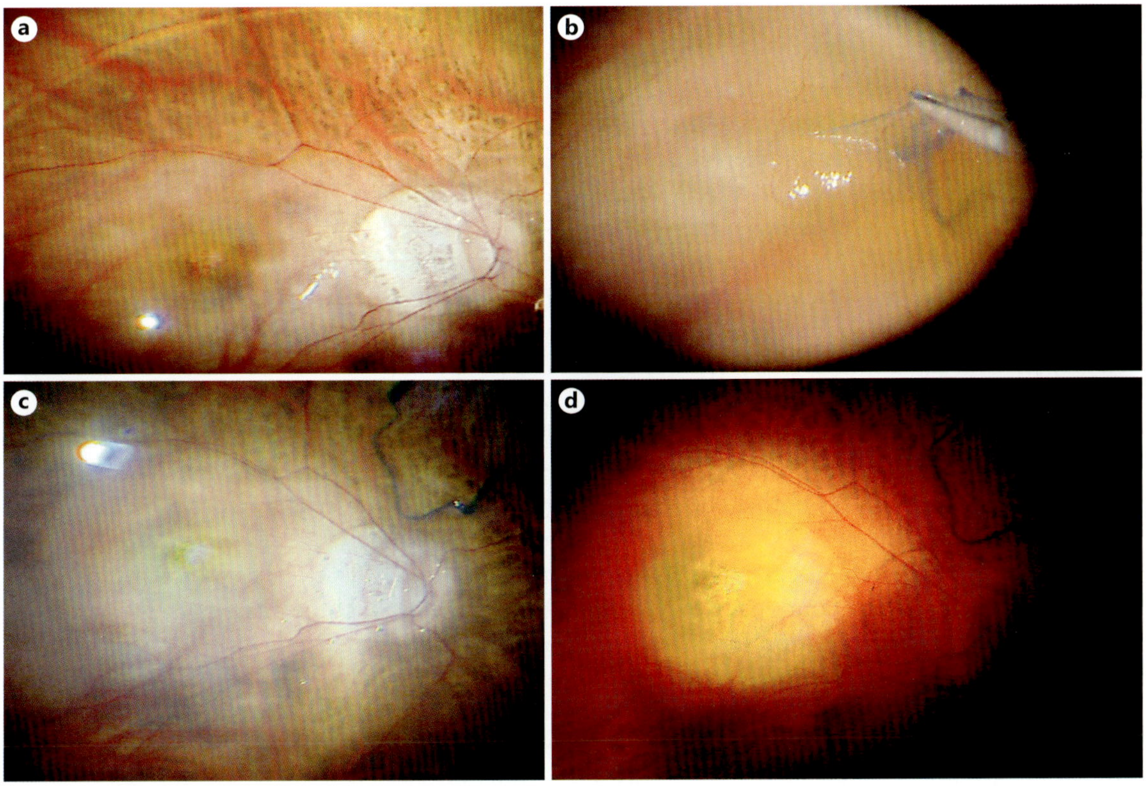

Fig. 5. a MHRD; liquid perfluorocarbon injection over the posterior pole. **b** ILM peeling using a 23-gauge microsurgical forceps; liquid perfluorocarbon can facilitate peeling of the membrane without exertion of excessive retinal traction. **c** Macular buckle under the macular area. **d** Illuminated macular buckle with an internal 30-gauge chandelier optical fiber; this technique allows placing it correctly under the fovea.

than in conventional rhegmatogenous retinal detachment, and reoperations are often necessary [38]. There is no standard technique for the treatment of MHRD, and as for MF [36, 39], OCT is key both in the diagnosis and as a follow-up tool.

The main causative factors in MHRD are vitreous and retinal tractions over the macular area; therefore, its removal is crucial. Fang et al. [40] achieved up to 88% retinal reattachment after one surgery in 34 eyes, removing all epiretinal tissue and posterior hyaloid assisted with triamcinolone. Most patients also showed an improvement in visual acuity without an increase in intraocular pressure. However, MH closure could only be confirmed by OCT in 46% of the patients. Other studies have shown better anatomic results after ILM peeling [41, 42] since this guarantees complete removal of all epiretinal tractions and a more flexible retina [41].

The dyes used in vitreoretinal surgery are potentially toxic. Thus, the combination of the dye with a viscoelastic substance may help to prevent migration into the subretinal space through the MH. Kadonosono et al. [41] used a viscoelastic material containing indocyanine green to stain the ILM. Another option is to place a small drop of perfluorocarbon liquid over the MH before using the dye; however, the complex anatomy of the posterior staphyloma can turn this procedure into a challenging one [43].

Gas or Silicone Oil?
According to Mancino et al. [44], C_3F_8 tamponade after vitrectomy and ILM peeling offers better results, both functional and anatomic, than silicone oil. Silicone oil offers some advantages, such as faster visual recovery and a long-acting tamponade effect, and is therefore preferred for patients who are unable to remain in a face-down position. The drawback of silicone oil is that, due to its toxicity and elevation of intraocular pressure, it will have to be removed in most patients, requiring a new surgical procedure with its potential complications. Mete et al. [45] found similar results in terms of visual gain and retinal reapplication for both 1,000 cSt silicone oil and heavy silicone oil, retrospectively. On the other hand, Avitabile et al. [46] defended the use of Densiron as the tamponade of choice, maintaining retinal reapplication in 87% of the cases after Densiron extraction compared to 53% after standard silicone oil extraction. A fundamental step when using microincision vitrectomy surgery is choosing a low-viscosity silicone oil to facilitate both injection and extraction.

Photocoagulation around the Macular Hole?
Kwok et al. [47] found no visual or anatomic differences between endolaser around the MH or no laser associated with vitrectomy and gas tamponade. On the other hand, Yu et al. [48] found that patients treated with laser showed better visual results than those who did not receive laser treatment during the vitrectomy (100 vs. 53.8% improvement). Laser is a destructive treatment that may increase the size of previous scar tissue and limit visual prognosis. Therefore, it should only be used in eyes with a poor visual prognosis.

Combined Scleral Buckle?
Given the results of Ghoraba et al. [49], the use of a 360° encircling band in combination with pars plana vitrectomy and silicone oil offers no additional effect on either the anatomical success or the rate of MH closure in the management of myopic MHRD.

Macular Buckling?
Macular buckling is a surgical technique that pretends to counteract the pulling effect of the progressive staphyloma. Different techniques have been used together with modern vitrectomy techniques [50–52]. Pars plana vitrectomy is useful for removing two of the main tractions that cause myopic traction maculopathy: vitreous traction and an abnormally rigid ILM. However, vitrectomy does not address the pulling effect exerted by the stretched retinal vessels nor the posterior staphyloma. Macular buckling offers better visual and anatomic results in cases of MHRD in eyes with a high axial length since it is capable of addressing a major cause of traction over the macula: posterior staphyloma [53]. MH closure in eyes with high axial length is difficult to obtain by vitrectomy alone due to the disproportion between the retina and the pronounced staphyloma [42]. Alkabes et al. [52] obtained excellent anatomic and visual outcomes in the treatment of MHRD with macular buckling. Though the results were positive in previously vitrectomized eyes as well as untreated eyes, the results were superior when macular buckling was the first-choice technique.

References

1 Panozzo G, Mercanti A: Optical coherence tomography findings in myopic traction maculopathy. Arch Ophthalmol 2004;122:1455–1460.

2 Takano M, Kishi S: Foveal retinoschisis and retinal detachment in severely myopic eyes with posterior staphyloma. Am J Ophthalmol 1999;128:472–476.

3 Benhamou N, Massin P, Haouchine B, Erginay A, Gaudric A: Macular retinoschisis in highly myopic eyes. Am J Ophthalmol 2002;133:794–800.

4 Kobayashi H, Kishi S: Vitreous surgery for highly myopic eyes with foveal detachment and retinoschisis. Ophthalmology 2003;110:1702–1707.
5 Ishida M, Yamazaki K, Shinoda K, et al: Macular hole retinal detachment in highly myopic eyes: ultrastructure of surgically removed epiretinal membrane and clinicopathologic correlation. Retina 2000;20:176–183.
6 Ikuno Y, Sayanagi K, Ohji M, Kamei M, Gomi F, Harino S, Fujikado T, Tano Y: Vitrectomy and internal limiting membrane peeling for myopic foveoschisis. Am J Ophthalmol 2004;137:719–724.
7 Akiba J, Konno S, Sato E, et al: Retinal detachment and retinoschisis detected by optical coherence tomography in a myopic eye with macular hole. Ophthalmic Surg Lasers 2003;31:240–242.
8 Yeh SI, Chang WC, Chen LJ: Vitrectomy without internal limiting membrane peeling for macular retinoschisis and foveal detachment in highly myopic eyes. Acta Ophthalmol 2008;86:219–224.
9 Ikuno Y, Gomi F, Tano Y: Potent retina arteriolar traction as possible cause of myopic foveoschisis. Am J Ophthalmol 2005;139:462–467.
10 Bando H, Ikuno Y, Choi JS, Tano Y, Yamanaka I, Ishibashi T: Ultrastructure of internal limiting membrane in myopic foveoschisis. Am J Ophthalmol 2005; 391:197–199.
11 Sayanagi K, Ikuno Y, Tano Y: Tractional internal limiting membrane detachment in highly myopic eyes. Am J Ophthalmol 2006;142:850–852.
12 Hirakata A, Hida T: Vitrectomy for myopic posterior retinoschisis or foveal detachment. Jpn J Ophthalmol 2006;50: 53–61.
13 Panozzo G, Mercanti A: Vitrectomy for myopic traction maculopathy. Arch Ophthalmol 2005;125:767–772.
14 Smiddy WE, Kim SS, Lujan BJ, Gregori D: Myopic traction maculopathy: spectral domain optical coherence tomographic imaging and a hypothesized mechanism. Ophthalmic Surg Lasers Imaging 2009;40:169–173.
15 Phillips CI: Retinal detachment at the posterior pole. Br J Ophthalmol 1958;42: 749–753.
16 Kanda S, Uemura A, Sakamoto Y, Kita H: Vitrectomy with internal limiting membrane peeling for macular retinoschisis and retinal detachment without macular hole in highly myopic eyes. Am J Ophthalmol 2003;136:177–180.
17 Baba T, Ohno-Matsui K, Futagami S, et al: Prevalence and characteristics of foveal retinal detachment without macular hole in high myopia. Am J Ophthalmol 2003;135:338–342.
18 Polito A, Lanzetta P, Del Borrello M, et al: Spontaneous resolution of a shallow detachment of the macula in a highly myopic eye. Am J Ophthalmol 2003;135: 546–547.
19 Kwok KH, Lai TY, Yip WW: Vitrectomy and gas tamponade without internal limiting membrane peeling for myopic foveoschisis. Br J Ophthalmol 2005;89: 1180–1183.
20 Cha DM, Woo SJ, Park KH, Chung H: Intraoperative iatrogenic peripheral retinal break in 23-gauge transconjunctival sutureless vitrectomy versus 20-gauge conventional vitrectomy. Graefes Arch Clin Exp Ophthalmol 2013;251:1469–1474.
21 Ikuno Y, Asai T, Yano S, Nishida K: Small gauge vitrectomy in macular surgery for myopic complications (in Japanese). Nihon Ganka Gakkai Zasshi 2012;116:1130–1136.
22 Gao X, Ikuno Y, Nishida Y: Long-shaft forceps for membrane peeling in highly myopic eyes. Retina 2013;33:1475–1476.
23 Kuhn F: Internal limiting membrane removal for macular detachment in highly myopic eyes. Am J Ophthalmol 2003;135:547–549.
24 Wollensak G, Spoerl E, Grosse G, Wirbelauer C: Biomechanical significance of the human internal limiting lamina. Retina 2006;26:965–968.
25 Kwok AK, Lai TY: Internal limiting membrane removal in macular hole surgery of severely myopic eyes: a case-control study. Br J Ophthalmol 2003;87: 885–889.
26 Baba T, Tanaka S, Maesawa A, Teramatsu T, Noda Y, Yamamoto S: Scleral buckling with macular plombe for eyes with myopic macular retinoschisis and retinal detachment without macular hole. Am J Ophthalmol 2006;142:483–487.
27 Mateo C, Gómez-Resa MV, Burés-Jelstrup A, Alkabes M: Surgical outcomes of macular buckling techniques for macular retinoschisis in highly myopic eyes. Saudi J Ophthalmol 2013;27:235–239.
28 Mateo C, Burés-Jelstrup A, Navarro R, Corcóstegui B: Macular buckling for eyes with myopic foveoschisis secondary to posterior staphyloma. Retina 2012;32: 1121–1128.
29 Burés-Jelstrup A, Alkabes A, Gómez-Resa M, Ríos J, Corcóstegui B, Mateo C: Visual and anatomical outcome after macular buckling for macular hole with associated foveoschisis in highly myopic eyes. Br J Ophthalmol 2014;98: 104–109.
30 Iida Y, Hangai M, Yoshikawa M, Ooto S, Yoshimura N: Local biometric features and visual prognosis after surgery for treatment of myopic foveoschisis. Retina 2013;33:1179–1187.
31 Kim KS, Lee SB, Lee WK: Vitrectomy and internal limiting membrane peeling with and without gas tamponade for myopic foveoschisis. Am J Ophthalmol 2012;153:320–326.
32 Ikuno Y, Sayanagi K, Soga K, Oshima Y, Ohji M, Tano Y: Foveal anatomical status and surgical results in vitrectomy for myopic foveoschisis. Jpn J Ophthalmol 2008;52:269–276.
33 Fujimoto S, Ikuno Y, Nishida K: Postoperative optical coherence tomographic appearance and relation to visual acuity after vitrectomy for myopic foveoschisis. Am J Ophthalmol 2013;156:968–973.
34 Gaucher D, Haouchine B, Tadayoni R, Massin P, Erginay A, Benhamou N, Gaudric A: Long-term follow-up of high myopic foveoschisis: natural course and surgical outcome. Am J Ophthalmol 2007;143:455–462.
35 Gao X, Ikuno Y, Fujimoto S, Nishida K: Risk factors for development of full-thickness macular holes after pars plana vitrectomy for myopic foveoschisis. Am J Ophthalmol 2013;155: 1021–1027.
36 Shimada N, Sugamoto Y, Ogawa M, Takese H, Ohno-Matsui K: Fovea-sparing internal limiting membrane peeling for myopic traction maculopathy. Am J Ophthalmol 2012;154:693–701.
37 Gonvers M, Machemer R: A new approach to treating retinal detachment with macular hole. Am J Ophthalmol 1982;94:468–472.
38 Ortisi E, Avitabile T, Bonfiglio V: Surgical management of retinal detachment because of macular hole in highly myopic eyes. Retina 2012;32:1704–1718.
39 Kuriyama S, Hayashi H, Jingami Y, Kuramoto N, Akita J, Matsumoto M: Efficacy of inverted internal limiting membrane flap technique for the treatment of macular hole in high myopia. Am J Ophthalmol 2013;156:125–131.

40 Fang X, Weng Y, Xu S, Chen Z, Liu J, Chen B, Wu P, Ni H, Yao K: Optical coherence tomographic characteristics and surgical outcome of eyes with myopic foveoschisis. Eye 2009;23:1336–1342.
41 Kadonosono K, Yazama F, Itoh N, Uchio E, Nakamura S, Akura J, Sawada H, Ohno S: Treatment of retinal detachment resulting from myopic macular hole with internal limiting membrane removal. Am J Ophthalmol 2001;131: 203–207.
42 Ichibe M, Yoshizaka T, Murakami K, Ohta M, Oya Y, Yamamoto S, Funaki S, Funaki H, Ozawa Y, Baba E, Abe H: Surgical management of retinal detachment associated with myopic macular hole: anatomic and functional status of the macula. Am J Ophthalmol 2003;136: 277–284.
43 Facino M, Mochi B, Lai S, Terrile R: A simple way to prevent indocyanine green from entering the subretinal space during vitrectomy for retinal detachment due to myopic macular hole. Eur J Ophthalmol 2004;14:269–271.
44 Mancino R, Ciuffoletti E, Martucci A, Aiello F, Cedrone C, Cerulli L, Nucci C: Anatomical and functional results of macular hole retinal detachment surgery in patients with high myopia and posterior staphyloma treated with perfluoropropane gas or silicone oil. Retina 2013; 33:586–592.
45 Mete M, Parolini B, Maggio E, Pertile G: 1000 cSt silicone oil vs heavy silicone oil as intraocular tamponade in retinal detachment associated to myopic macular hole. Graefes Arch Clin Exp Ophthalmol 2001;249:821–826.
46 Avitabile T, Bonfiglio V, Buccoliero D, Castiglione F, Reibaldi M, Castaing M, Mistretta A: Heavy versus standard silicone oil in the management of retinal detachment with macular hole in myopic eyes. Retina 2011;31:540–546.
47 Kwok A, Cheng L, Gopal L, Sharma T, Lam D: Endolaser around macular hole in the management of associated retinal detachment in highly myopic eyes. Retina 2000;20:439–444.
48 Yu J, Wang F, Cao H, Fan Y, Zhang X: Combination of internal limiting membrane peeling and endophotocoagulation for retinal detachment related to high myopia in patients with macular hole. Ophthalmic Surg Lasers Imaging 2010;41:215–221.
49 Ghoraba HH, Mansour HO, Elgouhary SM: Effect of 360° episcleral band as adjunctive to pars plana vitrectomy and silicone oil tamponade in the management of myopic macular hole retinal detachment. Retina 2013;0:1–9.
50 Mitamura Y, Takeuchi S, Tsuruoka M: Macular buckling combined with pars plana vitrectomy for complicated retinal detachment due to macular hole. Retina 2000;20:669–672.
51 El Rayes EN: Supra choroidal buckling in managing myopic vitreoretinal interface disorders: 1-year data. Retina 2014; 34:129–135.
52 Alkabes M, Burés-Jelstrup A, Salinas C, Dutra Medeiros M, Rios J, Corcóstegui B, Mateo C: Macular buckling for previously untreated and recurrent retinal detachment due to high myopic macular hole: a 12-month comparative study. Graefes Arch Clin Exp Ophthalmol 2014;252:571–581.
53 Ripandelli G, Coppé AM, Fedeli R, Pairi V, D'Amico DJ, Stirpe M: Evaluation of primary surgical procedures for retinal detachment with macular hole in highly myopic eyes. Ophthalmology 2001;108: 2258–2265.

Carlos Mateo
Instituto de Microcirugía Ocular (IMO)
C/Josep María Lladó, No. 3
ES–08035 Barcelona (Spain)
E-Mail carlosmateo@me.com

Oh H, Oshima Y (eds): Microincision Vitrectomy Surgery. Emerging Techniques and Technology.
Dev Ophthalmol. Basel, Karger, 2014, vol 54, pp 213–222 (DOI: 10.1159/000360469)

Subretinal Hemorrhage

Glenn Yiu · Tamer H. Mahmoud
Department of Ophthalmology, Duke University Medical Center, Durham, N.C., USA

Abstract
Large submacular hemorrhage (SMH) is a devastating complication of neovascular age-related macular degeneration (AMD) that cannot be effectively managed with anti-vascular endothelial growth factor injections alone. While SMH is not common, AMD patients with existing coagulopathies or taking anticoagulant medications are particularly susceptible. Today, various techniques are available for the management of SMH, including pneumatic displacement with or without intravitreal tissue plasminogen activator (tPA), pars plana vitrectomy with subretinal tPA and gas tamponade, and submacular surgery with vitrectomy and retinotomy for clot extraction. While no consensus exists, the preferred technique is often determined by the extent or duration of the hemorrhage and surgeon preference. This chapter reviews treatment options for managing SMH, as well as the current evidence for supporting their use.

Natural History of Subretinal Hemorrhage

The natural course of submacular hemorrhage (SMH), if left untreated, is severe, progressive, and often irreversible vision loss. A review of 16 eyes with subfoveal hemorrhages that did not meet criteria for laser treatment showed a mean deterioration of 3.5 ETDRS (Early-Treatment Diabetic Retinopathy Study) lines after 36 months [1]. A larger series of 60 eyes with SMH >1 disc area (DA) showed that 80% suffered worsened vision over 24 months, with a mean visual acuity (VA) decline from 20/240 to 20/1,250 [2]. Factors that contributed to this included recurrence of SMH, fibrous tissue proliferation, atrophic scar formation, and retinal pigment epithelium (RPE) tears [2].

Prognostic factors include the thickness and diameter of the hemorrhage [1–3], although no consensus exists for defining these parameters. One classification scheme defines hemorrhages <2 DA as 'small', those ≥2 DA up to the vascular arcades as 'medium', and those extending past the arcades as 'large' (fig. 1) [4]. The prognosis is particularly poor with 'massive' SMH, often defined as thick subretinal blood that extends past the equator in ≥2 quadrants, where visual outcomes even after surgery is no better than count fingers [5].

The prognosis of SMH correlates with duration as well, since subretinal blood damages the retina and RPE in a short amount of time. Early studies in rabbits by Glatt and Machemer [6] demonstrated irreversible retinal injury with photoreceptor edema and pyknosis of the outer

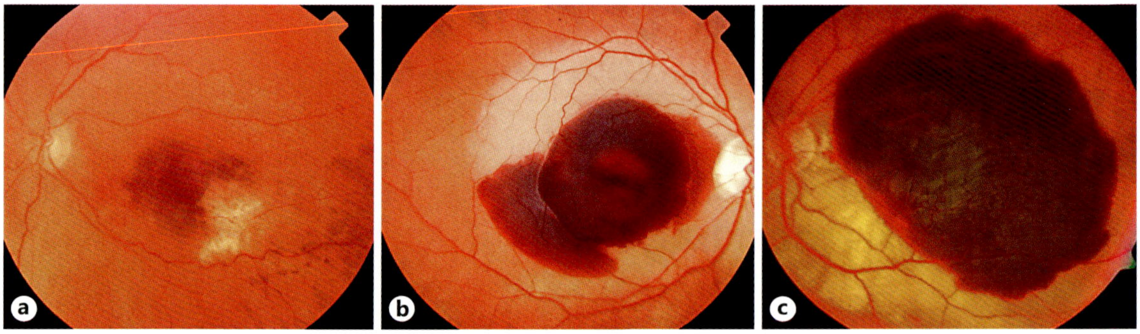

Fig. 1. Size classification of SMH: those that are <2 DA are generally classified as 'small' (**a**), those ≥2 DA up to the vascular arcades are 'medium' (**b**), and those extending past the arcades are considered to be 'large' (**c**). Picture **b** is courtesy of Dr. Brooks W. McCuen II, MD.

nuclear layer within 24 h after subretinal injections of autologous blood. Later studies by Toth et al. [7] supported these findings in cats. At 7 days, there is more severe degeneration with shearing of photoreceptor outer segments and RPE cells showing shortened apical microvilli and mitochondrial distortion. At 14 days, the outer retina and RPE exhibit atrophy and disorganization with vacuolization, accompanied by an influx of phagocytic cells. The mechanism of damage was postulated to be multifactorial, including a barrier effect limiting diffusion of nutrients, retraction of the fibrin clot causing shearing of photoreceptors [6], and toxicity from fibrin [7], iron [8], and hemosiderin [9]. The use of tissue plasminogen activator (tPA) prevented clot organization and retraction of fibrin strands [7], leading to the concept of using tPA to facilitate fibrinolysis in SMH.

Use of Tissue Plasminogen Activator

tPA is a thrombolytic agent that activates plasminogen into plasmin, which catalyzes the lysis of fibrin to liquefy blood clots. Early animal studies in rabbits and cats demonstrated the feasibility of injecting recombinant tPA subretinally to facilitate removal of experimental SMH [10, 11]. Clot removal within 7 days reduced outer retinal degeneration on histology. In contrast, subretinal tPA alone without removal of the hemorrhage improved anatomical clearance, but did not protect against retinal degeneration [12–14]. Similarly, intravitreal tPA injection also enhanced fibrinolysis and clearance in rabbits and pig eyes, although electroretinogram amplitudes did not recover, suggesting that retinal damage could not be prevented [15, 16]. Together, these animal studies suggest that intravitreal or subretinal tPA may be clinically useful for SMH treatment, but only as an adjunct to displacement or extraction. Recombinant tPA was found to be safe when injected subretinally at doses up to 25–50 μg/0.1 ml in rabbits [12], while irreversible toxic effects were documented at 100 μg/0.1 ml in cats [11]. These results provided the parameters for the use of tPA in humans.

The use of tPA for surgical evacuation of subretinal hemorrhages in humans was first reported by Peyman et al. [17] in 1991. The technique involved the use of a micropipette to fashion a small retinotomy through which tPA was injected into the subretinal space and through which the dissolved clot was removed. VA improved in 3 out of 5 patients from count fingers to 20/50–20/400, and remained stable in the other two [17]. Since then, various techniques have been developed using tPA to help remove SMH.

Submacular Surgery

Early reports of surgical extraction of large SMH emerged in the 1990s. Vander et al. [18] reported the outcomes of 11 patients who underwent pars plana vitrectomy (PPV) with retinotomy for mechanical SMH removal. While technically feasible, the results were dismal, with postoperative VA ranging from 20/200 to light perception, and 36% of patients suffering retinal detachment. Ibanez et al. [19] later compared two different surgical approaches retrospectively in 47 patients. In group 1, patients underwent PPV with retinotomy and mechanical clot extraction with a silicone-tip extrusion needle or vitreoretinal forceps. In group 2, tPA was injected through the retinotomy after PPV, then drained using either a Lewis double-lumen subretinal irrigator-aspirator or a 30-gauge subretinal cannula. Although patients with tPA-assisted drainage performed better (92 vs. 57% showing improved VA), the results were not statistically significant. Nevertheless, 21% of all patients combined improved by ≥2 ETDRS lines, which is significantly better than the natural history of the condition.

A few years later, Kamei et al. [20] added perfluorocarbon liquid to assist in expressing SMH. After injecting tPA subretinally using a 27- or 30-gauge cannula and waiting 20 min for fibrinolysis, a 1-mm retinotomy was created with vitreoretinal scissors at the injection site. Perfluorocarbon was then applied until it reached the retinotomy, allowing the SMH to be squeezed out with a rocking motion. In a series of 22 patients, 73% achieved VA ≥20/100. The surgical techniques were further refined by Claes and Zivojnovic [21], who showed that clot lysis required up to 45 min, and that larger retinotomies were required for evacuation of large SMH.

The Submacular Surgery Trials (SST) Group B study was the first major randomized clinical trial to evaluate submacular surgery in a prospective manner. This study evaluated patients with subfoveal choroidal neovascularization (CNV) lesions ≥3.5 DA and composed of >50% blood, with a best-corrected visual acuity (BCVA) of 20/100 to light perception [22]. Of 336 patients enrolled, half were assigned to observation while the remainder underwent surgical removal of blood and any associated CNV. The technique was similar to the larger SST Group N trial evaluating submacular surgery for all subfoveal CNV secondary to AMD [23], and involved standard 3-port PPV with retinotomy and microforceps for CNV and clot removal. Subretinal tPA was given at the surgeon's discretion. At 24 months, there was no significant difference in percentage of eyes with ≥2 ETDRS lines VA loss (56% of surgery vs. 52% of observation eyes). Although surgery more often prevented severe vision loss (≥8 lines VA loss), with 21% in the surgery and 36% in the observation arms, there were also more eyes that developed retinal detachment after surgery (16 vs. 2%). While these results did not support surgical intervention for SMH, the outcomes may have been limited by the trauma of subretinal manipulations and clot extraction, resulting in higher rates of retinal detachment and possibly proliferative vitreoretinopathy. Given the potential complications of submacular surgery, studies were underway to evaluate less invasive techniques to displace SMH without extraction.

Pneumatic Displacement

There were reports of pneumatic displacement combined with intravitreal tPA even prior to the SST studies. In 1996, Heriot [24] proposed intravitreal injection of tPA and an expansile gas as a minimally invasive outpatient procedure for displacing SMH. A retrospective series of 15 AMD patients with large SMH showed encouraging results, with complete displacement from the fovea in all 15 eyes, and BCVA improvement of ≥2 ETDRS lines in 14 eyes (93%) after a mean of 4.6 months [25]. The procedure was performed with topical anesthesia, 25–100 μg tPA in 0.1–0.2 ml injected into the vitreous cavity through the pars plana, followed by a 0.3- to 0.4-ml injection of perfluoropropane (C_3F_8) or sulfur hexafluoride (SF_6) gas and 24-hour prone positioning. However, subsequent case series from Germany [26–30], Austria [31], China [32], Thailand [33], and Australia [34] using similar techniques were less impressive, with results ranging from 38 to 64% demonstrating a ≥2 ETDRS line gain. Larger series from Asia also included idiopathic polypoidal choroidal vasculopathy, retinal macroaneurysms, and pathologic myopia, although the outcomes were similar to those reported for AMD patients [35, 36].

Pneumatic displacement of SMH without concurrent use of tPA has also been described [37–39]. A series of 20 patients undergoing pneumatic displacement with C_3F_8 gas and prone positioning reported a final mean VA ≥20/63 in 10 eyes (50%), which was comparable to combining pneumatic displacement with tPA [40]. The fact that tPA may not be required raised the question of whether intravitreal tPA is even capable of reaching the subretinal space. tPA has a molecular weight of 70 kDa, which prevents its diffusion across intact retina, where the pore size of the external limiting membrane limits passage of molecules to around 50–60 kDa [41]. To study this, Kamei et al. [42] injected fluorescein-labeled tPA into rabbit eyes, and found no signal in the retina or subretinal space except in eyes with concurrent vitreous hemorrhage. The authors postulated that microperforations associated with SMH may increase susceptibility to intravitreal tPA. A study by Hillenkamp et al. [43] further addressed this by comparing the efficacy of PPV with intravitreal versus subretinal tPA retrospectively in 47 patients. Eyes treated with subretinal tPA demonstrated higher rates of complete displacement (55 vs. 22%), but were also associated with more complications, including retinal detachment, vitreous hemorrhage, and SMH recurrence. Nevertheless, vitrectomy surgery not only provides a means to deliver tPA directly to the subretinal space, but also allows for a complete air or gas fill to enhance pneumatic displacement.

Vitrectomy with Gas Tamponade

The combination of vitrectomy and subretinal tPA with a full gas tamponade for displacing thick SMH was described by Haupert et al. [44] in 2001. The technique involved PPV, subretinal tPA (25–50 μg in 0.1 ml), and fluid-air exchange with SF_6 and prone positioning. In all 11 eyes in the series, the SMH was displaced from the fovea, with postoperative BCVA ranging from 20/30 to 5/200 after a mean of 6.5 months, with ≥2 ETDRS lines improvement in 6 eyes (55%). Despite the small sample size and lack of a control group, the technique was implemented by others. Olivier et al. [45] employed a lower concentration of subretinal tPA (12.5 μg in 0.1 ml) in 29 patients, and found similar efficacy with 17 eyes (59%) showing ≥2 lines vision gain. Interestingly, a comparison of PPV with subretinal tPA and gas versus forceps-removal of the SMH favored the latter approach, with ≥3 lines VA gain in 48% in the submacular surgery group and 13% in the PPV/tPA/gas group at 1 year [46]. The authors attributed this difference to continuing VA decline in the tPA group, although the comparison was not a randomized study, and the tPA group did not do as well as in previous reports. Nevertheless, the combination of vitrectomy, subretinal tPA, and gas tamponade continued to grow in popularity, and has shown moderate success even in cases of thick, massive SMH where the prognosis without intervention is poor [5].

One aspect of pneumatic displacement that remains uncertain is whether the primary mechanism involves a 'steam-rolling' mechanism of a partial tamponade, or a gravitational effect within a complete air or gas fill. Stopa et al. [47] analyzed the forces acting upon SMH in pneumatic displacement. According to the Archimedes principle, a body immersed in a fluid experiences a

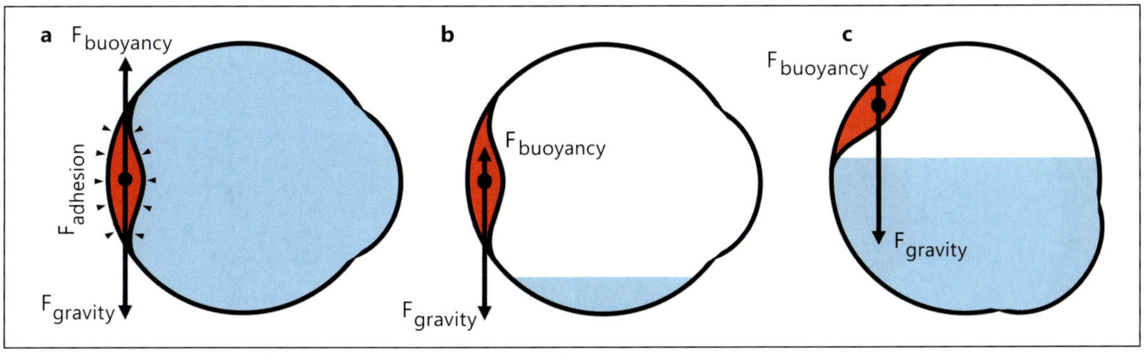

Fig. 2. Forces acting on SMH in pneumatic displacement. **a** Without intervention, adhesive forces keep a submacular hemorrhage attached to the retina and RPE, while the downward gravitational and upward buoyancy forces are relatively balanced. **b** Optimal SMH displacement requires tPA to reduce the adhesive forces, upright positioning to maximize the gravitational force, and gas to minimize the buoyancy force. **c** With a partial gas fill, as in pneumatic displacement without vitrectomy, a 40° downward gaze is preferred. Adapted from Stopa et al. [47] and Lincoff et al. [48].

buoyant force equal to the weight of the fluid it displaces. While the density of blood is similar to that of vitreous, it is roughly 830 times more dense or less buoyant in gas than vitreous fluid. Thus, optimal displacement occurs when the hemorrhage is completely immersed in gas and the patient is positioned upright, not face down, to maximize the gravitational force (fig. 2). In cases where a complete fill is not possible, as in pneumatic displacement without vitrectomy, Lincoff advocates a 40% gas bubble with a 40° gaze-down position [48]. In a series of 17 patients undergoing PPV, subretinal tPA, and partial fluid-air exchange with upright positioning, Singh et al. [49] found 88% of patients had stable or improved VA, with 9 patients showing total clearing and 8 with partial clearing of the SMH.

Subretinal Pneumatic Displacement

Recently, Martel and Mahmoud [50, 51] described a technique of subretinal pneumatic displacement by coinjection of subretinal tPA and bevacizumab with subretinal air. Based on the physical principles that justify intravitreal pneumatic displacement, a subretinal air bubble allows direct displacement of the blood in the subretinal space, without requiring transmission of forces across the retina. The direct exposure of the subretinal blood to air allows further reduction in buoyancy, reduced adhesion to the neurosensory retina and RPE, and possibly even improved oxygenation to the deprived photoreceptors and prevent potential efflux of subretinal tPA and bevacizumab into the vitreous cavity. The technique involves injecting 50 μg tPA in 0.4 ml, 2.5 mg bevacizumab in 0.1 ml, and 0.2–0.5 ml of filtered air into the subretinal space. This is followed by a partial fluid-air exchange and then 20% SF_6 and upright positioning, which keeps the subretinal air bubble in the macula and prevents its migration into the superior periphery (fig. 3, 4). Due to the large volume delivered, the authors advocate injecting near the superonasal edge of the hemorrhage to avoid creating a full thickness macular hole. In their experience, the subretinal air resolved in a few days with no reported complications.

Cotreatment with Anti-VEGF Therapy

Even after successful displacement of SMH and initial VA improvement, vision often deteriorates postoperatively, likely due to progression of the

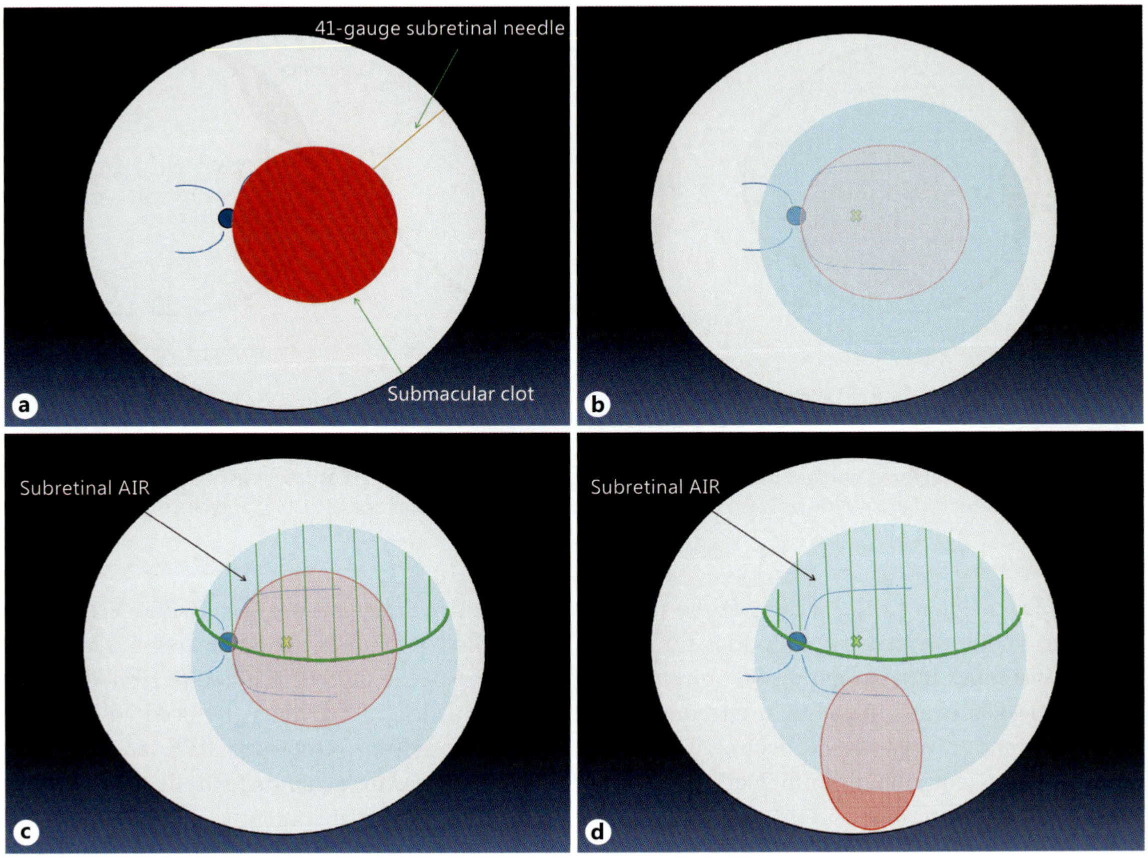

Fig. 3. Technique for subretinal pneumatic displacement. A 41-gauge needle is inserted into a large subretinal hemorrhage (**a**), followed by injection of tPA and an anti-VEGF agent to allow liquefaction of the hemorrhage (pink) and the formation of a subretinal fluid bleb (blue) with expansion of the area of retinal detachment (**b**). Subretinal air (green) is also added to minimize the buoyancy of the liquefied hemorrhage (**c**), facilitating inferior displacement of the blood (**d**). From Martel and Mahmoud [51].

underlying CNV. While evaluating the clinical course of SMH from various etiologies, Berrocal et al. [52] identified the presence of CNV to be associated with poorer visual outcomes. Such findings provide support for combination therapy with anti-VEGF therapy as an adjunct to promote CNV regression and prevent recurrence of SMH.

Currently, intravitreal anti-VEGF therapy is the standard of care for managing neovascular AMD, with evidence from large clinical trials supporting their safety [53, 54]. Meyer et al. [55] described consecutive intravitreal injections of tPA (50 μg/0.05 ml), SF_6 gas (0.3 ml), and bevacizumab (1.25 mg/0.1 ml) in 19 patients with small SMH, and reported successful displacement in 17 eyes, with a mean BCVA gain of 20/133–20/74 after 3 months. Similar positive results were obtained using a lower dose of tPA (12.5 μg/0.05 ml), SF_6 (0.5 ml), and ranibizumab (0.5 μg/0.05 ml) instead of bevacizumab [56]. The inclusion of tPA appeared to be important, as anti-VEGF monotherapy [57] or anti-VEGF with gas [58] did not produce the same level of visual improvement. When compared with in-

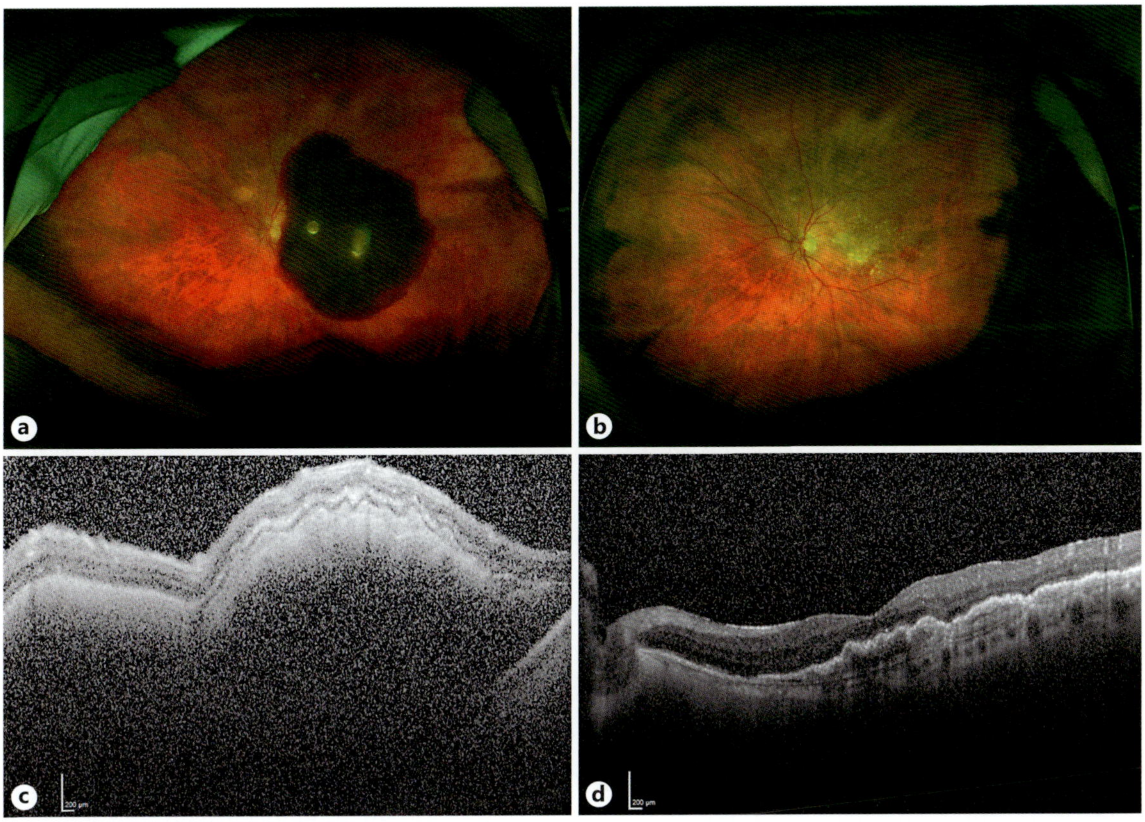

Fig. 4. Surgical subretinal pneumatic displacement of a large SMH. Fundus photos demonstrating a large SMH before (**a**) and 3 months after (**b**) vitrectomy, subretinal tPA, bevacizumab, and subretinal air with partial fluid-air exchange with SF_6. Preoperative (**c**) and postoperative (**d**) optical coherence tomography demonstrates successful SMH displacement. From Martel and Mahmoud [51].

travitreal tPA/gas alone, the combination of anti-VEGF/tPA/gas also produced greater VA outcomes [59]. While these studies suggest that this triple intravitreal therapy may be favored, most of the studies included only small to medium-sized hemorrhages, and intravitreal anti-VEGF was continued on a regular basis after displacement. Previous studies have also shown that eyes with small SMH can spontaneously improve without intervention [1, 52]. Hence, in cases with small or medium hemorrhages, the advantage of intravitreal tPA with pneumatic displacement over anti-VEGF monotherapy remains uncertain.

Like tPA, the ability of anti-VEGF agents such as bevacizumab (149 kDa) and ranibizumab (48 kDa) to penetrate intact retina has also been questioned, especially in the setting of SMH, which may impede their ability to reach the CNV. With large or massive SMH where vitrectomy with subretinal tPA is likely necessary, concurrent subretinal delivery of the anti-VEGF agent may therefore reduce the rate of hemorrhage recurrence. Compatibility studies with subretinal bevacizumab (1.25 mg/0.05 ml) and tPA (20 µg/0.1 ml) have shown efficacy with no evidence of toxicity [60, 61]. Treumer et al. [62] evaluated the long-term outcomes of 41 eyes after vitrectomy with subretinal tPA, bevacizumab, and SF_6 gas, followed by continued intravitreal anti-VEGF using a VA-driven retreatment regimen. The study showed ≥2 ETDRS lines of BCVA improvement in 30 eyes (73%) at 3 months, but BCVA decreased in 12 of 26 eyes after a mean follow-up of 17 months. These studies highlight the potential need for more sensitive retreatment parameters with anti-VEGF to improve long-term visual outcome after surgery for SMH.

Conclusion

Despite the wide range of techniques for managing SMH, there is still no consensus among vitreoretinal specialists on the optimal approach. Most studies have been either uncontrolled retrospective case series with limited patients, or non-randomized comparative retrospective studies with a low level of evidence. A literature review by van Zeeburg and van Meurs [63] identified 38 studies evaluating tPA use in SMH, and noted inconsistent reporting of inclusion criteria and outcome measures which preclude accurate cross comparisons between studies or a statistical meta-analysis to be performed.

Nevertheless, trends from the available evidence provide some guidelines for managing SMH. For small or medium-sized hemorrhages, the risk-benefit profile supports a more conservative approach with either continued anti-VEGF therapy alone, or in combination with pneumatic displacement with intravitreal tPA. For large or massive hemorrhages, submacular surgery has largely been abandoned in favor of less-invasive displacement by vitrectomy with subretinal tPA and anti-VEGF followed by gas tamponade and upright positioning. Subretinal pneumatic displacement further enhances the forces involved to ensure a more complete displacement. Given the rapid onset of retinal damage in the first 7–14 days [7], as well as evidence suggesting greater liquefaction of subretinal hemorrhage within 7 days or less [64], early intervention is paramount to maximize visual recovery. And while anti-VEGF agents in standard doses appear safe, recombinant tPA no greater than 50 μg should be given to minimize potential toxicity.

The specific choice of technique and reagents will depend on the etiology, duration, size, and location of the SMH, as well as surgeon experience and preference. No matter which method is employed, careful monitoring with continued intravitreal anti-VEGF therapy may be important to minimize potential complications like breakthrough vitreous hemorrhage and recurrent SMH. Future prospective, randomized trials and long-term studies are required to better evaluate the safety and efficacy of these various interventions.

References

1 Avery RL, Fekrat S, Hawkins BS, Bressler NM: Natural history of subfoveal subretinal hemorrhage in age-related macular degeneration. Retina 1996; 16:183–189.
2 Scupola A, Coscas G, Soubrane G, Balestrazzi E: Natural history of macular subretinal hemorrhage in age-related macular degeneration. Ophthalmologica 1999;213:97–102.
3 Bennett SR, Folk JC, Blodi CF, Klugman M: Factors prognostic of visual outcome in patients with subretinal hemorrhage. Am J Ophthalmol 1990;109:33–37.
4 Bopp S: Subretinal hemorrhage. Natural course and staging (in German). Ophthalmologe 2012;109:635–643.
5 Fine HF, Iranmanesh R, Del Priore LV, et al: Surgical outcomes after massive subretinal hemorrhage secondary to age-related macular degeneration. Retina 2010;30:1588–1594.
6 Glatt H, Machemer R: Experimental subretinal hemorrhage in rabbits. Am J Ophthalmol 1982;94:762–773.
7 Toth CA, Morse LS, Hjelmeland LM, Landers MB 3rd: Fibrin directs early retinal damage after experimental subretinal hemorrhage. Arch Ophthalmol 1991;109:723–729.

8 Bhisitkul RB, Winn BJ, Lee OT, et al: Neuroprotective effect of intravitreal triamcinolone acetonide against photoreceptor apoptosis in a rabbit model of subretinal hemorrhage. Invest Ophthalmol Vis Sci 2008;49:4071–4077.
9 el Baba F, Jarrett WH 2nd, Harbin TS Jr, et al: Massive hemorrhage complicating age-related macular degeneration. Clinicopathologic correlation and role of anticoagulants. Ophthalmology 1986;93:1581–1592.
10 Johnson MW, Olsen KR, Hernandez E: Tissue plasminogen activator thrombolysis during surgical evacuation of experimental subretinal hemorrhage. Ophthalmology 1992;99:515–521.
11 Benner JD, Hay A, Landers MB 3rd, Hjelmeland LM, Morse LS: Fibrinolytic-assisted removal of experimental subretinal hemorrhage within seven days reduces outer retinal degeneration. Ophthalmology 1994;101:672–681.
12 Lewis H, Resnick SC, Flannery JG, Straatsma BR: Tissue plasminogen activator treatment of experimental subretinal hemorrhage. Am J Ophthalmol 1991;111:197–204.
13 Johnson MW, Olsen KR, Hernandez E: Tissue plasminogen activator treatment of experimental subretinal hemorrhage. Retina 1991;11:250–258.
14 Morse LS, Benner JD, Hjelmeland LM, Landers MB 3rd: Fibrinolysis of experimental subretinal haemorrhage without removal using tissue plasminogen activator. Br J Ophthalmol 1996;80:658–662.
15 Coll GE, Sparrow JR, Marinovic A, Chang S: Effect of intravitreal tissue plasminogen activator on experimental subretinal hemorrhage. Retina 1995;15:319–326.
16 Boone DE, Boldt HC, Ross RD, Folk JC, Kimura AE: The use of intravitreal tissue plasminogen activator in the treatment of experimental subretinal hemorrhage in the pig model. Retina 1996;16:518–524.
17 Peyman GA, Nelson NC Jr, Alturki W, et al: Tissue plasminogen activating factor assisted removal of subretinal hemorrhage. Ophthalmic Surg 1991;22:575–582.
18 Vander JF, Federman JL, Greven C, Slusher MM, Gabel VP: Surgical removal of massive subretinal hemorrhage associated with age-related macular degeneration. Ophthalmology 1991;98:23–27.
19 Ibanez HE, Williams DF, Thomas MA, et al: Surgical management of submacular hemorrhage. A series of 47 consecutive cases. Arch Ophthalmol 1995;113:62–69.
20 Kamei M, Tano Y, Maeno T, Ikuno Y, Mitsuda H, Yuasa T: Surgical removal of submacular hemorrhage using tissue plasminogen activator and perfluorocarbon liquid. Am J Ophthalmol 1996;121:267–275.
21 Claes C, Zivojnovic R: Efficacy of tissue plasminogen activator (t-PA) in subretinal hemorrhage removal. Bull Soc Belge Ophtalmol 1996;261:115–118.
22 Bressler NM, Bressler SB, Childs AL, et al: Surgery for hemorrhagic choroidal neovascular lesions of age-related macular degeneration: ophthalmic findings: SST report no. 13. Ophthalmology 2004;111:1993–2006.
23 Hawkins BS, Bressler NM, Miskala PH, et al: Surgery for subfoveal choroidal neovascularization in age-related macular degeneration: ophthalmic findings: SST report no. 11. Ophthalmology 2004;111:1967–1980.
24 Heriot WJ: Intravitreal gas and tPA: an outpatient procedure for submacular hemorrhage. AAO Annual Vitreoretinal Update, Chicago, 1996.
25 Hassan AS, Johnson MW, Schneiderman TE, et al: Management of submacular hemorrhage with intravitreous tissue plasminogen activator injection and pneumatic displacement. Ophthalmology 1999;106:1900–1906, discussion 6–7.
26 Hesse L, Schmidt J, Kroll P: Management of acute submacular hemorrhage using recombinant tissue plasminogen activator and gas. Graefes Arch Clin Exp Ophthalmol 1999;237:273–277.
27 Meier P, Zeumer C, Jochmann C, Wiedemann P: Management of submacular hemorrhage by tissue plasminogen activator and SF(6) gas injection (in German). Ophthalmologe 1999;96:643–647.
28 Buhl M, Scheider A, Schonfeld CL, Kampik A: Intra-vitreal rt-PA and gas introduction in submacular hemorrhage (in German). Ophthalmologe 1999;96:792–796.
29 Framme C, Toukhy HE, Sachs HG, et al: Clinical results of intravitreal administration of tissue-type plasminogen activator (tPA) and gas for removal of subretinal hemorrhage in senile macular degeneration (in German). Klin Monbl Augenheilkd 2000;216:33–39.
30 Hattenbach LO, Klais C, Koch FH, Gumbel HO: Intravitreous injection of tissue plasminogen activator and gas in the treatment of submacular hemorrhage under various conditions. Ophthalmology 2001;108:1485–1492.
31 Krepler K, Kruger A, Tittl M, Stur M, Wedrich A: Intravitreal injection of tissue plasminogen activator and gas in subretinal hemorrhage caused by age-related macular degeneration. Retina 2000;20:251–256.
32 Tsai SC, Lin JM, Chen HY: Intravitreous recombinant tissue plasminogen activator and gas to treat submacular hemorrhage in age-related macular degeneration. Kaohsiung J Med Sci 2003;19:608–616.
33 Ratanasukon M, Kittantong A: Results of intravitreal tissue plasminogen activator and expansile gas injection for submacular haemorrhage in Thais. Eye (Lond) 2005;19:1328–1332.
34 Chen CY, Hooper C, Chiu D, Chamberlain M, Karia N, Heriot WJ: Management of submacular hemorrhage with intravitreal injection of tissue plasminogen activator and expansile gas. Retina 2007;27:321–328.
35 Kung YH, Wu TT, Hong MC, Sheu SJ: Intravitreal tissue plasminogen activator and pneumatic displacement of submacular hemorrhage. J Ocul Pharmacol Ther 2010;26:469–474.
36 Wu TT, Kung YH, Hong MC: Vitreous hemorrhage complicating intravitreal tissue plasminogen activator and pneumatic displacement of submacular hemorrhage. Retina 2011;31:2071–2077.
37 Ohji M, Saito Y, Hayashi A, Lewis JM, Tano Y: Pneumatic displacement of subretinal hemorrhage without tissue plasminogen activator. Arch Ophthalmol 1998;116:1326–1332.
38 Daneshvar H, Kertes PJ, Leonard BC, Peyman GA: Management of submacular hemorrhage with intravitreal sulfur hexafluoride: a pilot study. Can J Ophthalmol 1999;34:385–388.
39 Shiraga F, Matsuo T, Yokoe S, et al: Surgical treatment of submacular hemorrhage associated with idiopathic polypoidal choroidal vasculopathy. Am J Ophthalmol 1999;128:147–154.
40 Gopalakrishan M, Giridhar A, Bhat S, Saikumar SJ, Elias A, NS: Pneumatic displacement of submacular hemorrhage: safety, efficacy, and patient selection. Retina 2007;27:329–334.

41 Kamei M, Estafanous M, Lewis H: Tissue plasminogen activator in the treatment of vitreoretinal diseases. Semin Ophthalmol 2000;15:44–50.
42 Kamei M, Misono K, Lewis H: A study of the ability of tissue plasminogen activator to diffuse into the subretinal space after intravitreal injection in rabbits. Am J Ophthalmol 1999;128:739–746.
43 Hillenkamp J, Surguch V, Framme C, Gabel VP, Sachs HG: Management of submacular hemorrhage with intravitreal versus subretinal injection of recombinant tissue plasminogen activator. Graefes Arch Clin Exp Ophthalmol 2010;248:5–11.
44 Haupert CL, McCuen BW 2nd, Jaffe GJ, et al: Pars plana vitrectomy, subretinal injection of tissue plasminogen activator, and fluid-gas exchange for displacement of thick submacular hemorrhage in age-related macular degeneration. Am J Ophthalmol 2001;131:208–215.
45 Olivier S, Chow DR, Packo KH, MacCumber MW, Awh CC: Subretinal recombinant tissue plasminogen activator injection and pneumatic displacement of thick submacular hemorrhage in age-related macular degeneration. Ophthalmology 2004;111:1201–1208.
46 Thompson JT, Sjaarda RN: Vitrectomy for the treatment of submacular hemorrhages from macular degeneration: a comparison of submacular hemorrhage/membrane removal and submacular tissue plasminogen activator-assisted pneumatic displacement. Trans Am Ophthalmol Soc 2005;103:98–107, discussion.
47 Stopa M, Lincoff A, Lincoff H: Analysis of forces acting upon submacular hemorrhage in pneumatic displacement. Retina 2007;27:370–374.
48 Lincoff H, Kreissig I, Stopa M, Uram D: A 40 degrees gaze down position for pneumatic displacement of submacular hemorrhage: clinical application and results. Retina 2008;28:56–59.
49 Singh RP, Patel C, Sears JE: Management of subretinal macular haemorrhage by direct administration of tissue plasminogen activator. Br J Ophthalmol 2006;90:429–431.
50 Mahmoud TH: Displacement of subretinal hemorrhage. A proposed new technique! Vail Vitrectomy Meeting, Vail, 2013.
51 Martel JN, Mahmoud TH: Subretinal pneumatic displacement of subretinal hemorrhage. JAMA Ophthalmol 2013;131:1632–1635.
52 Berrocal MH, Lewis ML, Flynn HW Jr: Variations in the clinical course of submacular hemorrhage. Am J Ophthalmol 1996;122:486–493.
53 Heier JS, Brown DM, Chong V, et al: Intravitreal aflibercept (VEGF trap-eye) in wet age-related macular degeneration. Ophthalmology 2012;119:2537–2548.
54 Group CR, Martin DF, Maguire MG, et al: Ranibizumab and bevacizumab for neovascular age-related macular degeneration. N Engl J Med 2011;364:1897–1908.
55 Meyer CH, Scholl HP, Eter N, Helb HM, Holz FG: Combined treatment of acute subretinal haemorrhages with intravitreal recombined tissue plasminogen activator, expansile gas and bevacizumab: a retrospective pilot study. Acta Ophthalmol 2008;86:490–494.
56 Matt G, Sacu S, Stifter E, Prunte C, Schmidt-Erfurth U: Combination of intravitreal rTPA, gas and ranibizumab for extensive subfoveal haemorrhages secondary to neovascular age-related macular degeneration (in German). Klin Monbl Augenheilkd 2010;227:221–225.
57 Sacu S, Stifter E, Vecsei-Marlovits PV, et al: Management of extensive subfoveal haemorrhage secondary to neovascular age-related macular degeneration. Eye (Lond) 2009;23:1404–1410.
58 Mayer WJ, Hakim I, Haritoglou C, et al: Efficacy and safety of recombinant tissue plasminogen activator and gas versus bevacizumab and gas for subretinal haemorrhage. Acta Ophthalmol 2013;91:274–278.
59 Guthoff R, Guthoff T, Meigen T, Goebel W: Intravitreous injection of bevacizumab, tissue plasminogen activator, and gas in the treatment of submacular hemorrhage in age-related macular degeneration. Retina 2011;31:36–40.
60 Klettner A, Puls S, Treumer F, Roider J, Hillenkamp J: Compatibility of recombinant tissue plasminogen activator and bevacizumab co-applied for neovascular age-related macular degeneration with submacular hemorrhage. Arch Ophthalmol 2012;130:875–881.
61 Treumer F, Klatt C, Roider J, Hillenkamp J: Subretinal coapplication of recombinant tissue plasminogen activator and bevacizumab for neovascular age-related macular degeneration with submacular haemorrhage. Br J Ophthalmol 2010;94:48–53.
62 Treumer F, Roider J, Hillenkamp J: Long-term outcome of subretinal coapplication of rtPA and bevacizumab followed by repeated intravitreal anti-VEGF injections for neovascular AMD with submacular haemorrhage. Br J Ophthalmol 2012;96:708–713.
63 van Zeeburg EJ, van Meurs JC: Literature review of recombinant tissue plasminogen activator used for recent-onset submacular hemorrhage displacement in age-related macular degeneration. Ophthalmologica 2013;229:1–14.
64 Lewis H: Intraoperative fibrinolysis of submacular hemorrhage with tissue plasminogen activator and surgical drainage. Am J Ophthalmol 1994;118:559–568.

Tamer H. Mahmoud, MD, PhD, Associate Professor, Program Director, Vitreoretinal Surgery Fellowship
Vitreoretinal Surgery, Department of Ophthalmology, Duke University Medical Center
2351 Erwin Road, Box 3802
Durham, NC 27710 (USA)
E-Mail tamer.mahmoud@duke.edu

Oh H, Oshima Y (eds): Microincision Vitrectomy Surgery. Emerging Techniques and Technology.
Dev Ophthalmol. Basel, Karger, 2014, vol 54, pp 223–233 (DOI: 10.1159/000360470)

Surgical Management of Retinopathy of Prematurity

Michael A. Klufas · Samir N. Patel · R.V. Paul Chan

Department of Ophthalmology, Weill Cornell Medical College/NewYork-Presbyterian Hospital, New York, N.Y., USA

Abstract

The surgical treatment and management of retinopathy of prematurity (ROP) has evolved significantly over the last decade. The introduction of new techniques, instrumentation, and surgical adjuvants has added to the repertoire of options vitreoretinal surgeons have to treat complex surgical ROP cases. This chapter focuses on a review of the clinical outcomes, indications, techniques, and adjuncts for the surgical treatment of ROP.

The management of advanced retinopathy of prematurity (ROP) has undergone significant strides over the last decade. Major paradigm shifts for the surgical management of ROP have included an evidence-based trend towards lens-sparing vitrectomy (LSV) over scleral buckling (SB), newer microincision vitrectomy instrumentation, and surgical adjuncts including autologous plasmin and anti-vascular endothelial growth factor (VEGF) therapy. Although the management of ROP hinges primarily upon peripheral ablative laser for treatment-requiring disease, surgical management continues to play a role in the subset of children who develop retinal detachment (RD) despite laser therapy. In spite of improved anatomic outcomes, functional results remain disappointing in many cases, especially for stage 5 disease. This chapter describes the clinical outcomes, indications, techniques, and adjuncts for the surgical treatment of ROP.

Pathophysiology

ROP follows a biphasic pattern: from birth to 32 weeks there is suppression of VEGF with relative hyperoxia, and after 32 weeks there is a hypoxia-induced rise in VEGF that leads to abnormal vessel growth. The vasoproliferative drive is diminished by ablation of the ischemic peripheral retina. However, the subsequent regressed vasoproliferative cicatricial membranes may induce traction upon the retina that may require incisional surgery. The underlying vitreous traction is thought to be best addressed from a pathophysiologic standpoint with vitrectomy rather than SB.

Surgical Outcomes

In the Early Treatment of Retinopathy of Prematurity (ETROP) study, despite timely and adequate peripheral laser ablation, initial results showed nearly 1 in 10 infants developed structurally unfavorable outcomes [1, 2]. Although treatment of RD was not specifically part of the ETROP study, eyes with RD were treated at the discretion of the investigator physician. At the 6-year follow-up, among the 401 patients in the ETROP study, 15.2% (63 patients, 89 eyes) experienced RD (40% stage 4A, 20% stage 4B, 13% stage 5, 21% not classified) [1]. Overall, macular reattachment was achieved in 36% of eyes (25/70) with success varying by treatment technique: 34% (17/50) after vitrectomy with or without scleral buckle, 67% (6/9) after SB alone, and 18% with observation only (2/11). Six years after the initial vitreoretinal surgery, macular attachment was seen in 31, 60, and 0% of stage 4A, stage 4B, and stage 5 eyes, respectively. Favorable visual acuity classified as ETDRS visual acuity ≥20/200 was seen in 9% of subjects with RD (6/70 eyes: 5 with stage 4A, 1 unclassified). Among ETROP eyes that developed RD, vitrectomy for stage 4A detachments was not as successful as reported in other single-institution case series [3–7]. This may be explained by variable timing to surgery and physician-dependent factors in a multicenter cohort involving many different vitreoretinal surgeons.

Surgical Principles

RD from ROP is complex and surgical management of these unique pediatric cases have evolved over time. One of the overarching principles with ROP surgery to optimize the chance of a successful outcome is to pursue surgery once neovascular activity wanes and plus disease resolves, which often coincides with the child's due date [8]. Performing vitrectomy at the peak of the vasoproliferative process may induce bleeding, promote proliferation, and vasoproliferative membrane contraction. Observation until the optimal time for surgery may not be possible in cases of aggressive posterior ROP, which can progress rapidly to RD and continue to have signs of plus disease despite laser therapy.

Lens-Sparing Vitrectomy versus Scleral Buckling

Recent clinical studies have favored LSV over SB [4, 9–11]. Good anatomic outcomes after SB for ROP are achieved in approximately 70% of the cases and at the cost of an additional procedure to divide the band, induced myopia/anisometropia, and often poor visual outcomes [3]. A single report of 22 patients with stage 4 ROP found that after a single procedure, LSV was more than twice as effective (72 vs. 31.5%) at achieving retinal attachment at 1 month follow-up [12]. However, at the end of 6 months of follow-up, after one or more procedures there was no difference in the retinal attachment rate between LSV and SB as the first procedure.

From a pathophysiology standpoint, SB may have the benefit of supporting the vitreous base and reducing cortical vitreous traction. In ROP-related detachments, there are tractional forces on the retina which can be difficult to neutralize completely in the setting of a firmly attached posterior hyaloid in children. To further determine the role of SB in reducing tractional forces in ROP-related RD repair, Sears and Sonnie [13] investigated the use of SB in combination with LSV as the initial procedure for stage 4 detachments and found no additional benefit of SB either prior to or at the time of LSV.

LSV is an effective and safe technique for RD repair in ROP with a low incidence of complications for experienced pediatric vitreoretinal surgeons. Potential complications of vitrectomy include endophthalmitis, rhegmatogenous RD, glaucoma, and development of cataract [3]. Following LSV for all types of pediatric conditions, cataract may be seen in approximately 15% of children after this intraocular procedure [14].

Surgical Techniques

Early reports of surgical therapy for eyes with advanced ROP were reported by Machemer and colleagues [15–17], Tasman et al. [18], and Trese [19, 20]. Prior to the surgical technique reported by Maguire and Trese in 1992 [21], lensectomy was routinely performed in infants undergoing vitrectomy. This study described a two-port pars plicata vitrectomy with one instrument serving the dual function of infusion and endoillumination. Ten children 2.5 weeks to 3.75 years of age (median age: 4.25 months) were included, and 5 of these patients had ROP-related detachments [21]. Excluding stage 5 eyes, favorable outcomes were reported [21]. A multitude of other series evaluated the safety and efficacy of LSV for ROP surgery with positive results [3, 5, 7, 22–31], although less impressive results have been reported with progressive posterior-type stage 4A ROP [30] and with stage 5 eyes [29]. Other studies have reported on modified techniques including the use of three-port vitrectomy, smaller-gauge instrumentation [23, 32], and other approaches [33].

Viewing Systems

Visualization systems utilized intraoperatively include contact and non-contact systems. In contact systems, special attention is paid to the size of the contact lens [34, 35] so as not to interfere with the more anteriorly placed sclerotomies, given the pediatric ocular anatomy. Non-contact viewing systems such as the binocular indirect ophthalmic microscope (BIOM) have also been utilized in ROP surgery.

Sclerotomies

The distance sclerotomies are placed posterior to the surgical limbus has been investigated and is based upon anatomic properties of the developing eye including growth of the ciliary body and relatively larger crystalline lens in proportion to the vitreous cavity in young children [36, 37]. A useful approximate 'rule of thumb' to place sclerotomies for pars plicata vitrectomy in pediatric patients is to have incisions 0.5–1.5 mm posterior to the surgical limbus in neonates (fig. 1). Careful selection and placement of sclerotomies at specific clock hours is also of paramount importance and needs to be tailored to the intraocular pathology in each case. Likewise, surgeon position (superior vs. temporal) is an important consideration preoperatively.

Gauge Selection

Vitrectomy gauge selection has varied among studies and is important given the cohesive properties of the pediatric vitreous and unique anatomic constraints in ROP-related RD. Newer instrumentation such as 25+-gauge short (Alcon, Fort Worth, Tex., USA) (fig. 2) and endoscopy are being investigated to benefit surgical management of ROP surgery.

Early Surgery for Aggressive Posterior Retinopathy of Prematurity

Early surgery for aggressive posterior ROP (APROP), previously known as 'rush' disease, has also been suggested to be of benefit [38]. A study by Azuma et al. [38] was undertaken given

Table 1. Surgical outcomes in ROP (excluding stage 5)

Study	Eyes, n	Stage	Surgery	Follow-up	Anatomic success[1]	Visual outcome	Complications
Choi et al. [29]	13	stage 4B	LSV	5.6 years	62%	3 NLP, 4 LP, 6 form vision	corneal opacity, glaucoma, esotropia, retinal break
Choi et al. [30]	11	progressive posterior-type stage 4A (73% plus disease at time of vitrectomy)	LSV	4.6 years	27% attached, 73% TRD at final examination	2 eyes with attached retina favorable VA, with detached retina 68% NLP	cataract, corneal opacity, glaucoma
Singh et al. [31]	32	stage 4A (n = 23) and 4B (n = 9)	LSV ± SB	7.1 years	91% stage 4A, 88% stage 4B	mean logMAR 0.92 for stage 4A, mean logMAR 1.63 for stage 4B	not reported
Wu et al. [33]	26	stage 4	modified 23-gauge vitrectomy	13.9 months	77% achieved reattachment after single operation, 88% after multiple procedures	not reported	disc dragging (19%), cataracts (15%), glaucoma (8%), persistent vitreous hemorrhage (4%), posterior synechia (4%)
Shah et al. [66]	19	stage 4A (n = 10), stage 4B (n = 9)	LSV, vitrectomy with lensectomy ± SB	19.1 months	90% for stage 4A, 44.4% for stage 4B (defined as partial residual RD)	5 eyes had VA of 6/24 (2: stage 4A, 1: stage 4B), 1 eye 3/50 (stage 4A), 5 eyes HM (3: stage 4A, 2: stage 4B)	posterior retinotomy (66.7% in stage 4B, 21.1% overall), dialysis (9.1%), giant retinal tear (3%)
El Rayes et al. [71]	56	stage 4B	LSV (42.9%) or c ombined vitrectomy and lensectomy (57.1%)	3 years	73.2% overall (75% LSV)	ambulatory vision (VA better than 20/1900) achieved in 97.4%, near reading vision (VA better than 20/800) achieved in 42.8%	iatrogenic breaks (4.5%), cataract (3.4%), glaucoma (32.1%)
Kychenthal and Dorta [23]	13	stage 4A	25-gauge LSV	17 months	92%	not reported	postoperative hypotony with small choroidal detachment that resolved spontaneously
Sears and Sonnie [13]	21	stage 4	LSV alone (n = 9) vs. LSV + SB (n = 12)	range: 6 months to 5 years	86% overall – SB added little to success or failure of LSV	78% of stage 4A fix and follow, 57% of stage 4B fix and follow	macular hole progressing to inoperable RD (n = 1)

Table 1. Continued

Study	Eyes, n	Stage	Surgery	Follow-up	Anatomic success[1]	Visual outcome	Complications
Gonzalez et al. [26]	13	stage 4A (n = 11), stage 4B (n = 2)	25-gauge vitrectomy ± lensectomy	4.6 months	73% retinal reattachment after one or more surgery at last follow-up	not reported	vitreous hemorrhage (2 eyes), cataract (1 eye)
Lakhanpal et al. [72]	108	stage 4A (n = 32), stage 4B (n = 76)	LSV	32 months	85.2% of eyes were reattached after single LSV, overall 94.4% eyes ultimately achieved at least partial posterior pole reattachment, 100% stage 4A, 92.1% stage 4B (partial or complete retinal reattachment)	not reported	5.6% stage 4B eyes remained detached despite additional procedures – 66.7% of these eyes had intraoperative retinal breaks
Hartnett et al. [12]	27	stage 4	LSV (n = 11) vs. SB (n = 16) (first procedure)	last follow-up 6 months	when LSV first procedure 72%, when SB first procedure 31%, at last follow-up with additional procedures there was no difference between LSV first eyes (82%) vs. SB first eyes (69%)	not reported	7 eyes inoperable RDs, 1 eye vitreous hemorrhage
Hubbard et al. [5]	37	stage 4A (n = 25), stage 4B (n = 12)	LSV	13 months	86%: stage 4A 84%, stage 4B 92%	78% able to fix and follow	3 eyes glaucoma, 2 eyes retinal breaks
Capone et al. [3]	40	stage 4A	LSV	12 months	90%	90% fixation behavior	2 eyes with glaucoma with edematous corneas and tearing
Trese [11]	60	stage 4A (n = 27), stage 4B (n = 43)	SB	range: 6-40 months	70% stage 4A, 67% stage 4B complete retinal attachment or dry folds	not reported	none reported
Noorily et al. [73]	15	stage 4B	SB	10 months	66.67% achieved macular reattachment with single SB procedure	3 eyes fix and follow, 11 eyes LP, 1 eyes NLO	1 eye unable to be reattached despite SB and vitreous procedure, 1 eye complicated by lens opacification with pupillary block requiring cataract extraction

LP = Light perception; NLP = no light perception; TRD = tractional retinal detachment; VA = visual acuity. [1] Complete retinal attachment unless otherwise noted.

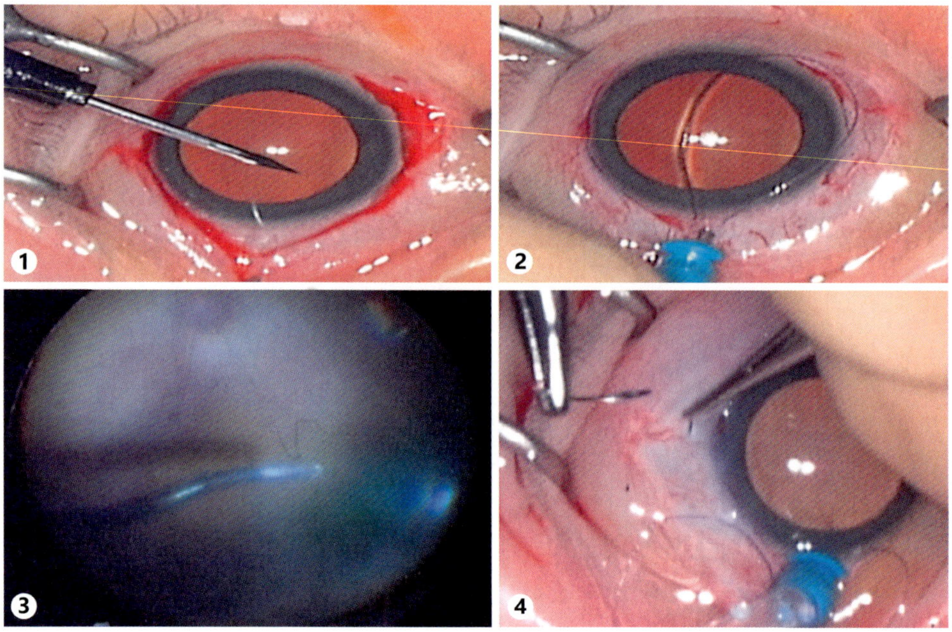

Fig. 1. Conjunctival peritomy performed and 23-gauge microvitreoretinal blade used to make sclerotomies approximately 1 mm posterior to the limbus for this 3-port approach.
Fig. 2. After preplacement of scleral suture, 25+-gauge (Alcon, Fort Worth, Tex., USA) sutured infusion (3.2 mm) secured in place.
Fig. 3. Fluorecein dye from prior fluorescein angiography stains vitreous here. 25+-gauge short vitrectomy cutter used. This length of the 25+-gauge cutter is 18 mm, allowing good access in these smaller neonatal eyes.
Fig. 4. All sclerotomies are closed with sutures at the end of the surgery.

that retinal photocoagulation, which is effective for less severe forms of ROP, often fails to prevent progressive detachment in APROP. In this series, 22 eyes (15 patients) with APROP underwent vitrectomy with or without lens sparing when retinal photocoagulation failed to prevent continued fibrovascular proliferation. The fovea was well formed in 56% as detected by clinical exam, and a favorable visual outcome (central, steady fixation) was achieved in all but two eyes. A follow-up study from this group on longer-term visual outcomes, found visual acuity ranged from 20/250 to 20/40 in 68.9% of the eyes with successful retinal reattachment [39]. The authors suggest surgical removal of the vitreous scaffold not only reduces tractional forces from fibrovascular tissues, but may also suppress growth of new vessels by removing inflammatory mediators; however it may also decrease abnormal blood vessel growth as traction itself can promote neovascularization. In these neonates at high risk of complications, protocols have been reported to optimize perioperative management by anesthesia [40].

Surgical Adjuncts

Early studies by Blacharski and Charles [41] investigated surgical adjuncts such as thrombin infusion to control hemorrhage during vitrectomy for stage 5 detachments. The use of perfluorocar-

Table 2. Selected surgical outcomes in stage 5 ROP

Study	Eyes, n	Stage	Surgery	Follow-up, months	Anatomic success (%)	Visual outcome	Complications
Shah et al. [66]	14	stage V: narrow-narrow (43%), open-narrow (50%), open-open (7%)	LSV, vitrectomy with lensectomy ± SB	32.1	14.3% (reattachment of posterior pole only)	not reported	complete retinal reattachment after stage 5 was seen in only 1 eye which later redetached after 2 years
Wu et al. [50]	80	stage V	autologous or maternal plasmin enzyme-assisted vitreoretinal surgery	49	68.8% (complete zone 1 reattachment of retina)	7.5% (6 eyes) achieved 20/60 to 20/600 vision, 73.8% (59 eyes) worse than 20/600 to LP vision, 13.8% (11 eyes) NLP vision, 5% (4 eyes) uncertain results	reproliferation of fibrovascular tissues (10–53.3%), glaucoma (7.5%), corneal decompensation (5%), phthisis bulbi (5%), vitreous hemorrhage (5%), band keratopathy (3.8%), papillary membrane (3.5%), cataract (2.5%), conjunctival cyst (1.3%)
Tsukahara et al. [49]	6	stage V: closed-closed (4 eyes), open-open (2 eyes)	vitrectomy with lensectomy and autologous plasmin	range: 11–14	100% reattachment of posterior pole	not reported	none reported
Lakhanpal et al. [74]	33	stage V: open-open (21 eyes), open-narrow (12 eyes)	LSV	48	45.5%, open-open configuration had a statistically significantly higher anatomic success rate than eyes with open-narrow configuration	not reported	intraoperative retinal tears, vitreous haze, ocular hypertension
Lakhanpal et al. [63]	21	stage V	vitrectomy with lensectomy with (11 eyes) or without (10 eyes) intravitreal triamcinolone acetonide	28 (range: 6–42)	28.6%	all 6 eyes that maintained posterior pole attachment were able to fix and follow light	vitreous hemorrhage, phthisis
Gonzales et al. [26]	2	stage V	vitrectomy with lensectomy	4.6	0%	not reported	vitreous hemorrhage, cataract
Gopal et al. [75]	96	stage V	vitrectomy with lensectomy (lens spared in 1 case)	15.8	22.5% (reattachment of posterior pole)	only 2 infants obtained mobile vision	reproliferation and secondary glaucoma
Choi and Yu [76]	38	stage V	vitrectomy with lensectomy (encircling band in 1 case)	24.1	29% (anatomic reattachment of posterior pole) – better success with open funnel type vs. closed funnel type (44.4% vs. 15%)	30% fix and follow vision	18.4% vitreous hemorrhage, 10.5% underwent additional vitrectomy due to persistent TRD
Trese [20]	45	stage V	vitrectomy with lensectomy ± SB	6	45% (anatomic reattachment of posterior pole)	30% functional success	not available

LP = Light perception; NLP = no light perception; TRD = tractional retinal detachment.

bon intraopertiavely [42, 43] or silicone oil tamponade [44] have been described in surgical reports in the past. More recent advances have focused on the use of enzymatic vitreolysis, perioperative anti-VEGF, and use of other adjuncts such as intravitreal steroids and dyes.

Vitreolysis

The idea of enzymatic vitreolysis to assist with vitrectomy has been considered for a number of years. However, complications including high rates of dissolution of lenticular zonules with frequent dislocation of crystalline lenses have been presented [45]. More recently, the use of autologous plasmin and ocriplasmin (Jetrea®; ThromboGenics NV, Leuven, Belgium) has been described [46]. Studies have shown the posterior hyaloid and vitreous cortex are more firmly adherent to the internal limiting membrane in children [47], making induction of a mechanical posterior vitreous detachment difficult in this population. Compounds used to disrupt the vitreous have been broadly grouped into 'liquefactants' (which liquefy the vitreous), and 'interfactants' (which disrupt the vitreoretinal interface).

Plasmin enzyme has both liquefactant and interfactant effects [48], and is used in both autologous [49] and heterologous [50] forms as a surgical adjunct. Of note, in the series utilizing autologous plasmin, anatomic reattachment was achieved in all six eyes treated. This is in comparison to a previous series from the same surgeon where anatomic reattachment was only achieved in 47% of stage 5 eyes [51]. Collected inactive human plasminogen requires activation in vitro with streptokinase to form enzymatically active plasmin, which has a limited shelf life. To overcome these onerous preparation barriers, a recombinant compound, ocriplasmin, has been evaluated in multiple trials in adults [52–54]. A phase II, single-center, randomized, placebo-controlled study (ClinicalTrials.gov NCT00986362) investigating the safety and efficacy of a single 175-μg dose of ocriplasmin in children (age <16 years) undergoing vitrectomy has been completed, but the results and outcomes have yet to be published in the literature.

Anti-Vascular Endothelial Growth Factor

There is a significant interest in anti-VEGF therapy as a primary treatment for ROP, including one prospective trial [55]. Intravitreal administration of anti-VEGF compounds prior to surgical intervention for ROP have also been reported [8, 56–60]. Use of anti-VEGF agents, most commonly bevacizumab, may facilitate surgery on a vascularly active eye. Adverse effects of anti-VEGF therapy include 'ROP crunch' via a paradoxical reaction whereby rapid contraction of fibrovascular membranes worsen tractional elements and forces [61, 62]. The use of these medications may be most effective in select cases with careful patient selection. Safety, proper dosing, and optimal administration time prior to surgery remain to be defined.

Steroids

Perioperative use of intravitreal steroids to promote vascular regression and improve surgical outcomes in advanced ROP, particularly in stage 5 eyes, has been investigated [63, 64]. One series reported use of 2.0 mg/0.5 ml of intravitreal triancinolone at the end of surgery on 10 vascularly active eyes with stage 5 ROP and found the anatomic success rate to be 60% [49], which is superior to success rates of 28% or lower in other large series of stage 5 eyes [24, 65–67] or equivalent to results in other series [68]. A case series for stage 4 ROP cases treated with 0.03 ml of preservative-free triancinolone after core vitrectomy reported anatomic success in all 4 patients [64].

Dyes

To better visualize the vitreous around fibrovascular tissue in surgical cases, investigators have compared the use of staining the vitreous with fluorescein versus triamcinolone [69]. The study included 45 eyes with stage 4A aggressive posterior ROP, and found that fluorescein dye produced homogenous and full-thickness staining of the vitreous including around fibrovascular tissues and the vitreous base while still allowing the vitreous to remain transparent. In contrast, triamcinolone only stained the cut surface of the vitreous. In the fluorescein group, the rate of complete retinal reattachment was 85% compared to 67% in the triamcinolone group. There were no systemic abnormalities intraoperatively or postoperatively and no allergic reactions reported. The authors have noted that fluorescein may leak from fibrous tissues and subsequently into the vitreous in active ROP when a fluorescein angiogram is performed, and that this diagnostic imaging modality has been used safely in evaluation of ROP [70] (Fig. 3). Improved staining of the vitreous may improve surgical outcomes by allowing a more complete vitrectomy and also reduce the chance of iatrogenic intraoperative breaks.

Conclusion

Although seminal studies such as ETROP have resulted in improved detection, earlier intervention and reduced unfavorable anatomic outcomes in treatment-requiring ROP, some children continue to experience RD and require surgical intervention despite appropriate treatment. Surgical techniques have evolved over the past decade with a trend to multiple studies supporting the use of LSV as the preferred surgical technique. Newer instrumentation, three-port vitrectomy, and surgical adjuncts such as autologous plasmin, ocriplasmin, steroids, anti-VEGF, and dyes continue to add to the pediatric vitreoretinal surgeon's armamentarium of tools to improve outcomes in these complex surgical ROP cases.

References

1 Repka MX, Tung B, Good WV, et al: Outcome of eyes developing retinal detachment during the Early Treatment for Retinopathy of Prematurity Study. Arch Ophthalmol 2011;129:1175–1179.
2 Repka MX, Tung B, Good WV, et al: Outcome of eyes developing retinal detachment during the Early Treatment for Retinopathy of Prematurity Study (ETROP). Arch Ophthalmol 2006;124: 24–30.
3 Capone A Jr, Trese MT: Lens-sparing vitreous surgery for tractional stage 4A retinopathy of prematurity retinal detachments. Ophthalmology 2001;108: 2068–2070.
4 Hinz BJ, de Juan E Jr, Repka MX: Scleral buckling surgery for active stage 4A retinopathy of prematurity. Ophthalmology 1998;105:1827–1830.
5 Hubbard GB 3rd, Cherwick DH, Burian G: Lens-sparing vitrectomy for stage 4 retinopathy of prematurity. Ophthalmology 2004;111:2274–2277.
6 Prenner JL, Capone A Jr, Trese MT: Visual outcomes after lens-sparing vitrectomy for stage 4A retinopathy of prematurity. Ophthalmology 2004;111: 2271–2273.
7 Moshfeghi AA, Banach MJ, Salam GA, Ferrone PJ: Lens-sparing vitrectomy for progressive tractional retinal detachments associated with stage 4A retinopathy of prematurity. Arch Ophthalmol 2004;122:1816–1818.
8 Hubbard GB 3rd: Surgical management of retinopathy of prematurity. Curr Opin Ophthalmol 2008;19:384–390.
9 Chuang YC, Yang CM: Scleral buckling for stage 4 retinopathy of prematurity. Ophthalmic Surg Lasers 2000;31:374–379.
10 Ricci B, Santo A, Ricci F, et al: Scleral buckling surgery in stage 4 retinopathy of prematurity. Graefes Arch Clin Exp Ophthalmol 1996;234(suppl 1):S38–S41.
11 Trese MT: Scleral buckling for retinopathy of prematurity. Ophthalmology 1994;101:23–26.
12 Hartnett ME, Maguluri S, Thompson HW, McColm JR: Comparison of retinal outcomes after scleral buckle or lens-sparing vitrectomy for stage 4 retinopathy of prematurity. Retina 2004;24:753–757.
13 Sears JE, Sonnie C: Anatomic success of lens-sparing vitrectomy with and without scleral buckle for stage 4 retinopathy of prematurity. Am J Ophthalmol 2007; 143:810–813.
14 Ferrone PJ, Harrison C, Trese MT: Lens clarity after lens-sparing vitrectomy in a pediatric population. Ophthalmology 1997;104:273–278.

15 Treister G, Machemer R: Results of vitrectomy for rare proliferative and hemorrhagic diseases. Am J Ophthalmol 1977;84:394–412.
16 Machemer R, deJuan E: Retinopathy of prematurity: approaches to surgical therapy. Aust NZ J Ophthalmol 1990;18:47–56.
17 Chong LP, Machemer R, de Juan E: Vitrectomy for advanced stages of retinopathy of prematurity. Am J Ophthalmol 1986;102:710–716.
18 Tasman W, Borrone RN, Bolling J: Open sky vitrectomy for total retinal detachment in retinopathy of prematurity. Ophthalmology 1987;94:449–452.
19 Trese MT: Two-hand dissection technique during closed vitrectomy for retinopathy of prematurity. Am J Ophthalmol 1986;101:251–252.
20 Trese MT: Surgical results of stage V retrolental fibroplasia and timing of surgical repair. Ophthalmology 1984;91:461–466.
21 CATT Research Group, Martin DF, Maguire MG, Ying GS, et al: Ranibizumab and bevacizumab for neovascular age-related macular degeneration. N Engl J Med 2011;364:1897–1908.
22 Chan-Kai BT, Lauer AK: Transconjunctival, sutureless 25-gauge lens sparing vitrectomy for stage 4 retinopathy of prematurity-related retinal detachments. Retina 2009;29:854–859.
23 Kychenthal A, Dorta P: 25-gauge lens-sparing vitrectomy for stage 4A retinopathy of prematurity. Retina 2008;28(3 suppl):S65–S68.
24 Yu YS, Kim SJ, Kim SY, et al: Lens-sparing vitrectomy for stage 4 and stage 5 retinopathy of prematurity. Korean J Ophthalmol 2006;20:113–117.
25 Lakhanpal RR, Davis GH, Sun RL, et al: Lens clarity after 3-port lens-sparing vitrectomy in stage 4A and 4B retinal detachments secondary to retinopathy of prematurity. Arch Ophthalmol 2006;124:20–23.
26 Gonzales CR, Boshra J, Schwartz SD: 25-gauge pars plicata vitrectomy for stage 4 and 5 retinopathy of prematurity. Retina 2006;26(7 suppl):S42–S46.
27 Luna JD, Caribaux LJ, Reviglio VE, Juarez CP: Lens-sparing surgery for retinopathy of prematurity. Ophthalmology 2003;110:1669.
28 Shah PK, Narendran V, Kalpana N: Lens-sparing pars plicata vitrectomy for stage 4 retinopathy of prematurity. Indian J Ophthalmol 2010;58:255.
29 Choi J, Kim JH, Kim SJ, Yu YS: Long-term results of lens-sparing vitrectomy for stages 4B and 5 retinopathy of prematurity. Korean J Ophthalmol 2011;25:305–310.
30 Choi J, Kim JH, Kim SJ, Yu YS: Long-term results of lens-sparing vitrectomy for progressive posterior-type stage 4A retinopathy of prematurity. Korean J Ophthalmol 2012;26:277–284.
31 Singh R, Reddy DM, Barkmeier AJ, et al: Long-term visual outcomes following lens-sparing vitrectomy for retinopathy of prematurity. Br J Ophthalmol 2012;96:1395–1398.
32 Gonzales CR, Singh S, Schwartz SD: 25-gauge vitrectomy for paediatric vitreoretinal conditions. Br J Ophthalmol 2009;93:787–790.
33 Wu WC, Lai CC, Lin RI, et al: Modified 23-gauge vitrectomy system for stage 4 retinopathy of prematurity. Arch Ophthalmol 2011;129:1326–1331.
34 Peyman GA, Canakis C, Livir-Rallatos C, Whalen P: Small-size pediatric vitrectomy wide-angle contact lens. Am J Ophthalmol 2003;135:236–237.
35 Chalam KV, Shah VA: Small contact surface minified wide-angle contact lens for pediatric vitreous surgery. J Pediatr Ophthalmol Strabismus 2004;41:109–111.
36 Lemley CA, Han DP: An age-based method for planning sclerotomy placement during pediatric vitrectomy: a 12-year experience. Retina 2007;27:974–977.
37 Lemley CA, Han DP: An age-based method for planning sclerotomy placement during pediatric vitrectomy: a 12-year experience. Trans Am Ophthalmol Soc 2007;105:86–89, discussion 89–91.
38 Azuma N, Ishikawa K, Hama Y, et al: Early vitreous surgery for aggressive posterior retinopathy of prematurity. Am J Ophthalmol 2006;142:636–643.
39 Azuma N, Ito M, Yokoi T, et al: Visual outcomes after early vitreous surgery for aggressive posterior retinopathy of prematurity. JAMA Ophthalmol 2013;131:1309–1313.
40 Aoyama K, Kondou Y, Suzuki Y, et al: Anesthesia protocols for early vitrectomy in former preterm infants diagnosed with aggressive posterior retinopathy of prematurity. J Anesth 2010;24:633–638.
41 Blacharski PA, Charles ST: Thrombin infusion to control bleeding during vitrectomy for stage V retinopathy of prematurity. Arch Ophthalmol 1987;105:203–205.
42 Millsap CM, Peyman GA, Ma PE, Greve MD: The surgical management of retinopathy of prematurity using a perfluorocarbon liquid. Int Ophthalmol 1994;18:97–100.
43 Devenyi RG: The use of perfluorocarbon liquid in the surgical repair of stage 5 retinopathy of prematurity. Can J Ophthalmol 1993;28:294–295.
44 Scott IU, Flynn HW Jr, Azen SP, et al: Silicone oil in the repair of pediatric complex retinal detachments: a prospective, observational, multicenter study. Ophthalmology 1999;106:1399–1407, discussion 1407–1408.
45 Moorhead LC, Radtke N: Enzyme-assisted vitrectomy with bacterial collagenase. Pilot human studies. Retina 1985;5:98–100.
46 Wong SC, Capone A Jr: Microplasmin (ocriplasmin) in pediatric vitreoretinal surgery: update and review. Retina 2013;33:339–348.
47 Sebag J: Age-related differences in the human vitreoretinal interface. Arch Ophthalmol 1991;109:966–971.
48 Gandorfer A: Objective of pharmacologic vitreolysis. Dev Ophthalmol 2009;44:1–6.
49 Tsukahara Y, Honda S, Imai H, et al: Autologous plasmin-assisted vitrectomy for stage 5 retinopathy of prematurity: a preliminary trial. Am J Ophthalmol 2007;144:139–141.
50 Wu WC, Drenser KA, Lai M, et al: Plasmin enzyme-assisted vitrectomy for primary and reoperated eyes with stage 5 retinopathy of prematurity. Retina 2008;28(3 suppl):S75–S80.
51 Fujisawa K, Tsukahara Y, Yamamoto M: Vitrectomy for retinopathy of prematurity. Jpn Rev Clinc Ophthalmol 1999;92:174–176.
52 Stalmans P, Benz MS, Gandorfer A, et al: Enzymatic vitreolysis with ocriplasmin for vitreomacular traction and macular holes. N Engl J Med 2012;367:606–615.
53 de Smet MD, Gandorfer A, Stalmans P, et al: Microplasmin intravitreal administration in patients with vitreomacular traction scheduled for vitrectomy: the MIVI I trial. Ophthalmology 2009;116:1349–1355.e1–e2.
54 Benz MS, Packo KH, Gonzalez V, et al: A placebo-controlled trial of microplasmin intravitreous injection to facilitate posterior vitreous detachment before vitrectomy. Ophthalmology 2010;117:791–797.

55 Mintz-Hittner HA, Kennedy KA, Chuang AZ: Efficacy of intravitreal bevacizumab for stage 3+ retinopathy of prematurity. N Engl J Med 2011;364:603–615.
56 Xu Y, Zhang Q, Kang X, et al: Early vitreoretinal surgery on vascularly active stage 4 retinopathy of prematurity through the preoperative intravitreal bevacizumab injection. Acta Ophthalmol 2013;91:e304–e310.
57 Kychenthal A, Dorta P: Vitrectomy after intravitreal bevacizumab (Avastin) for retinal detachment in retinopathy of prematurity. Retina 2010;30(4 suppl):S32–S36.
58 Sun HJ, Choi KS, Lee SJ: Adjunctive effect of intravitreal bevacizumab prior to lens-sparing vitrectomy in aggressive posterior retinopathy of prematurity: a case report. Jpn J Ophthalmol 2012;56:476–480.
59 Choovuthayakorn J, Ubonrat K: Intravitreal bevacizumab injection in advanced retinopathy of prematurity. J Med Assoc Thai 2012;95(suppl 4):S70–S75.
60 Law JC, Recchia FM, Morrison DG, et al: Intravitreal bevacizumab as adjunctive treatment for retinopathy of prematurity. J AAPOS 2010;14:6–10.
61 Zepeda-Romero LC, Liera-Garcia JA, Gutierrez-Padilla JA, et al: Paradoxical vascular-fibrotic reaction after intravitreal bevacizumab for retinopathy of prematurity. Eye (Lond) 2010;24:931–933.
62 Honda S, Hirabayashi H, Tsukahara Y, Negi A: Acute contraction of the proliferative membrane after an intravitreal injection of bevacizumab for advanced retinopathy of prematurity. Graefes Arch Clin Exp Ophthalmol 2008;246:1061–1063.
63 Lakhanpal RR, Fortun JA, Chan-Kai B, Holz ER: Lensectomy and vitrectomy with and without intravitreal triamcinolone acetonide for vascularly active stage 5 retinal detachments in retinopathy of prematurity. Retina 2006;26:736–740.
64 Shah PK, Narendran V, Kalpana N: Triamcinolone acetonide-assisted vitrectomy for stage 4 retinopathy of prematurity. Int Ophthalmol 2011;31:237–238.
65 Cusick M, Charles MK, Agron E, et al: Anatomical and visual results of vitreoretinal surgery for stage 5 retinopathy of prematurity. Retina 2006;26:729–735.
66 Shah PK, Narendran V, Kalpana N, Tawansy KA: Anatomical and visual outcome of stages 4 and 5 retinopathy of prematurity. Eye (Lond) 2009;23:176–180.
67 Capone A Jr, Trese MT: Stage 5 retinopathy of prematurity: then and now. Retina 2006;26:721–723.
68 Fuchino Y, Hayashi H, Kono T, Ohshima K: Long-term follow up of visual acuity in eyes with stage 5 retinopathy of prematurity after closed vitrectomy. Am J Ophthalmol 1995;120:308–316.
69 Kobayashi Y, Yokoi T, Yokoi T, et al: Fluorescein staining of the vitreous during vitrectomy for retinopathy of prematurity. Retina 2011;31:1717–1719.
70 Nishina S, Yokoi T, Yokoi T, et al: Effect of early vitreous surgery for aggressive posterior retinopathy of prematurity detected by fundus fluorescein angiography. Ophthalmology 2009;116:2442–2447.
71 El Rayes EN, Vinekar A, Capone A Jr: Three-year anatomic and visual outcomes after vitrectomy for stage 4B retinopathy of prematurity. Retina 2008;28:568–572.
72 Lakhanpal RR, Sun RL, Albini TA, et al: Visual outcomes after 3-port lens-sparing vitrectomy in stage 4 retinopathy of prematurity. Arch Ophthalmol 2006;124:675–679.
73 Noorily SW, Small K, de Juan E Jr, et al: Scleral buckling surgery for stage 4B retinopathy of prematurity. Ophthalmology 1992;99:263–268.
74 Lakhanpal RR, Sun RL, Albini TA, et al: Anatomical success rate after primary three-port lens-sparing vitrectomy in stage 5 retinopathy of prematurity. Retina 2006;26:724–728.
75 Gopal L, Sharma T, Shanmugam M, et al: Surgery for stage 5 retinopathy of prematurity: the learning curve and evolving technique. Indian J Ophthalmol 2000;48:101–106.
76 Choi WC, Yu YS: Surgical management for stage 5 retinopathy of prematurity. Korean J Ophthalmol 1994;8:37–41.

Paul Chan, MD, FACS
Weill Cornell Medical College
NewYork-Presbyterian Hospital
1305 York Ave, 11th Floor
New York, NY 10021 (USA)
E-Mail roc9013@med.cornell.edu

Oh H, Oshima Y (eds): Microincision Vitrectomy Surgery. Emerging Techniques and Technology.
Dev Ophthalmol. Basel, Karger, 2014, vol 54, pp 234–242 (DOI: 10.1159/000360471)

Dropped Lens Fragment, Dislocated Intraocular Lens

Manish Nagpal · Pravin Jain

Retina Foundation, Ahmedabad, India

Abstract

Management of posteriorly dislocated crystalline lens has traditionally been performed with a standard 20-gauge vitrectomy system. The latest surgical platforms integrate multiple devices into single systems and feature advanced fluidics, vitreous cutting technology, and intraocular pressure control along with continued improvements in small-gauge instrumentation and wide-angle viewing systems. This allows truly robust removal of core vitreous and outstanding control of the surgical field on par with its 20-gauge predecessor, resulting in an expanded spectrum of complex vitreoretinal maneuvers feasible with 23- or 25-gauge systems. Posteriorly dislocated crystalline lens/intraocular lens is one such indication which can be safely and effectively managed by a 23- or 25-gauge vitrectomy system alone or combined with the 20-gauge fragmatome/forceps with lesser complications and early recovery.

Nucleus drop/retained lens material (RLM) in the vitreous cavity is a potentially serious complication of modern cataract surgery, estimated to occur in 0.3–1.1% of cases [1]. The potential risk factors for RLM include hypermature, dense brunescent, or posterior polar cataracts; zonular compromise; pseudoexfoliation; previous vitrectomy; floppy iris syndrome; miotic pupil, and an inexperienced (trainee) surgeon [2]. Eyes with nucleus drop/RLM or vitreous loss can develop elevated intraocular pressure (IOP), uveitis, corneal edema, vitreous hemorrhage, retinal detachment (RD), and cystoid macular edema (CME), which usually leads to poor visual acuity [3]. When managed properly, however, the risk of further complications can be minimized, and the results can be as good as if it had never happened.

The many publications investigating risk factors associated with posterior capsule rupture and vitreous loss have allowed surgeons to more accurately predict complications prior to surgery, plan more effectively, and counsel patients who are at risk [2]. Early recognition of posterior capsular rupture or zonular dehiscence is key to preventing further problems as surgery progresses; it allows the surgeon to try to avoid certain maneuvers that can upset a precariously perched nucleus. In most cases the nucleus will sit supported by the vitreous if undisturbed; however, vitreous with more syneresis will allow easier passage of the nucleus into the posterior segment. High aspiration and a postocclusion surge due to high vacuum settings and turbulence created by phacoemulsification, however, are identified as contributing factors in shifting vitreous support allowing the nucleus to drop [4].

Historically, achieving good visual acuity outcomes after pars plana vitrectomy (PPV)/lensectomy for RLM has been a challenge because complication rates were high. Smiddy et al. [5] reported an RD rate of 8% and final visual acuity of 20/40 or better in 54% of eyes. Scott et al. [6] reported an RD rate of 13% and final visual acuity of 20/40 or better in 56% of eyes. Efforts to optimize the final outcomes of PPV/lensectomy for RLM have focused on surgical techniques to minimize complications, in particular CME, corneal edema, and RD.

Management of /Nucleus Drop/Retained Lens Material

Reducing complications associated with RLM removal by PPV/lensectomy involves not only the surgery, but also management throughout the entire perioperative period, beginning with the cataract surgeon. There is evidence that the clinical course for patients with RLF begins the instant the fragments enter the vitreous and is affected by the cataract surgeon's decisions and actions. The underlying principle of complication management in any surgical setting must be to reduce the risk of further complications [7].

Anterior Segment Management

The primary goal for the surgeon following early posterior capsular rupture or zonular dehiscence is to remove as much of the remaining nucleus as possible, but not without considering the risks that this involves. It is dangerous to continue to phaco (ultrasound plus vacuum/aspiration) in the presence of vitreous in order to remove nuclear fragments at this stage. The phaco tip cannot cut vitreous gel and would instead aspirate, leading to vitreoretinal traction via the vitreous base and creating a high risk of retinal tear. An ophthalmic viscosurgical device, preferably dispersive, can be injected to coat and tamponade the vitreous while also supporting the nucleus, allowing the phaco needle to be withdrawn without letting the vitreous surge forward toward the wound. The surgeon can then remove vitreous by performing bimanual vitrectomy through two paracenteses with a low bottle height, low vacuum (100–150 mm Hg), and highest cut rate possible, using triamcinolone acetonide for visualization. This allows further surgical maneuvers to be performed in a vitreous-free environment, reducing or eliminating vitreous traction. Residual soft lens matter can then be removed using the vitrector in aspiration mode, but blind or aggressive maneuvers should be avoided. In the case of a dense nucleus, an alternative strategy is to enlarge the wound and remove nuclear fragments directly.

Vitreous loss/retained cortical matter during phacoemulsification can also be managed intraoperatively under topical anesthesia via a pars plana approach using 25-gauge vitrectomy instrumentation [8]. In the event of vitreous prolapse, the corneal wound is sutured without further cortical clean up. An additional self-sealing limbal side port is made and an infusion cannula (not opened) is introduced. The clear corneal wound (tunnel) is cleared of vitreous strands with an iris spatula inserted through the other side port. The infusion cannula is subsequently opened. The irrigating fluid increases the IOP making the eye firm, and pushes the vitreous back towards the posterior segment, away from the cornea. A transconjunctival 25-gauge sclerotomy through the pars plana is made [8]. The high-speed 25-guage transconjunctival vitrectomy system under topical anesthesia is introduced and a partial core vitrectomy to debulk the vitreous is

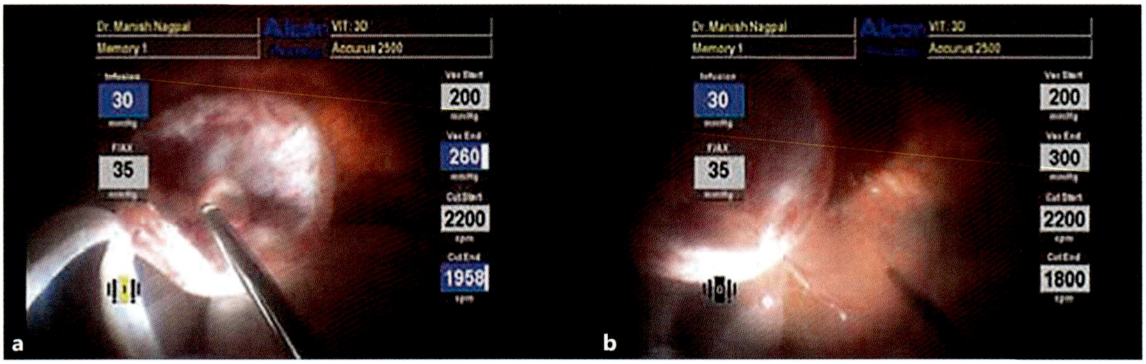

Fig. 1. Lens matter in the posterior segment along with a giant retinal tear. **a** When the nucleus was displaced, the referring surgeon tried to chase it with the phaco tip, and resulting traction probably caused the giant tear. **b** As PFCL is used to flatten the retina, a linear retinal tear extending almost up to the optic disc is also seen, which is along the probable line of the phaco probe approach.

performed. The anterior chamber is also cleared of vitreous and residual cortical matter, and the epinucleus (if present) is removed simultaneously. A foldable intraocular lens is subsequently inserted. This technique is performed in a closed chamber avoiding IOP fluctuations and thus reducing related complications. The high-speed cutter exerts minimal traction on the vitreous. The accessibility to the vitreous improves through the pars plana route, ensuring more complete removal of the vitreous and restoration of normal anatomy. Topical anesthesia avoids the risks of globe perforation, retrobulbar hemorrhage, and prolonged postoperative akinesia of the eye.

In eyes with increased posterior pressure, the pars plana approach is better than an anterior approach as it reduces the amount of vitreous prolapsed into the anterior chamber. Vitreous incarceration, dragging of the retina, entry site retinal dialysis and tears, injury to the ciliary body, fibrovascular downgrowth, suture protrusion, wound dehiscence, difficulty in maintaining stable IOP during closure, and postoperative hypotony (wound leakage) are some of the complications related to a large sclerotomy and are avoided.

If the nucleus has drifted out of reach, an attempt at retrieval via the anterior chamber is ill-advised and should be converted to PPV (fig. 1). In cases managed by an anterior segment surgeon who lacks the experience and equipment, the eye should be closed and the patient referred to a vitreoretinal surgeon. It is especially important to check for vitreous to the wound, which tends to increase the risk of complications, including endophthalmitis.

Considerations of Intraocular Lens Placement at Primary Surgery and Timing of Vitreoretinal Intervention

The question of whether to implant an IOL at the time of nucleus drop if no PPV is undertaken is contentious. Most vitreoretinal surgeons currently agree that placement of a secure IOL at the time of primary surgery is advisable as long as it is stable. With an intact capsulorrhexis, a three-piece IOL can be placed using optic capture with the haptics in the sulcus but the optic behind the capsulorrhexis, resulting in a stable IOL position. A one-piece IOL should not be used in this situation.

Lack of immediate availability of an experienced vitreoretinal surgeon and the necessary equipment usually precludes a same-day vitrectomy, which most vitreoretinal surgeons suggest might be the optimal time for RLF removal in the current era [9–11]. Visualization was often a challenge during PPV/lensectomy for RLM as the cornea may not be clear due to edema, and the pupil may be small because of inflammation. The wide-field viewing systems and wide-angle illumination probes available for today's surgical platforms are an asset in situations like this. If required, the pupil can be manually stretched to aid visibility. Several authors have reported better visual acuity and lower rates of complications (RD, corneal edema, elevated IOP, CME, and intraocular inflammation/infection) among immediate/same-day vitrectomy patients [9–11].

Perhaps immediate vitrectomy prevents time-dependent inflammation and the accompanying choroidal congestion that occurs due to RLF and may take advantage of a clear cornea and minimally inflamed eye to enable better removal with fewer complications. Lower rates of elevated IOP and/or CME may be related to less intraocular inflammation/infection [11]. Moreover, a trend toward increasing concurrent RDs (before/during PPV) has been found with increasing intervals between cataract surgery and PPV [12].

Today, patients expect a rapid visual recovery after cataract surgery and most patients of RLM remain very dissatisfied with poor vision postoperatively. Same-day vitrectomy, when feasible, could mitigate patient dissatisfaction, prevent the need for a second procedure, and hasten visual recovery. However, in cases where vitrectomy is delayed, close monitoring is required and if visibility is limited, a B-scan should be done to make sure the retina is not detached. If it is, the intervention should be done immediately. In high-risk situations, such as unstable traumatic cataracts and posterior polar cataracts, where the risk of posterior capsular rupture and nucleus displacement is significant, it may be best for the vitreoretinal surgeon to see the patient preoperatively. This drives home the importance of potential complications and emphasizes that good pathways for professional collaboration are in place to deal with any complications that may occur.

Pars Plana Vitrectomy: Intraoperative Tips and Techniques

The underlying principle of PPV for displaced nuclear fragments is to perform a complete vitrectomy, including removal of the vitreous base as far as possible, employing a standard three-port pars plana approach with the goals of reducing IOP and inflammation, repairing any retinal breaks or RD, and ultimately restoring visual acuity. In cases where only a small amount of cortical material has gone in the vitreous cavity, vitreoretinal surgery may not be necessary, as these fragments often dissolve on their own.

When larger amounts of lens material or nuclear fragments are retained, a three-port PPV/lensectomy is required to remove the fragments, with a conventional 20-gauge system [6, 9, 10, 12] or with a microincision sutureless system (23- or 25-gauge) [13, 14]. A 20-gauge vitrectomy, however, most often requires a conjunctival peritomy, a larger sclerotomy, and suture closure of the wounds, leading to longer operative and healing time, postoperative discomfort, and refractive changes [15]. Decreased healing and operative time, faster visual recovery, and reduced postoperative inflammation illustrate the benefits of smaller-gauge vitrectomy systems. Compared with the conventional 20-gauge vitrectomy, the aspiration and infusion rate through the 23-gauge instruments will inevitably be lower due to smaller port size and narrower inner diameter of the vitrector handpiece. The main difference between the early-generation 25-gauge and 23-gauge systems is the greater stiffness and fluidics of the 23-gauge system that mirror the 20-gauge system, leading to a preference for the 23-gauge system by an increasing number of vitreoretinal surgeons.

If the RLM to be addressed consists of small fragments and does not include much nuclear material, it is often possible to remove it using only the 23-/25-gauge vitrectomy cutting probe with relatively lower cut rates and higher vacuum settings. When only the vitrector is used to remove the lens material, a bimanual technique can be used in which the light pipe guides the lens material into the vitreous cutter port.

For moderate-sized or denser nucleus material, the vitrector cutter alone may be inadequate for removing, and emulsification with a phacofragmatome is necessary. The superotemporal 23-/25-gauge sclerotomy can be enlarged in such cases for the 20-gauge fragmatome. The advantages of this 'hybrid technique' include having only one incision to suture at the end of a case, being able to perform faster surgery, and speeding up postoperative healing [16]. Phaco in the posterior segment increases the risk for retinal tears and detachments. Also, smaller-gauge vitrectomy systems require high infusion pressures and high flow rates to meet the demand of the aspiration through the wider-bore fragmatome, which might lead to more vitreous traction and intraoperative hypotony. Therefore, ensuring the vitrectomy is complete and the hyaloid is lifted from the retinal surface are key factors to success. Triamcinolone is a useful adjunct for improving visualization of vitreous gel and confirming complete vitrectomy has been achieved. The newer-generation platforms like Constellation have integrated pressurized infusion which constantly monitors infusion pressure with flow-sensing capabilities, resulting in more stable IOP. This IOP compensation feature on the Constellation system automatically adjusts for the pressure drop that occurs due to imbalance between aspiration from the fragmatome and inflow from the 23-/25-gauge infusion line. In other machines, it can be avoided by raising the infusion pressure.

Regardless of the surgical platform and phacofragmentation technology being employed, having a good hold of the lens material at the tip is crucial. When the fragments are not too dense, standard phaco settings do the job adequately. Also, because there is no counterresistance by the capsular bag, it is essential to use a pulse or micropulse setting on the fragmatome, with low-to-moderate vacuum, to avoid bouncing the nuclear fragments around the vitreous cavity due to the repulsion caused by ultrasound energy. However, if emulsification is not progressing in a timely manner and the lens fragments are not holding well to the tip, gradually increase vacuum and phaco power. Under suction, engage the fragments and bring them to the midvitreous, away from ocular structures, to emulsify them.

Perfluorocarbon liquid (PFCL) can be used to cover the macula and float the nucleus away from the retina prior to engaging the fragment with either the vitrector or the fragmatome. This helps to protect the macula during removal of the lens fragments in the midvitreous cavity. After it appears that all RLM is removed, the anterior chamber should be irrigated to remove any fragments that may be trapped in the angle. Prior to closure, it is important to remove all PFCL and to carefully inspect for residual fragments and iatrogenic retinal tears. It is particularly important to inspect the vitreous base with sclera indentation, as tiny retinal breaks close to the ora serrata are easy to miss but can cause subsequent RD. If any are present, they should be treated on the spot with laser.

Another option for lensectomy in RLM cases is to use the INFINITI® Vision System (Alcon) with the OZil® torsional phaco handpiece. It can be used when dealing with dense and hard RLM. Torsional phaco tends to be more efficient than traditional phaco. It creates less turbulence in the eye and draws lens fragments to the phaco tip rather than repulsing them, which helps to protect the retina and decrease the risk of breaks [17]. The OZil® torsional handpiece recently became available with the Constellation® system as well.

Intraocular Lens Dislocation

Dislocation of an IOL is an infrequent but serious complication of cataract surgery and estimated to occur in 0.2–3% of cases [18]. The most common etiologies include pseudoexfoliation, prior vitreoretinal surgeries, trauma, increased axial length, various surgical complications, white mature cataract, and secondary implantation [19, 20]. This can happen in the early or late postoperative period and the best approach for a dislocated IOL must be determined individually for each patient and is based on factors such as clinical circumstances and coexisting complications. The most common indications for surgery would include decreased visual acuity, persistent CME, increased IOP, inflammation, coexisting RD, monocular diplopia, halo phenomenon, and fluctuating vision caused by a shifting IOL.

During surgical intervention, an important consideration is whether to remove, reposition, fixate with suture, or exchange the dislocated IOL after performing a PPV. In patients who are poor surgical candidates and have good visual function in the fellow eye, observation of a dislocated IOL in the vitreous cavity may be a reasonable option [21]. If there is adequate capsular support, the same IOL may be repositioned to the ciliary sulcus. IOL removal with or without exchange is usually performed for IOL with damaged haptics, small optics, or highly flexible haptics unsuitable for suture support or in eyes with coexisting complex RD [22]. Numerous techniques and IOLs are available if exchange is required in eyes with inadequate capsular support. The posterior iris claw IOL can be anchored to the posterior surface of the iris. Otherwise, the IOL may be anchored to the sclera, using one of several possible techniques, like transscleral suture fixation, externalization of one or both haptics, and glue fixation.

The majority of patients with posterior IOL dislocations are treated surgically by either a limbal or a pars plana approach. If the IOL is still supported to some degree by the capsular remnants, a limbal approach may be considered. However, when the patient is supine on the operating table, the IOL frequently falls further posteriorly, making a limbal approach more difficult. PPV techniques offer several advantages to a limbal approach, including more complete and controlled removal of formed vitreous, better access to the posterior vitreous cavity, and better ability to address potential intraoperative complications, such as retinal tear, suprachoroidal hemorrhage, and progressive IOL dislocation into the posterior vitreous.

A complete three-port PPV is essential. The vitreous has to be removed from the anterior chamber, from around the capsule and from the vitreous base. If it is not, the manipulation of instruments inside the vitreous may cause traction on the vitreous and the retina and its attendant complications. A complete vitrectomy around the capsular remnants also ensures that the vitreous does not tend to push the IOL and reduces the chances of redislocation. Also, the IOL has to be freed from all of the vitreous gel enveloping it (fig. 2a).

The IOL is retrieved from the retinal surface and brought anteriorly with the help of end-gripping forceps grasping the haptic optic junction (where the shadow of one of the haptics cast on the retinal surface by the light from the endoillumination probe, thus showing that it was above the level of the retina). The IOL is then either repositioned in the sulcus or removed through the limbal incision (fig. 3a, b). Although removal and exchange of a dislocated PC IOL using the limbal approach may be easier than repositioning the lens, the former approach often induces intraoperative fluctuation in IOP, iris prolapse, postoperative astigmatism, and corneal endothelial damage [22]. However, managing a posteriorly dislocated IOL completely in the posterior segment reduces the risk of several intraoperative complications, is more efficient, and offers patients a more comfortable recovery period.

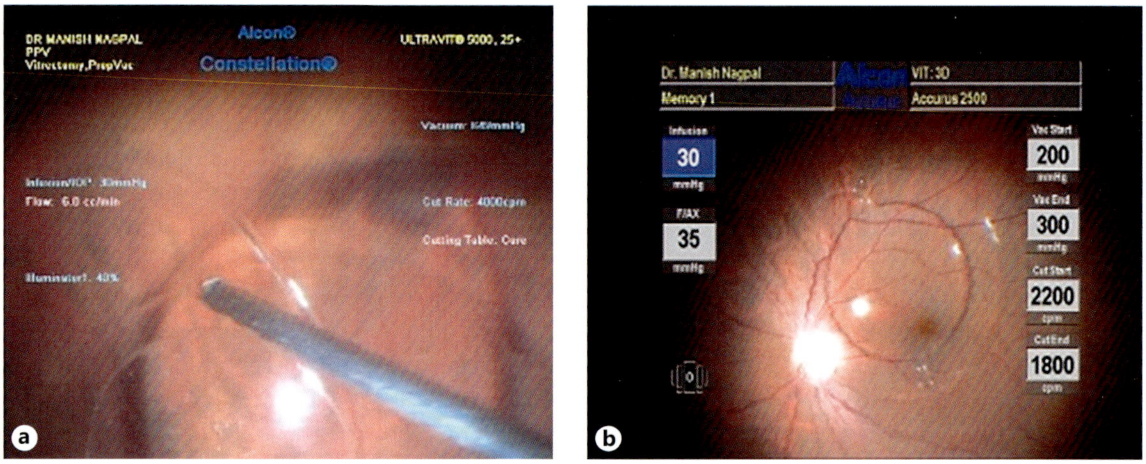

Fig. 2. a After a thorough vitrectomy the IOL is free from all its vitreous adhesions and lying flat on the retinal surface. **b** Heavy liquid PFCL buffers the IOL from touching the macular surface.

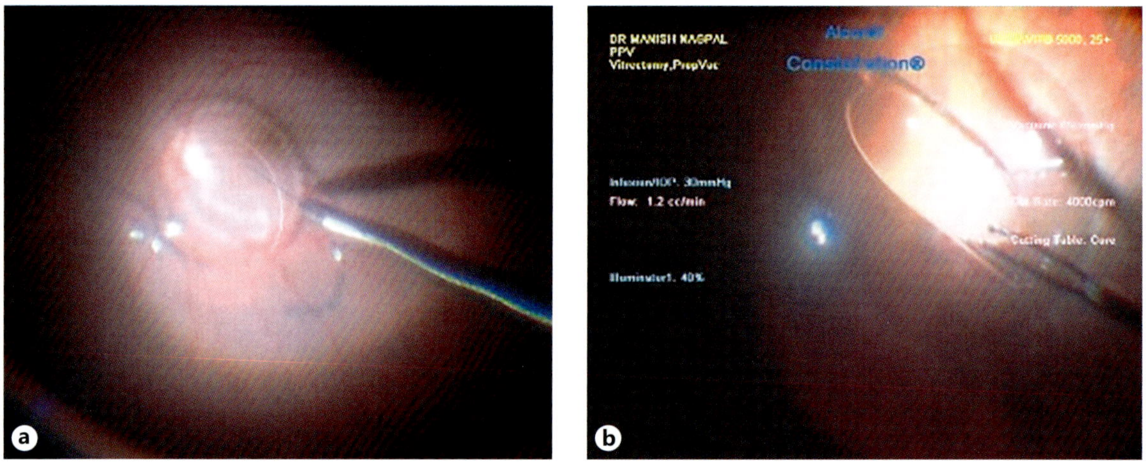

Fig. 3. a, **b** IOL being grasped with end-gripping forceps in order to bring it up for either reposition or extraction from the limbal area.

A newer technique for managing a dislocated IOL completely in the posterior segment involves a standard three-port 20-gauge vitrectomy with a chandelier light and BIOM® wide angle viewing system. It important to accomplish a complete vitrectomy so the IOL is free of vitreous, especially near the sclerotomies. The 10-o'clock sclerotomy (right-hand side) is enlarged to accommodate a pair of Packer/Chang IOL Cutters (MST, Redmond, Wash., USA). These microscissors are designed for cataract surgeons to use through the paracentesis and have exceptional cutting ability. The IOL is safely grasped with forceps and elevated into the midvitreous cavity. With forceps in the left hand and the scissors in the right hand, the IOL is cut into several thin strips. When it is in sections, the same enlarged sclerotomy is used to remove the pieces one at a time with forceps. One caveat worth mentioning: this procedure will not work with a polymethyl methacrylate lens – only silicone and acrylic lenses are flexible enough to be cut with scissors. Rigid polymethyl methacrylate lenses must be removed as a single unit, and this is most easily done through a limbal incision. While the new technique could also be performed with the Accurus® Surgical System or other state-of-the-art vitrectomy systems with chandelier lighting (to free up both hands for grasping and cutting), the chandelier lighting system available for the Constellation® system is brighter and has a broad illumination angle of 106°, providing excellent visualization for the necessary IOL manipulations described.

When the IOL is on the retinal surface, flexible, silicone plate haptic IOLs may be difficult to grasp. The use of active suction with a vitrector to engage the IOL, or PFCL to 'float' the IOL anteriorly, may be helpful (fig. 2b). At the end of case, inspection of peripheral retina with sclera depression is necessary to avoid subsequent RD.

Following PPV/lensectomy for RLM or a dislocated IOL, it is important to closely monitor patients for inflammation, elevated IOP, and signs of peripheral retinal tears or detachments. Topical steroids and topical nonsteroidal anti-inflammatory drops, which are tapered slowly over 6–8 weeks, or longer if necessary, are prescribed. If visual acuity does not improve as expected by the 4-week visit, OCT scans should be obtained to check for CME. If CME is detected, it should be treated aggressively with a sub-Tenon's or intravitreal injection of triamcinolone, as necessary.

References

1 Scott IU, Flynn HW: Retained lens fragments after cataract surgery. Ophthalmol Clin North Am 2001;14:675–679.
2 Mahmood S, von Lany H, Cole MD, et al: Displacement of nuclear fragments into the vitreous complicating phacoemulsification surgery in the UK: incidence and risk factors. Br J Ophthalmol 2008;92:488–492.
3 von Lany H, Mahmood S, James CR, et al: Displacement of nuclear fragments into the vitreous complicating phacoemulsification surgery in the UK: clinical features, outcomes and management. Br J Ophthalmol 2008;92:493–495.
4 Osher RH, Yu BC, Koch DD: Posterior polar cataracts. A predisposition to intraoperative posterior capsular rupture. J Cataract Refract Surg 1990;16:157–162.
5 Smiddy WE, Guererro JL, Pinto R, Feuer W: Retinal detachment rate after vitrectomy for retained lens material after phacoemulsification. Am J Ophthalmol 2003;135:183–187.
6 Scott IU, Flynn HW, Smiddy WE, et al: Clinical features and outcomes of pars plana vitrectomy in patients with retained lens fragments. Ophthalmology 2003;110:1567–1572.
7 Stewart MW: Managing retained lens fragments: raising the bar. Am J Ophthalmol 2009;147:569–570.
8 Shah VA, Gupta SK, Chalam KV: Management of vitreous loss during cataract surgery under topical anesthesia with transconjunctival vitrectomy system. Eur J Ophthalmol 2003;13:693–696.
9 Romero-Aroca P, Fernandez-Ballart J, Mendez-Marin I, Salvat-Serra M, Baget-Bernaldiz M, Buil-Calvo JA: Management of nucleus loss into the vitreous: long term follow up in 63 patients. Clin Ophthalmol 2007;1:505–512.
10 Chen CL, Wang TY, Cheng JH, Tai MC, Lu DW, Chen JT: Immediate pars plana vitrectomy improves outcome in retained intravitreal lens fragments after phacoemulsification. Ophthalmologica 2008;222:277–283.
11 Gonvers M: New approach to managing vitreous loss and dislocated lens fragments during phacoemulsification. J Cataract Refract Surg 1994;20:346–349.
12 Margherio RR, Margherio AR, Pendergast SD, et al: Vitrectomy for retained lens fragments after phacoemulsification. Ophthalmology 1997;104:1426–1432.
13 Minhee Cho, Paul Chan RV: 23-gauge pars plana vitrectomy for management of posteriorly dislocated crystalline lens. Clin Ophthalmol 2011;5:1737–1743.
14 Ho LY, Walsh MK, Hassan TE: 25-gauge pars plana vitrectomy for retained lens fragments. Retina 2010;30:843–849.
15 Chang CJ, Chang YH, Chiang SY, Lin LT: Comparison of clear corneal phacoemulsification combined with 25-gauge transconjunctival sutureless vitrectomy and standard 20-gauge vitrectomy for patients with cataract and vitreoretinal diseases. J Cataract Refract Surg 2005;31:1198–1207.
16 Khanifar AA, Roux HK, Paul Chan RV: Pars plana vitrectomy and lensectomy with a 23-gauge vitrectomy system. Retina Today 2010;5:34–36.

17 Garg SJ, Lane RG: Pars plana torsional phacoemulsification for removal of retained lens material during pars plana vitrectomy. Retina 2011;31:804–805.

18 Mönestam EI: Incidence of dislocation of intraocular lenses and pseudophakodonesis 10 years after cataract surgery. Ophthalmology 2009;116:2315–2320.

19 Hayashi K, Hirata A, Hayashi H: Possible predisposing factors for in-the-bag and out-of-the-bag intraocular lens dislocation and outcomes of intraocular lens exchange surgery. Ophthalmology 2007;114:969–975.

20 Davis D, Brubaker J, Espandar L, et al: Late in-the-bag spontaneous intraocular lens dislocation: evaluation of 86 consecutive cases. Ophthalmology 2009;116:664–670.

21 Mello MO Jr, Scott IU, Smiddy WE, Flynn HW, Feuer W: Surgical management and outcomes of dislocated intraocular lenses. Ophthalmology 2000;107:62–67.

22 Lee SC, Chen FK, Tseng SH, Cheng HC: Repositioning a subluxated sutured intraocular lens in a vitrectomized eye. J Cataract Refract Surg 2000;26:1577–1580.

Dr. Manish Nagpal, DO, MS, FRCS
Retina Foundation
Near Shahibaug Underbridge, Rajbhavan Marg
Ahmedabad, Gujarat 380004 (India)
E-Mail drmanishnagpal@yahoo.com

Subject Index